A Fresh Start

Accelerate Fat Loss

& Restore

Youthful Vitality

D1111753

Susan Smith Jones, Ph.D.

CELESTIALARTS

Berkeley Toronto

CELESTIALARTS

P.O. Box 7123
Berkeley, California 94707
www.tenspeed.com

Distributed in Australia by Simon and Schuster Australia, in Canada by Ten Speed Canada, in New Zealand by Southern Publishers Group, in South Africa by Real Books, in Southeast Asia by Berkeley Books, and in the United Kingdom by Airlift Book Company.

Designed by Greene Design

Libraray of Congress Cataloging-Publication-Data
On file with the Publisher

First printing, 2002
Printed in Canada

1 2 3 4 5 6 7 8 9 10 - 05 04 03 02

Other Books by Susan S. Jones

Choose to Live Peacefully

For children, ages 2 to 10
Vegetable Soup/The Fruit Bowl (co-authored with Dianne Warren)

Audio Cassette Albums

Celebrate Life!
*Choose to Live a Balanced Life
*A Fresh Start: Rejuvenate Your Body
*Making Your Life a Great Adventure: SoulCaring
Wired to Meditate (Audio Book)
Choose to Live Peacefully (Audio Book)

For more information on Susan's books and audio cassette programs, or to purchase her books and tapes, please call (800) 843-5743 or log onto: www.susansmithjones.com

*Recorded live from her popular workshops.

Disclaimer

The health suggestions and recommendations in this book are based on the training, research, and personal experiences of the author. Because each person and each situation is unique, the author and publisher encourage the reader to check with his or her holistic physician or other health professional before using any procedure outlined in this book. Neither the author nor the publisher is responsible for any adverse consequences resulting from a change in diet or from the use of any of the other suggestions in this book.

Dedication

This book is dedicated, in loving memory, to my mother, June: You have been God's richest gift and blessing in my life. As proud as you always were of me, I was even more proud of you. Through your invincible courage, resplendent spirit, and shining example, you taught me how to love deeply, live fully, and celebrate life. I love you always and forever.

and

In loving memory to my brother, Reid, who loved life and lived each day fully with vivacity and valor and who, along with my mother, taught me the most important lesson in life—love is the greatest healer, starting with loving yourself.

Gratitudes

As I strive to live my dream with as much heart and grace as possible, there are many people who have enriched my life and assisted me in following my heart. So I would like to take this opportunity to express my gratitude . . .

To my family, June, Reid, Jamie and Tony, Tyler and Bryce, June and Ad, and Jackie, for your special love and for reminding me that love is always the answer and that life is meant to be lived fully—one day at a time.

To Lynn Carroll, Helen Guppy, Lisa Ray, Diana Feinberg, Eileen Lawrence, Ralph Rudser, Aurora Berbecaru, Mary A. Tomlinson, Ron Hromadka, Donica Beath, Dianne Warren, Bonnie Ross, and Rev. John Strickland, all angels in human form, for helping me to move in the direction of my dreams and not settle for less than the best in every area of my life.

To Torri Randall and Caroline Pincus, my editors, for bringing life to my words and energy to this book.

To Rose Marie Stack, Brian Sievers, Mamiko Matsuda, Don Macri, Jackie Day, Susan Kulick, Lane Gray, Lynn and Morris Walker, Christine Fields, Dr. Peter Brown, Richard Thompson, Mike Richman, Karen McGuire, Walter Martinez, James M. Lennon, Marti Townsend, Dee and Arch Wilkie, Gilli Stuppel, Dr. Edger Maeyens, Kim Nguyen, Darlene Dahl Keller, Charlie Fox, Gina Otto, Mary Jo Irwin, Dr. Nancy Schort, Paulette Suzanne, Victoria Moran, Jodie Villanueva, Tahayra Manjra, Junia Chambers, Kim Phongsa, Jean and Bob Macy, Bev and Doug Beath, Melinda Grubbauer, and Gary Peattie, my dear friends who have blessed and enriched my life with laughter, kindness, munificence, encouragement, and loving support.

To Jo Ann Deck, Veronica Randall, Mary Ann Anderson, and everyone involved at Celestial Arts, for sharing and supporting my vision and heart's desire.

To Christ, Paramahansa Yogananda, White Eagle, my guardian angels, guides, and celestial companions—all who nurture my spiritual side, enrich my life, and guide me along this magnificent journey with their gentle touch, wise counsel, and loving presence. Thank you for being the wind beneath my wings and showing me that with enough love, faith, trust, and patience, all challenges can be overcome and dreams can become reality.

Table of Contents

Introduction vi

**Part I: Sure-Fire Tips to Accelerate Fat Loss
& Restore Youthful Vitality**

S Chapter 1 StressLess Living: Keys to Success 1

U Chapter 2 Understand & Utilize Mind Power 28

C Chapter 3 Choose the Optimum Diet 53

C Chapter 4 Create a Toned, Fit Body—Fitness
for Life! 86

E Chapter 5 Enhance Your Metabolism 117

S Chapter 6 SuperFoods & Supplements that Heal
& Rejuvenate the Body 145

S Chapter 7 Simple Ways to Detoxify and Rejuvenate
Your Body & Your Life 169

Part II: Savory Recipes

Chapter 8 Juices & Smoothies 199

Chapter 9 Breakfasts & Brunches 223

Chapter 10 Spreads, Sauces, Dips & Marinades 234

Chapter 11 Salads 252

Chapter 12 Dressings & Special Treats 273

Chapter 13 Soups 298

Chapter 14 Vegetable Entrées 316

Chapter 15 Grain & Bean Recipes 336

Chapter 16 Side Dishes & Snacks 370

Chapter 17 Meals Kids Love 385

Chapter 18 Desserts 401

Part III: Retreats & Resources

Chapter 19 3-Day Rejuvenation Retreat 417

Chapter 20 7-Day Detox & Rejuvenate Retreat 445

Resource Directory 457

About the Author 461

Index 462

INTRODUCTION

Cherish Your Vision

Cherish the music that stirs in your heart, the beauty that forms in your mind, the loveliness that drapes in your purest thoughts, for out of them will grow all delightful conditions, all heavenly environments; of these, if you but remain true to them, your world will at last be built.
—James Allen

Oh, while I live to be the ruler of life, not a slave; to meet life as a powerful conqueror, and nothing exterior shall ever take command of me.
—Walt Whitman

What a joy it is to have this opportunity to share my thoughts, experiences, and research on being fit and vibrantly healthy, youthful, and fully alive. As you read this book, I want you to feel like we're sitting across from each other while I talk to you personally. I already know that we have lots in common since you've chosen to read a book on radiant health and vitality and to strive to be the best you can be. I am eager to share with you this program that has created SUCCESS for thousands of people. I know it can do the same for you.

For those of you who are new to me and my work, I first want to share with you something about my background in holistic health, my strongly held belief that our spiritual selves must be healed before we can heal physically, the undeniably powerful influence of love, and some of the life lessons that have influenced how I now view my world. I hope my odyssey will inspire and motivate you to make the necessary choices to bring more health, joy, passion, and peace into your life.

More than two decades ago, I fractured my back in an automobile accident. The doctor told me that I would have to get used to a life of pain, inactivity, and difficulty, as I would never be able to carry anything heavier than a light purse. Of course I was devastated when I heard this prognosis. All I could see was a closed door. I was filled with depression, self-pity, and confusion. I felt like a victim. Little did I know at the time that this accident would turn out to be one of the richest blessings of my life. It served as a "wake-up call" and became one of those moments in life when the universe got my attention in a big way.

A month after the accident, I went to a favorite inspirational spot overlooking the Santa Monica Bay for a heart-to-heart talk with myself. The life my doctor had described as the best I could expect was simply unacceptable. I knew I had a choice to make and I made it. Helen Keller once wrote: "When one door closes, another opens; but often we look so long at the closed door that we do not see the one which has opened for us." Although I didn't know how I could change my physical condition, I knew that there was a Higher Power within me that would guide me toward the answers. So I made a deep commitment to let go, live from inner guidance, and accept only vibrant, radiant health.

The power of choice is ours. It's up to each of us to create a meaningful life for ourselves. We are all made in God's image and have the potential to make our lives extraordinary. We can choose to be radiantly healthy, with a fit, strong body, and filled with joy and thanksgiving. We can choose to be at peace with life. We have the power and ability to make our dreams a reality, to manifest our heart's best desires.

The value of life is what we bring to it. Henry David Thoreau knew this when he said, "There is no value in life except what you choose to place upon it, and no happiness in any place except what you bring to it yourself." I no longer look to other people, things, or circumstances as my source of happiness and fulfillment.

Of course, it hasn't been easy. I have made many mistakes, or what I prefer to think of as simply lessons in what didn't work for me.

After my conversation with myself, a series of events began that set me on the road to self-healing: First, I found some perfect books and tapes. Then, I attended some great lectures. Finally, I met some special people who taught me about healing, salutary foods, visualization, and meditation—much of which, admittedly, sounded kind of weird to me at first.

During the months following the accident, and right up to this day, I have continued to make crucial changes in my lifestyle, behavior, thoughts, and attitude. I have learned to bring more consciousness to my everyday living, to pay attention to and observe patterns; to use the ones that support me and to get rid of or change the ones that don't. I now choose to live more deeply, to find the intention beneath my intentions, and to always talk things over with God before making any decisions. Commitments link me, both mind and heart, to people, aspirations, and goals. When I give myself wholeheartedly to a relationship, my work, or some plan, I do well. However, when my first commitment is to be God-centered, I bring a greater measure of love, energy, understanding, and imagination to all of my commitments. When I am God-centered, I do my best in a new or long-standing relationship. When I am God-centered, I bring love and compassion to all my interactions with others, and inspiration to every activity I undertake.

I have the following poem by Johann Wolfgang von Goethe framed in my home so I can read it often. It so beautifully expresses the impact commitment can have on your life.

Until one is committed there is hesitancy,
the chance to draw back, always ineffectiveness.
Concerning all acts of initiative and creation there is one
*   elementary truth*
the ignorance of which kills countless ideas and splendid plans:
that the moment one definitely commits oneself
then Providence moves too.
All sorts of things occur to help one
that would never otherwise have occurred.
A whole stream of events issues from the decision,
raising in one's favor all manner of unforeseen incidents and
meetings and material assistance,
which no man could have dreamed would come his way.
Whatever you can do or dream, begin it!
Boldness has genius, power, and magic to it.

During my six-month checkup following the accident, the doctor shook his head in bewilderment and said, "This just can't be. There is no sign of a fracture and you seem to be in perfect health, free of pain. There must be some mistake. It's just miraculous."

Perhaps it was. Yet I've since discovered that miracles are a natural part of being healthy, happy, and peaceful. Every day we are surrounded with miracles waiting for our awareness. Life-giving fresh fruits and vegetables are miracles. So are sunsets and the buds on a rose, puppies and horses, and our magnificent bodies that house the loving Spirit within. Every situation, seen rightly, contains the seeds of freedom. You can be sure that it's there, just waiting for you to look at it from the right perspective. The profoundly spiritual guidebook *A Course in Miracles* says, "When any situation arises which tempts you to become disturbed, say: 'There is another way of looking at this.'"

Ultimately our choices are what separate us from everyone else. They set us on the road to becoming truly independent and vibrantly healthy and youthful: Choose what you want and how you want to live. Accept and expect the best. Learn to trust your ability to make decisions because the greatest lessons often come from the choices that appear to be wrong. Taking risks is our chance to find out what works for us, what we can do well. We must learn to choose what we want and to not worry about the rest, knowing it's all in God's hands.

In my time of crisis, I didn't just choose health. I chose to be the best I could be—physically, mentally, emotionally, and spiritually. That's what this book is about: tapping into your inner truth and power and choosing to be the best you can be. It's about living your truth and reclaiming your spirituality. And it's also about taking loving care of yourself (by eating healthy foods, exercising regularly, choosing to be positive, etc.), honoring the Divine within you, and bringing spirituality, health, and balance into your everyday life.

A Fresh Start is based on a program I've used for almost thirty years. Throughout this time I have been teaching fitness classes to students, staff, and faculty at UCLA, working as a fitness trainer and personal growth and wellness lifestyle coach, teaching vegetarian cooking classes, and counseling hundreds of people.

During my "Wellness Lifestyling" consultations, I visit people in their homes to see, first hand, how they live, what kinds of exercise they do (or don't do), and how they eat. Part of the process of working with them to help create greater health, fitness, and balanced living involves looking through kitchen cupboards and refrigerators and cleaning out the sabotaging elements that undermine optimum health.

We visit supermarkets and health food stores so they can relearn how to shop. I teach them how to choose a whole foods diet and to eat foods as close to the way nature made them as possible, with an emphasis on living (raw) foods. They learn to cook healthier meals and to live a more balanced holistic lifestyle with minimum stress that includes meditation, detoxification, and a more trusting, positive attitude about life. I also individualize one- to seven-day Personal Retreat Programs for my clients to help them achieve their health, fitness, and peaceful living goals and make their cherished visions come to fruition. This book is like your own customized retreat you can take any time you want.

With knowledge and determination, willingness and perseverance, you can make being out-of-shape and unhealthy a thing of the past. This book will provide the map, but it's up to you to make the healthy choice. The beauty of this *Fresh Start* program is that all the things that I recommend in this book that help accelerate fat loss, reshape your body, increase energy, and restore youthful vitality, also have the added bonus of helping to boost immunity, self-esteem, libido, prevent disease, and make you feel better and look younger.

You may find that I suggest things that are entirely new to you, such as meditation, visualization, solitude, certain foods and supplements, exercises, or a way of living that's different from your present lifestyle. The Resource Directory can help you find some of the products I mention. But don't just take my word for it. You have all the answers within you. Always consult your inner guidance on every decision and choice in your life. Deep within our hearts, each of us knows the truth. But remember that active participation is important in reading this book. It's not what we read that makes a difference in our lives; it's how we apply and experience the material that is of real value.

Like you, I have a lot of things I want to accomplish in this life and I have no interest in being slowed down in any way by health problems. You owe it to yourself to choose being healthy and fit because no one is going to do it for you. You must make health and fitness your top priorities. Don't give up. Don't ever give up! You can do anything to which you set your mind. Move in the direction of your dreams. I believe in you and your ability to be your best, and I salute your great adventure.

Namaste,
Susan S. Jones

If one advances confidently in the direction of his dreams, and endeavors to live the life which he has imagined, he will meet with a success unexpected in common hours. . . . If you have built castles in the air, your work need not be lost; that is where they should be. Now put foundations under them.
—Henry David Thoreau

To laugh often and much; to win the respect of intelligent people and the affection of children; to earn the appreciation of honest critics and endure the betrayal of false friends; to appreciate beauty; to find the best in others; to leave the world a bit better, whether by a healthy child, a garden patch or a redeemed social condition; to know even one life has breathed easier because you have lived. This is to have succeeded.
—Ralph Waldo Emerson

The natural force within each one of us is the greatest healer of all diseases.
—Hippocrates

Part I:

SURE–FIRE TIPS TO ACCELERATE FAT LOSS & RESTORE YOUTHFUL VITALITY

SUCCESS

Chapter 1

STRESSLESS LIVING: KEYS TO SUCCESS

Life is a paradise for those who love many things with passion.
—Leo Buscaglia

The lowest ebb is the turn of the tide.
—Longfellow

Not long ago I gave a talk in Los Angeles on "StressLess Living: The Power to Be Your Best." I shared the tips you'll be reading about in this chapter about putting inspiration back into your life because when you feel inspired, you feel purposeful, you feel empowered. I also shared that many women are currently experiencing a crisis of the spirit. They feel disconnected from their authentic selves or the real spiritual self within us that's connected with the divine. What's needed is a revolution of the spirit and that begins by taking loving care of yourself.

1

After my presentation I went into the ladies' room and noticed a woman crying. I remembered her because she had been sitting in the front row and had cried through much of my talk. Since I had no plans for dinner, I asked her to join me. Surprised, she gratefully accepted.

It turned out that Melissa's husband had recently left her for a woman half Melissa's age. Her two children had been taken away and given to a relative to care for. She was almost 100 pounds overweight, had no job, and was so depressed she was actually considering suicide. That morning when she was at her lowest, she took a walk and noticed a flier for my talk in the window of a natural food store. Something inside her told her she had to attend—even though she had never attended a motivational talk before.

Melissa believed in the ideas I discussed but wasn't sure how to implement them in her life. She knew she was falling downhill but she didn't know how to climb back up. She wanted more than anything to turn her life around—to find a job, get her children back, lose weight, and get back into shape. After hearing her story, I shared the thought with her that it seemed like the universe was taking everything away from her so that she could and would, for the first time in her life, put herself first. Like most women, she was so accustomed to putting everyone else's needs before her own that she took no time for herself. She was learning the hard way that you can't run on empty forever. She was being forced to learn that she had to take loving care of herself first before she could nurture, love, and take care of others.

I told Melissa that if she was willing to make a real commitment to do whatever it took to live her highest vision, then I'd be happy to work with her. For the rest of that evening, I had her share with me her highest vision and answer questions like: If she couldn't fail and if she were living her best self right now, what would that look like? I also gave her all my books and tapes and wrote out a walking and meditation program that she could start the very next morning.

Over the next month, I designed a nutrition program for Melissa and cleaned out her refrigerator and cupboards and all junk foods that didn't align with her new vision of herself. I taught her how to shop for healthy foods and products and customized a cardio-weights-and-stretching routine for her at the gym. Finally, I also taught her how to meditate and visualize her goals.

Melissa was and is an inspiration. Her dedication and commitment created miraculous results. Within three weeks, she found a part-time job that eventually led to full-time employment at a florist shop. Within four months she had saved enough money to move into a new, larger apartment and, happily, she got her children back.

Today, Melissa is down to her ideal weight, works out regularly, frequents natural food stores, is managing the florist shop, is engaged to be married, and is feeling empowered and divinely guided. When her ex-husband told her he wanted to get back together with her, she knew it wouldn't be for her highest good. She now lives with a sense of freedom, control, and power over her life, having learned, firsthand, that breakthroughs and miracles occur when you are willing to live from your vision and commitment.

Healing a Hasty Life

Stress is a major problem in modern life. Technological advances have increased the pressure to keep busy, even in our leisure hours. We talk on the telephone while we drive, watch television while we read, conduct business while we listen to the radio.

We are all overstimulated, receiving more information from television, computers, radio, satellites, etc., than our ancestors of several generations ago could ever have imagined! This year alone you will probably make more appointments, meet more people, and go more places than your grandparents did in their entire lives. All this rushing around creates a life filled with stress.

Given our current pace, we have little time to relax and cultivate relationships with our spouses, children, friends, and nature. Is it any wonder that stress-related diseases are now on the rise? Some studies even suggest that 80% to 90% of all doctor visits are for stress-related complaints.

I see this as a sickness of epidemic proportions—a "busyness" or "hurry" sickness. But you can choose to slow down and create a life of balance. We'll address this idea later in this chapter, but for now, let's see if you can find any of these signs of "hurry" sickness in your daily life.

Do You Suffer from Busyness Sickness?

1. Do you eat in a rush, often while standing or on the go, or in your car?
2. Does your busy life prevent you from spending much time at home? And when you finally get home, are you too tired to do much beyond collapse and "veg out" in front of the television?
3. Do you routinely drive too fast, run yellow lights, constantly change lanes, and jockey for position? Are you impatient with other drivers?
4. Do you talk fast, have problems communicating how you feel, and rarely find time to give emotional support to your family and friends?
5. Is your life so full of undone chores and responsibilities that relaxing has become almost impossible? When you're not doing something productive, do you experience anxiety and guilt? Have vacations become more trouble than they're worth?

Why We Have a Need to Rush

What causes our need to rush? We can blame it on economics: we must make enough money to pay for our chosen lifestyle. Or we can blame it on the fact that everything's moving so fast, and we have to, too. But the real cause, I believe, is something deeper. By crowding our schedule with "more"—more socializing, more eating, more work, more activity, more appointments—we may be trying to fill the emptiness we feel inside ourselves.

When you constantly direct your attention and energies outward, it's easy to lose the sense of inner wonder, beauty, and calmness where true happiness, joy, and peace originate. By slowing down and redirecting your energies inward, you will not only train your brain to relax, but also fill that emptiness with a new sense of yourself that can ultimately change your life. Let's take a closer look at the physiology of stress and how it affects you.

The Physiology of Stress

Stress can be defined as a "synergy of endocrinological impairments that creates a syndrome." Loosely translated, that means that stress comes about because you have an effect on your hormones and your hormones have an effect on you. According to John M. Kells in his superb book, *The HRT Solution* (which Christine Northrup, M.D., referred to as "the bible of hormone replacement"), "sometimes the things that go on in your life can put a burden on you physically by causing endocrine, or hormonal, events that go on in your body. Medical experts now believe that this is at the root of many degenerative disease processes. In other words, stress has a biological as well as an emotional effect on you and, over time, it can diminish your body's ability to fortify, protect, regenerate, and heal itself."

Stress can be triggered by emotions, such as anger, fear, worry, grief, or guilt. It can be the result of an injury or trauma, an accident or surgery. Everyday pressures, like family squabbles, impossible bosses, unfaithful spouses, unruly teens, or overdue bills cause stress. An extreme change in sleep patterns, diet, exercise, and even the climate you live in can also create stress. So can chronic illness, pain, allergies, and inflammation. And, as mentioned above, too much work or too much of anything can create stress that can lead to depression.

Stanford neuroendocrinologist and stress researcher, Robert Sapolsky, the author of the insightful book *Why Zebras Don't Get Ulcers*, recognizes how closely stress and depression are tied together, especially in women. Study after study has found that women suffer from both stress and depression more often than men. "Now we can begin to see how closely the two are linked. After all, depression is the archetypal stress-related illness," says Sapolsky.

For Lisa, one of my clients, depression made it difficult for her to get up in the morning and face each day. A single mother in her late thirties and close to becoming a partner in a law firm, Lisa traveled two hours daily in heavy traffic both to and from work, adding four stress-filled hours to her already long workday. She was usually greeted by screaming rap music blasting from her teenager's room every evening when she came home from work. With no time to call her own, Lisa felt like she always had an endless list of things to do that never got completed. Although she tried to watch her diet and tried to squeeze in two to three hours a week on her home treadmill, she seemed to be gaining weight monthly. Even more alarming, Lisa hadn't had a period in over a year, and she thought she was too young to be entering menopause, although she confessed she felt twenty years older than her actual age.

The first time she came to see me in the midst of uncontrollable tears, Lisa admitted that she was having a hard time just getting out of bed in the morning. She had been feeling this crippling despair for years, ever since she discovered her husband having an affair with his personal secretary. Just a few months after their divorce, when Lisa thought she was beginning to get her life back, her mother died of cancer and one of her children was in a serious automobile accident. Although her friends and neighbors all applauded her outward strength and ability to rise above these tragedies and challenges, inside she felt like she was losing herself and her life. As I listened to Lisa's story, it was clear that she was in the midst of a severe depression. I explained to her that the physiological root of depression is often the flood of hormones that is released during times of extreme stress. For millions of women like Lisa, finding ways to relieve stress can make the difference between waking up ready to face the day or wanting to hide under the weight of the bleakest kind of despair.

When Lisa fights rush-hour traffic or faces a wall of rap music at the end of a demanding day, her brain, with the best of intentions, sounds an alarm. Her heart rate accelerates, her blood sugar soars, and an army of endorphins marches out to dull potential pain. A wave of neurotransmitters—serotonin among them—spreads the alarm from cell to cell throughout her nervous system. The hypothalamus also gets in on the act, releasing a hormone called CRH that signals for the release of other hormones. Meanwhile, the adrenal glands atop the kidneys send out the stress hormones adrenaline, DHEA, and cortisol, also known as steroid hormones.

These substances are usually body-friendly and at our service to protect us by increasing our alertness and strength and to help us do what needs to be done. The problem comes when the stress is prolonged and the chemicals' normal routes change: serotonin tends to hasten away too quickly; DHEA can make itself sparse; cortisol can overstay its welcome.

Cortisol's Role in Stress & Hormone Balance

Produced by the adrenal glands and commonly known as the "stress hormone," cortisol helps the body cope with all types of stress, from infection to fright, from a major job or home move to divorce and even death. Whether you are facing an emergency, an accident, a confrontation, or just doing your job or getting some exercise, cortisol is there to get you up and going, to get you through the day.

Cortisol helps determine how the proteins, carbohydrates, and fats from your diet are utilized. For example, cortisol influences the breakdown of carbohydrates into glucose so the body can use them for energy. Cortisol also influences the breakdown of protein into amino acids. Amino acids are the building blocks of protein, and they are also the building blocks of the immune system, blood vessels, muscles, and other tissues. Thus, the immune system, blood vessels, and muscles all rely on cortisol for strength and proper function. Cortisol prevents the loss of too much sodium from the body and helps maintain blood pressure as well. It also helps to suppress reactions such as pain, allergic reactions, and inflammation.

Perhaps most interesting of all, cortisol helps the body protect itself from itself. For example, during a strenuous workout, the body breaks down fat and muscle tissue to produce energy. In order to prevent the immune system from recognizing all of these tissue molecules as foreign invaders, the body produces more cortisol and gently suppresses the immune response so that the body does not go on red alert when it doesn't have to.

The cortisol that can flood your system to assist you in emergencies helps to provide your body with the nutrients you need to cope with stress. That's why it's known as the stress hormone. Normally, once you have managed the stressful circumstances, the brain shuts off the production of cortisol, your physical reactions subside, and soon you are back to normal, according to Kells (see page 5).

But there is another side of the cortisol story. If the brain perceives that stress is ongoing or chronic, it can override the messages to shut off cortisol production. Cortisol production then stays elevated because the brain thinks the body needs it to cope with what it's experiencing. So, as important and necessary as cortisol is, you can have too much of it. If too much cortisol stays in the body for too long, a damaging cycle can begin that can lead to blood sugar problems, fat accumulation, compromised immune function, exhaustion, bone loss, even heart disease. If, like Lisa, you experience one major stress after another, and if you haven't created ways to reduce and release that stress, it can have a detrimental effect on your health.

Just like everything in nature, the body is in a continuous state of regeneration. It is constantly building itself up, tearing itself down, and rebuilding itself all over again. Cortisol levels go up to provide the body with the energy, but it breaks tissues down in order to do this. Once the job is done, the body has to rebuild and recuperate. That is when DHEA comes into play to help the body recuperate and get back to normal. DHEA and cortisol work together under normal conditions to handle stress.

Think back to the last time you felt a big rush of adrenaline. I felt it just recently when I was invited to appear on a popular national television talk show. We experience these adrenaline rushes when we react to something that excites us, frightens us, surprises us, or makes us angry. An adrenaline rush is the first in a chain reaction of hormonal events. It is the signal that sets in motion the release of cortisol and DHEA, which are the hormones that help us to take action, to get a job done, and even to get our point across.

However, if you are always "under the gun"—which can mean anything from a continual struggle to make ends meet to traveling all the time because you are at the peak of your success in your career— then you constantly have stress hormones flooding into your bloodstream. When this happens, your adrenal glands can become overworked and exhausted. Over time, this excess wear and tear on them can be very serious, creating major disease. Given how most people live these days, it's no wonder that 80% to 90% of diseases are stress-related.

The hallmark of adrenal compromise is a decrease in DHEA production. When the buffering effects of DHEA are in short supply or no longer available, then the negative effects of cortisol can go unchallenged, which can leave the body more susceptible to everything from hay fever to cancer. Low levels of DHEA are also associated with many of the chronic degenerative diseases commonly attributed to aging.

What endocrinologists have learned from studying women like my client, Lisa, who are depressed or experiencing extended periods of psychological trauma, is that continually elevated levels of cortisol can prevent them from ovulating. The cessation of regular ovulation means that not enough estrogen and progesterone are being produced. Low estrogen levels can increase the activity of the bone-metabolizing osteoclasts. To further complicate things, the cortisol that provides the extra calcium needed in a fight-or-flight situation also stimulates the bone-metabolizing osteoclasts. Left unchecked over a long period of time, high cortisol levels can cause the body to lose bone faster than it is able to replace it. Low levels of progesterone, the "air-traffic controller" hormone that can cascade into DHEA, estrogen, testosterone, and cortisol, can lead to weight gain, PMS symptoms, fluid retention, depression, low energy and libido, blood sugar and mineral imbalances, and osteoporosis, just to name a few.

In a natural rhythm, the body produces much more cortisol in the morning than in the evening. This helps you to get up and get going, and also helps you to get through your day. At the end of the day your cortisol level should be going down. One recent study demonstrated that when men come home from work, their cortisol levels go down. This is what is supposed to happen—when you come home and wind down. However, the same study showed that many women who work outside the home and have primary responsibility for taking care of their families, as Lisa does, have cortisol levels that stay elevated in the evening. This is the way their bodies respond to the stress of the "second shift." Women who have high cortisol and low DHEA levels can experience panic attacks and a strange feeling of being both anxious and exhausted at the same time.

Because of the role of all of these hormones on stress, health, weight, and vitality, before I begin counseling, I recommend that all of my clients do saliva hormone testing and urine deoxypyridinoline (Dpd) bond resorption tests, both of which are available from labs like Aeron Life Cycles and others. Standard blood tests, which are what most doctors would recommend, are not sensitive enough to pick up on important hormone imbalances. If you go to your doctor, the blood test is what you're likely to get. I recommend doing your own saliva test. These labs provide you with the collection supplies necessary to test your estradiol, estriol, estrone, progesterone, testosterone, DHEA, and cortisol levels, and your rate of bone loss. Once you have collected your saliva and urine samples at home, you simply send them to the lab of your choice for processing. Results can be sent to you and your doctor (see Resource Directory for information on contacting Aeron Life Cycles). I have myself tested at least a couple of times each year—and even more often when I'm under extended stress.

If my clients' hormones are out of balance, which is usually the case, I recommend that they consider using natural hormone creams, which are absorbed through the skin. The brand I use is *Life-Flo* (see Resource Directory for more information). Studies reveal that transdermal delivery is more effective than oral delivery because the hormones go directly to the bloodstream, initially bypassing the liver, which can mean that as much as 95% of the supplements get to the cells where they are needed. For comparison, testing on substances taken orally shows that in some cases as little as 5% make it to the cells where they are needed. This is because the stomach, liver, and digestive systems excrete and discard much of them. Check with your doctor concerning your own individual needs.

Cortisol Causes Food Cravings & Weight Gain

Everyday pressures, recent surveys reveal, cause 9 out of 10 of us to look to food for comfort. In fact, just today I read in *Prevention* magazine that almost 40% of Americans polled say that they always eat when they see food and this survey didn't even factor in how this pattern is affected when we're under stress. But if you're one of those people who turn to food during stressful periods in your life, don't be hard on yourself. What at first may seem like bad eating habits, writes Pamela Peeke, M.D., a former senior scientist at the National Institutes of Health and author of *Fight Fat After Forty*, are, in fact, "our body's natural reaction to stress. And strict dieting can actually make you more stressed out, and more prone to weight gain."

Peeke says that when you're wound up as tight as a spring, the brain sends out signals—in the form of hunger—to stockpile emergency fuel. But today, it's not because we're fleeing from tigers, it's our day-to-day stresses—"struggling" with overdue bills, unruly teens, inconsiderate neighbors, loud rap music, illness in the family, unending traffic, and other environmental stimulation. So we're left full of nervous tension, "which we often soothe by chewing," says Dr. Peeke. And that emergency fuel we stockpiled? It stays stockpiled—as fat, of course.

What's more, to create instant energy, the body drains its nutritional reserves. "Under extreme stress, we need as much protein as there is in four quarts of milk," says Stephen Langer, M.D., president of the American Nutritional Medical Association. What if we haven't eaten that much protein? The body uses its own protein-rich tissues—namely muscle. You'll read in Chapter 5 how important lean muscle tissue is to keeping metabolism revved, increasing fat burning enzymes, and burning more calories, even when sleeping. And for every pound of muscle destroyed through stress, our metabolisms drop, burning at least 42 fewer calories a day.

Do you ever wonder why some people appear to thrive on stress, while others suffer ill health? New studies suggest that it may not be the stress that lowers immunity, but whether you feel a sense of control over it. In one Dutch study scientists compared two groups of men taking a math test under a barrage of noise: those who could adjust the noise level had little change in immune function, while those who couldn't experienced a drop in immune-cell production. But feeling in control has less to do with your situation and more to do with your attitude. And as you'll see in the tips that follow, choosing to be positive and optimistic, always reminding yourself that you're doing the best you can, will do wonders toward keeping the negative repercussions of stress at bay.

So what can we do to break the stress-fat link cycle? Although stress can overwhelm us at times, we can choose to take the steps necessary to understand what it means to live a balanced life. Radiant health and peace of mind (the opposite of stress) go hand-in-hand—you can't reach your potential for physical health without being mentally fit as well. Making choices that integrate and heal the body, mind, and spirit is what living with balance is all about.

Susan's Top Stress–Busting Tips
Simple Reminder:

1. Practice the art of relaxation
2. Meditate
3. Exercise
4. Sleep
5. Drink water
6. Eat fresh fruits and vegetables
7. Be mindful
8. Consider massage, music, money, and color
9. Wear natural clothing
10. Enjoy nature time
11. Laugh as often as possible
12. Simplify and slow down
13. Nurture intuition
14. Live with integrity
15. Be positive and grateful
16. Act with love and kindness
17. Live with reverence

---

1. Practice the art of relaxation. One of the world's leading experts on the brain is a Harvard medical doctor, Herbert Benson, author of *The Relaxation Response* and *Your Maximum Mind*. What Benson calls "the relaxation response" is the body's ability to enter into a state characterized by an overall reduction of the metabolic rate and a lowered heart rate. According to Benson, this state of relaxation also acts as a door to a renewed mind and a changed life, a feeling of awareness. He describes the physiological changes that occur when you are relaxed as a harmonizing or increased communication between the two sides of the brain, resulting in feelings often described as well-being, unboundedness, infinite connection, and peak experience.

One way to cultivate calmness and peacefulness is to progressively relax your body, beginning with your toes and ending with your head. Breathe slowly and deeply and totally relax each part of your body, saying to yourself as you go along, "My toes, feet, legs [and so on] are relaxed," until you have gone through your entire body. Then rest for a while in the quiet and silence. Listening to a relaxation or meditation tape may also be helpful. (You can find out more about my own relaxation tapes by checking my Web site www.susansmithjones.com.)

My favorite way to do this relaxation exercise is on my BodySlant, where my head is lower than my heart and my feet higher. In this position, it's possible to reach a deeper level of relaxation. I often have my clients visualize themselves feeling relaxed and peaceful. Then I simply ask them to focus on their breath. That's it. Nothing else. New clients often report that they haven't felt so relaxed or calm in years. All it takes is giving yourself permission to relax and a little bit of time to do it.

Here's another great tip you can easily do at work or at home to help relax your mind and body: Look at a picture of a beautiful landscape. Yes, it's that simple. Two studies measured the effect of certain photographic images on emotional and physiological responses. The first study was designed to find ways of fighting the boredom and homesickness that astronauts experience during extended stays in space. Researchers projected a variety of slides on the walls of a room built to simulate a space station and recorded the subjects' responses to various scenes. The second study focused on hospital patients who were about to undergo surgery. In both groups, pictures of spacious views and glistening water lowered heart rates and produced feelings of calmness.

An easy and inexpensive way to look at a beautiful landscape is to get a poster. I have a Sierra Club poster in my meditation room that has a dazzling view of water, mountains, colorful wildflowers, etc. Every time I look at it, I feel more relaxed. This is the perfect solution if you work in an office without windows. Larger posters of beautiful nature scenes can transform a room and provide you with a mini fantasy vacation whenever you need it.

2. Meditate.   When you think of meditation, you may envision crossed legs and chants of "ommmm," but meditation can be anything that helps you focus your attention and increase your awareness of your body and the world around it (I describe all this in detail in my audiobook *Wired to Meditate*).

Meditation, along with deep, whole body progressive relaxation and visualization as described above, are the best ways to bring stress hormone levels back to normal quickly, especially after an adrenaline-producing, cortisol-raising experience. I know of no more effective way to bring about relaxation than through meditation—turning inward in silence and reconnecting with the peace and calmness that's always within you.

Nurture this inner peacefulness by book-ending your day with quiet meditation for 15 minutes first thing in the morning and again before you go to sleep at night. This quietude will remind you that you can make the choice every day to live in the world but not be caught up in the frenzy of it.

Part of the meditation process is focused, deep breathing. In fact, conscious breathing—inhaling and exhaling slowly and deeply—is itself a form of meditation. Take deep, clean breaths by breathing through the nose, filling the diaphragm first and then the lungs, then push out through the mouth. You can tell you've taken a deep breath in the proper way if your stomach expands and contracts (as opposed to your shoulders moving up and down as is often the case with shallow breathers).

In addition to practicing this type of breathing while meditating, take mini breathing breaks throughout your day. Perhaps every hour or two, for two to three minutes, take a deep breathing break to help you to see life from a higher perspective. While you're breathing, be sure to focus on your breath or a relaxing, peaceful thought and not on anything that might be stressful.

3. Exercise. Physical exercise is another effective means of reducing stress and tension. A single dose of exercise works even better than tranquilizers as a muscle relaxant among individuals with symptoms of anxiety and tension, but without any undesirable side effects.

In a classic study of tense and anxious people, Herbert de Vries, Ph.D., former director of the Exercise Physiology Laboratory at the University of Southern California, administered a 400-milligram dose of meprobamate, the main ingredient in many tranquilizers, to a group of patients. On another day, he had these same patients take a walk vigorous enough to raise their heart rates to more than one hundred beats per minute. Using an EMG (electromyogram) machine to measure the patients' tension levels as shown by the amount of electrical activity in their muscles, de Vries found that after exercise the electrical activity was 20% less than the patients' normal rate, indicating that their bodies were less tense. By contrast, the same patients showed little difference after the dose of meprobamate.

Yoga is the perfect exercise for reducing stress. A study of yoga-class beginners found that workouts left them less nervous and more energetic. Another study found that yogis go through life with lower stress hormone levels.

When you've determined an appropriate exercise program for yourself, stay with it, especially when extra stress has been added to your life.

4. Sleep. America is a chronically sleep-deprived nation, and lack of sleep undermines the body's inherent ability to deal with stress. One clear sign of sleep deprivation is needing an alarm clock to roust you out of bed in the morning. To dramatically improve your alertness, mood, appearance, and overall health, as well as help normalize stress hormones, try to get to bed 30 to 60 minutes earlier than you're used to.

If after reading all the sleep tips in Chapter 7 you're still not sleeping well, try this cue from infants. Babies often twiddle an earlobe as they fall asleep, and doctors say it actually promotes sleep. A nerve that regulates heartbeat radiates to the earlobe, and when the pulse slows, sleep comes more easily.

5. Drink water. You may be wondering what water has to do with reducing stress. Well, plenty, and that's why you'll find me mentioning the importance of drinking enough water several times throughout this book. When you don't get enough water, the result is added stress on all of the organs and cells in the body. Yet one-third of all Americans suffer from chronic dehydration. According to F. Batmanghelidj, M.D., author of the enlightening book *The Body's Many Cries for Water*, and considered one of the world's leading experts on water and health, over time even mild dehydration poses numerous health risks. Let's look at a few:

Cancer: Low fluid consumption is associated with increased risk for colon, breast, and urinary tract cancers. In a recent study, risk for colon cancer was substantially lower in women who drank more than five glasses of water daily than in those who drank two or fewer.

Constipation: Dehydration hardens stools and makes them difficult to pass.

Kidney stones: About 15% of Americans develop kidney stones at least once in their lives. Dehydration promotes the process, concentrating in the kidneys the calcium salts and other compounds that constitute stones. One recent study showed that individuals with a history of kidney stones could reduce the risk for recurrence by 15% just by drinking at least 4 more cups of water daily.

Diminished coordination and thinking: Without enough water, hand-eye coordination falters and reaction time slows. The mind is less nimble, and short-term memory flags. Many older people who consult a doctor fearing dementia may actually be suffering from dehydration.

Dehydration can also lead to frequent headaches, general fatigue, dizziness, and weight gain. That's right. A shortage of water will result in excess water weight, as too little H_2O causes our bodies to store water outside of our cells, making us feel bloated and heavy. Drinking plenty of water will actually help you lose or maintain a healthy weight, too. Water is calorie-free, suppresses the appetite naturally (drink a large glass 15 minutes before mealtime on an empty stomach), and helps metabolize fat.

Without enough water, your kidneys can't function properly, which forces them to send some of their workload to your liver. Since one of the liver's main functions is to metabolize stored fat, the added work from the kidneys means that the liver burns less fat, so that more fat remains in the body—usually in the hips and thighs for women and around the waist for men. If you desire to lose some fat, it's a good idea to drink at least three *extra* glasses of water every day.

You don't have to sauna daily or run twenty miles to experience dehydration. You lose water continuously simply through respiration, perspiration, and excretion. By the time thirst first sets in, you have already lost 2% of your body's weight in water. Signs of dehydration that you may notice right away are a slight headache, dry eyes, fatigue, and a burning sensation in the stomach. Check your urine. Unless you've just taken vitamins, it should be odorless and nearly colorless— no darker than straw. Caffeinated and alcoholic beverages do *not* count toward your daily water intake as they flush out some of the fluid they supply. For every cup of caffeinated (coffee, tea, soda) or alcoholic beverage you drink, you must offset it with at least 1 cup of water. And make sure to increase your water consumption by at least 2 cups if you consume a high-fiber diet (as I hope you will after reading Chapter 3), take diuretics, live at a high altitude or in a very dry or hot climate, are pregnant or nursing, are traveling (especially on planes) or, as I said above, you want to lose fat.

And for those of you who are exercising vigorously for 15 minutes or more, your need for extra water is even greater. The American College of Sports Medicine recommends that you drink 16 ounces of liquid 2 hours before exercise, 4 to 8 ounces every 15 minutes while you are exercising, and at least 16 ounces after you exercise. Endurance athletes who exercise for more than 1 hour may need replacement drinks. My favorite is Emer'gen-C because of its neutral pH and mineral ascorbates, which are efficiently and quickly assimilated into all the body's cells.

How much water does the average person need every day? Batmanghelidj recommends drinking a minimum of half your body weight in ounces. That means if you are a sedentary 128-pound woman, you'll need to drink at least 64 ounces of water (one-half gallon) daily. If you are an active 128-pound woman who exercises vigorously, takes saunas, travels on planes, drinks coffee, and lives in the desert, be aware: You'd need several more glasses than this each day.

I tell my clients to drink at least 80 ounces of water every day. Begin the day with two 8-ounce glasses of water. Then fill a half-gallon container and make it your goal to finish it before bedtime. If you try to remember to drink water, chances are you won't take in enough, but by filling your container each morning, you will see exactly how much you are drinking. When you leave your home for work, school, errands, etc., pour from your half gallon container into your personal bottle to take with you. In other words, keep purified water with you all the time to drink so you won't get close to dehydration. (See Chapter 7 for an added suggestion about AlkaLife drops.) Get in the habit of drinking throughout the day. Place some water next to your bed, take it with you in the car, have it at your desk, etc. (See Chapter 2 for ideas about establishing new habits.)

To give water a little zing and flavor, I sometimes add thin slices of cucumber, orange, lemon, lime, strawberries, fresh ginger juice, or combinations of any of these. Some water is replenished through the food you eat, especially if your diet is rich in fresh fruit and vegetables, fresh juices, smoothies, and noncaffeinated herbal teas.

Because of my vigorous exercise routine, regular saunas, and high-fiber diet, I try to consume 100 ounces daily. I find that it makes my skin look younger, my body more energetic and strong, my mind more focused and clear, and my meditations deeper.

6. *Eat fresh fruits, vegetables & other stress-busting foods.*

Because fruits and vegetables are the foods highest in water content, and because they are the foods easiest to digest, they take stress off your digestive system and are what I refer to as "body-friendly" foods. Keep the following three tips in mind when planning your meals.

1. Eat at least 8 servings of fruits and vegetables daily. Emphasize the vegetables, especially leafy greens like romaine lettuce and spinach.

2. Eat a variety of fruits and vegetables to attain the widest selection of nutrients and cancer-fighters.

3. Select produce with rich, diverse colors. Many of the beneficial antioxidants in fruits and vegetables are also the pigments responsible for making them red, orange, green, or yellow.

Besides being rich in fiber, phytonutrients, chlorophyll, antioxidants, minerals, and enzymes, life-giving fruits and vegetables provide vitamins that help the body when it's under stress. For example, numerous studies show that taking extra **vitamin A** when under chronic stress can keep the adrenal glands from overproducing cortisone—the hormone responsible for stress-related cravings and fat storage. Strive to get at least 5,000 IU of vitamin A each day and much more when under stress. The best sources are from food such as sweet potatoes, carrots, cantaloupe, spinach, and mangos. One 4-ounce sweet potato alone provides a slimming 28,000 IU.

Without sufficient amounts of **vitamin C**, the body struggles to respond to stress, which actually stresses it even more, sending it into a heightened (and very fattening!) state of emergency, notes the American Nutritional Medical Association's Dr. Stephen Langer. The more stress we experience, the more vitamin C we need. I take at least 3,000 mg when I'm under extra pressure and spread it out during the day. Since it's hard to get large doses of C from food alone, try Emer'gen-C, which makes it easy to get ample C in a form that does not cause an increase in acidity and is convenient to take. Good food sources of vitamin C include oranges, strawberries, tomatoes, grapefruit, and dark green leafy vegetables.

The body also has higher **protein** needs when it's under stress. Beans, soy products, nuts and seeds, sprouts, whole grains, dark leafy greens, such as romaine lettuce, chlorella, Barlean's Greens, and Living Food, are all good sources I would choose. If you eat animal products, fish is a good source of protein but select fish that's high in omega-3 fatty acids such as salmon or tuna. And don't fry your fish; bake, poach, or broil it. If you don't take in enough protein, your body will get what you need from its own protein-rich, metabolism-boosting muscle instead. Dr. Langer suggests an extra 3 ounces of protein daily, for a total of about 10 ounces daily in times of extra stress. This high quality protein reduces feelings of stress—the ones that lead to cravings. When I eat a little extra protein such as a protein shake or some black beans and tofu on my green salad, I feel more grounded.

Studies have found that people suffering from **selenium** deficiencies are more anxious than their well-nourished counterparts. So to keep yourself mellow and your metabolism high, it's important to eat about 100 mcg daily. A single Brazil nut boasts 120 mcg of selenium and they are also an excellent source of calcium. It's also one of the few nuts that offers a significant amount of vitamin C. For these reasons, I've included one Brazil nut in my daily diet for years.

Let's take a quick look at carbs. "**Carbohydrates** perform a simple trick: they enhance your brain's uptake of the amino acid tryptophan," says Judith Wurtman, Ph.D., author of *The Serotonin Solution*. In the brain, tryptophan becomes serotonin, a neurotransmitter that produces a sense of calm and decreases appetite. But don't start "carbo-loading" just yet. If you eat too many carbohydrates, you'll trigger enough serotonin to make you sleepy. That's why the grazing tip I offer in Chapter 5 is so effective. It's better to eat 3 to 4 ounces of unrefined, whole food carbs every three hours. That way you'll minimize feelings of stress, maximize energy, *and* cut cravings all at once!

Finally, for those chocolate lovers among you, a very little chocolate might just do the trick. Studies show that one 1 to 2 ounce serving tastes so good it stimulates the production of endorphins—brain chemicals that relieve stress. The result? By stopping stress-eating, a little chocolate actually saves you way more calories than it contains! And the darker and richer the chocolate, the stronger the effect. That's why I included a few recipes that incorporate a small amount of high quality organic cocoa powder.

7. Be mindful. Have you ever driven to work or run errands and not remembered how you got there? Check in with yourself every half hour. Are you slouching? How's your attitude? What are you thinking? Is your breathing shallow? Don't wait until your shoulders are up around your ears before you try to relax. Learn to be mindful about how you're feeling and what's happening around you. I usually describe mindfulness as developing the mind's capacity to attain a balanced, awake understanding of what's happening, knowing how you feel about it, and choosing your wisest response.

8. Consider massage, music, money & color. You're wondering how these all tie into stressless living, right? (Massage can cut cortisol levels, lower blood pressure, and boost immunity, as I explain in detail in Chapter 7.)

Have you ever felt depressed or stressed out and you put on some favorite music and noticed that within minutes your mood had lifted and you felt much less anxious? Studies have shown that the right kind of music (not heavy metal) reduces tension and anxiety while often improving performance. Make your home a place of music and sing a lot. When I'm under extra stress, I often forget to sing, so I have a reminder card on a centrally located mirror in my home to remind me to exercise my vocal cords. It's hard to feel stressed out and sing at the same time.

Live *below* your means. You can exercise regularly, eat healthy foods, have massages, and meditate daily, but if you can't pay your bills, your stress level is going to go up. Let go of your need to "keep up with the Jones" and do whatever it takes to manage your finances in a responsible way. See what you can release in your life that's draining you financially because it is also draining you mentally, emotionally, and spiritually. Some books that offer wise and helpful tips and have made positive differences in my life with organizing and uplifting my finances are Suze Orman's *The Courage to Be Rich* and David Bach's *Smart Women Finish Rich.*

Color is vibration, and different colors produce different vibrations that you can use to bring in specific energy levels that your body needs. Colors such as red, orange, and yellow tend to stimulate and energize, so these would be good colors to wear when working out or for your study, office, or kitchen. Blues, greens, and purples are more conducive to relaxing and cooling. One of my clients, Don, had trouble sleeping and would wake up several times during the night and have a hard time getting back to sleep. When I visited his home to do a "Wellness Lifestyle" makeover, I understood why he was sleep-deprived. His bedroom walls were painted red and yellow. I suggested the color green since it was his favorite color and green is believed to lower blood pressure and have calming sedative effects, and recommended 100% cotton bed linens. It worked. Two nights after the paint smell vanished, he was sleeping through the night.

9. Wear natural clothing. Fabrics can also have an adverse effect on your stress level. Studies now show that synthetic clothing and synthetic bedding can be as harmful as some synthetic food ingredients, causing allergies, respiratory problems, depression, distressing heart responses, slowing of mental responses, slower healing of irritations and wounds, poor sleep patterns, and distress intensified by magnification of air pollution.

Many people identify the problem without realizing it. We've all heard someone say, "I have a headache every time I wear this dress," or "It seems my sinuses act up every time I put on this shirt." A prime reason why many synthetics have undesirable effects has to do with electronics, and more specifically, ions.

Ions are created largely by natural forces: by wind or cosmic rays, by radioactive gases escaping from earth, by lightning and by falling water—any phenomenon with sufficient force to coax air molecules to dance. The molecule may be likened to an infinitesimally small golf ball. At its core are positive charged protons. Encircling these is a single negatively charged electron that weighs about 1,800 times less than the protons.

When jostled by the wind or other atmospheric friction, the electron, an unstable character at best, detaches itself and goes in search of a new home. Once it has departed, the original molecule assumes a positive charge; it becomes a positive ion. The electron, meanwhile, merges with another molecule, and in so doing imparts an additional negative charge. That molecule then becomes a negative ion.

We inhale ions when we breathe, and also absorb them through our skin. Then the fun—or havoc—begins. Clearly, ions affect us, but until recently scientists didn't understand how, or why. Much of the research on the effect of ions to our health has been done by former UC Berkeley professor Albert Paul Krueger, a physician-turned-biometerologist, and is reported in the book, *The Ion Effect* by Fred Soyka. The implications of his work are staggering.

Dr. Krueger discovered that the primary reason why ions affect us is that they alter the level of serotonin in the brain and body tissues. Positive ions increase the serotonin level; negative ions lower it. The powerful neurohormone has been dubbed "the ultimate downer." If the level gets too high (as can also be the case with overdoing refined carbs), the following symptoms have been reported: aching joints, insomnia, irritability, tension, tremors, migraines, suicidal impulses, dry throat, nausea, hot and cold flashes, hyperactivity, diarrhea, vertigo, respiratory ailments, fatigue, and depression. Pain is also felt more intensely. But when serotonin levels drop to a more balanced level, a sense of tranquil well-being occurs, pain sensations are reduced, and spirits are lifted.

You might be wondering what all this has to do with clothing. Plenty! The clothes you wear—your second skin—can carry electrical charges. In some materials these small charges can move around freely. This kind of material is called a conductor. Other materials, known as nonconductors, will restrict the charges' movements and they can become trapped. When one or more particles of the same charge are trapped on an object and cannot escape, the object is said to have an electrical charge.

Synthetic fabrics are woven from manmade fibers that are products straight from the chemistry lab. Under the microscope the synthetic fibers appear as solid plastic rods. They are nonconductors, which don't allow charges to escape, and so have what is called a positive potential.

Cotton, on the other hand, is a natural product and each fiber is of tubular design rather than the solid-rod structure of synthetics. Cotton fibers can absorb and hold even very small amounts of moisture. This small amount, even just the amount absorbed from the body, gives cotton the ability to drain away and rapidly lose any charge that might otherwise be trapped. Cotton fibers become neutral in the battle of the charges.

When we feel static electricity clinging to our clothing, it is due to an active electrical charge. And if the clothing you wear has a positive charge, it tends to attract the negative ions in the air we breathe to the clothing, thus diminishing the number available for inhalation.

Most of us are totally unaware of any effect, but asthmatics or people with emphysema and other respiratory ills often suffer additional agonies because of the clothes they wear. Many things in our environment can strip the negative ions out of the air, creating an unhealthy imbalance and leading to all sorts of problems.

To rectify the negative situation (no pun intended), furnish your home and workplace with items made of more natural materials. Select furniture made of wood rather than plastic. Choose wool carpeting and natural fabrics for draperies and curtains, and whenever possible, wear natural clothing fibers such as cotton, linen, wool, or silk. (See the next tip on nature time to learn more about the effect ions have on our bodies and well-being.)

10. Enjoy nature time. Being out in nature, where the air is filled with negative ions, lifts the spirits, relaxes the body, and gives us a sense of well-being. As mentioned above, the air all around us is electrically charged with positive and negative ions. Most of us live and work in environments dominated by technology—surrounded by computers, microwaves, air conditioners, heaters, TVs, and vehicular traffic. These and other "conveniences" of modern life emit excessive amounts of positive ions into the air we breathe, which can result in mental or physical exhaustion and affect overall wellness as described above. But when you're in nature, especially surrounded by water, like the ocean or a fountain, negative ions abound. In fact, the revolving water generated by fountains creates negative ions that cause air particles to achieve electrical (ionic) balance.

One way to increase the negative ions in your environment is to surround yourself with fountains. I have them all over my home—in my gardens and in several rooms, running 24/7 except in the bedroom, where I prefer quiet. Since ancient times, the sound created by moving or flowing water has been known to have great healing power. It has been said that the movement of water releases negative ions (chi energy) which, in turn, make you feel refreshed, bringing peace to your heart and mind. (See Fountainside in the Resource Directory.)

11. Laugh as often as possible. Along with my faith in God, laughter and faith are the two main things that help get me through life and help me deal with stress. It is okay to laugh, even when times are tough. Toxic worry almost always entails a loss of perspective and a sense of humor almost always restores it.

According to researchers, laughter releases endorphins into the body that act as natural stress beaters. And while you're grinning, take a second to note the actual physical sensation of smiling. The state of being happy, which is likely to be accompanied by a smile, produces a long-lasting pleasure buzz in the front part of the brain, say researchers at the University of Wisconsin in Madison. Laughter also aids most—and probably all—major systems of the body. A good laugh gives the heart muscles a good workout, improves circulation, fills the lungs with oxygen-rich air, clears the respiratory passages, stimulates alertness hormones that stimulate various tissues, alters the brain by diminishing tension in the central nervous system, counteracts fear, anger, and depression, all of which are linked to physical illness and stress, and helps relieve pain.

12. Simplify & slow down. Start by de-cluttering your personal environment—either work and/or home. Even something as simple as organizing your desk will make you more efficient and help to relieve stress. What makes a world of difference in my life is the 15 minutes I spend before I leave the office. I use that time to straighten my desk and make a list of all the things I want to do the next day. I can go home with my work left neatly behind me and the knowledge that tomorrow I can easily pick up where I left off.

Slow down the pace of your life. Find joy in simple pleasures like breathing deeply, smelling the flowers, talking to your pets, singing with the birds, being with friends, greeting the sun, scratching behind your dog's or kitty's ear, making someone smile, telling someone you love them, and laughing out loud—often!

Allow yourself one or two daily routines or rituals that make you feel good, and don't let them go. One of my favorites is starting my day with a dry skin brushing, a sauna, and a shower of cool to cold water as I ice my face with a couple of ice cubes. For me, this is the perfect start to the day. Especially after the sunrise hike I took a few hours before. I always try to have some fresh flowers in my home, for their beauty and fragrance inspire and relax me.

Living an uncluttered life gives me time for the things I really care about, like time to think, to read, to walk in nature, to meditate, and watch the sunset. Through simplification, I am more clear-minded and, I believe, a kinder, more sensitive person. Life becomes meditation and the divine becomes perfect simplicity. (Please refer to Peace Pilgrim in the Resource Directory to find out how to receive a free booklet, *Steps Toward Inner Peace.*)

13. Nurture intuition. Intuition is sometimes called a sixth sense, a hunch, a gut feeling, going on instinct, or just knowing deep inside. Psychologists define intuition as an obscure mental function that provides us with information so that we know without knowing how we know. The word "intuition" means to guide and protect. Intuition can be nurtured in a variety of ways—through contemplation, gazing out a window, relaxing, or by taking walks in nature. The best way is to be still and listen. The more we act on our intuitive hunches, the stronger and more readily available they become.

14. Live with integrity. To live with integrity means that who you appear to be is who you really are. Your inner realities—your beliefs, your commitments, your values—are all reflected in how you live your life on the outside. The more you live in synchronicity with what you believe, think, feel, say, and do, the more peace and happiness you will invite into your life. It takes a lot of energy to live without integrity. It is emotionally and intellectually exhausting when who you are on the inside and how you behave on the outside are not one and the same.

Honesty and integrity go hand-in-hand. To be honest is to be genuine, authentic, and real. To be dishonest is to be partly forged, fake, or fictitious. Honesty is best cultivated by being honest. The more you choose to be real and honest, the more it becomes a habit.

Make the effort to keep your word with yourself and others. Whether it's something as simple as calling someone on a certain day because you said you would or something bigger like remaining faithful to your partner because of the vow you made. It's all the same. Each time you don't keep your word, you disconnect a little bit from your Spirit and all the little bits add up.

15. Be positive & grateful. The link between mind and body has been contemplated since the time of Plato, but it's only recently that research has been done on the neurophysiology of the brain. Every thought transmits instructions to the body through some 70 trillion nerve cells, so when you think a negative thought, your immune system is immediately compromised. By the same token, when you think positive thoughts, your immune system is enhanced and your whole body benefits. Furthermore, an anxious or fearful mind instructs the body to be likewise—tense and nervous. A calm mind creates a calm body. And a mind emptied of ego-thought creates a space for divine healing and perfection.

So choose your thoughts wisely. A new report from the *Mayo Proceedings* suggests that individuals who profess pessimistic explanations for life events have poorer physical health and a higher mortality rate compared with either optimists or "middle-of-the-road" types, regardless of age or sex. In fact, every 10-point increase in the study's pessimism scores was associated with a 19% increase in the risk of death. Conversely, participants whose test scores indicated optimism had a survival rate significantly better than expected. The reason for this may be that pessimists may be more "passive" or have a "darker" outlook on life than other personality types, leaving them more prone to "bad life events"—such as illness, injury, and depression. The researchers concluded that pessimism itself is a "risk factor" for early death, and should be viewed in the same way as other risk factors, such as obesity or high cholesterol level, the key point being that a pessimistic view of life can lead to bad decision-making, affecting not only health but life in general.

One way to foster a positive attitude is to welcome an attitude of gratitude. Choose to be grateful for every aspect of your life—your ability to see, the food you eat, the air you breathe, your family, friends and animals, and the sunrise every morning. This simple act will help change your perspective about life and will transform your life for the better. A daily entry in a "gratitude journal" can help focus on the positive things, even when during the most difficult times of life.

16. Act with love & kindness. Being loving and kind improves health and reduces stress. It's a documented fact. We all need love—and I'm not just talking about romantic attraction. The warm, loving feeling you get from hugging a child, counseling a friend, being a good listener, or even treating yourself to a luxurious bubble bath boosts your self-esteem and your immune system. Petting a dog or watching fish in a tank lowers your blood pressure. In one study, people watching a film of Mother Theresa tenderly caring for sick children experienced the same heightened immune response as people who had recently fallen in love.

> *"The best portion of a good man's life is his little nameless unremembered acts of kindness and love."*
> — William Wordsworth

17. Live with reverence. Take time each day to meditate, pray, and talk to God. Studies have found lower rates of depression among those who believe in God. If you are not religious, meditate. Prayer and meditation help us keep things in perspective, keep our minds calm.

Many of us feel that we are at the mercy of other people or random circumstances, but we are not. By keeping our thoughts centered, we can understand any situation or "turbulence." So, take time every day to tap into, nurture, and protect that peacefulness and your stress will be manageable, you'll lose weight more easily, and you'll be healthier than ever. This will make your life more rewarding, you'll be more accomplished, and you'll have more fun in the process. Isn't that what living fully is all about? Celebrating life and being the best you can be.

SUCCESS

Chapter 2

UNDERSTAND & UTILIZE MIND POWER

How prompt we are to satisfy the hunger and thirst of our bodies, how slow to satisfy the hunger and thirst of our souls.

—Henry David Thoreau

Persistent thought patterns and unexpressed emotions ultimately manifest in our physical bodies. What you think and how you feel materialize in some form, whether as health or disease, in the physical body.

—James Van Praagh

One of the greatest truths of life is that it flows from the inside out. We are affected by what happens inside, by our feelings, and our thoughts and these, in turn, affect our emotions, the words we speak, and the actions we choose to take. What you feel or experience at any point in time is up to you. Change your thoughts and you change your life.

Easier said than done, right? Well, in this chapter, I will cover a variety of topics that help you understand your inner world better so that you can create more success with your health and every area of your life.

Take Loving Care of Yourself

Right this moment, stop reading and think about how truly remark-able your body is. Buckminster Fuller told us that 99% of who we are is invisible, untouchable, and unsmellable—because we are primarily spiritual beings living in a physical world. That's true, but the remaining 1%, the body in which you live, is a miracle, yet so often we take our bodies for granted.

The body is self-repairing, self-healing, and self-maintaining and, as a matter of course, persistently marshals its forces in a tireless quest to achieve and maintain radiant health. Health is the normal, natural state of the body. When you're healthy, the body automatically directs its efforts toward maintaining that state. When you're in a state of "dis-ease," living a life filled with stress and lack of balance, the body diligently strives to restore balance, to restore health.

As far back as 350 B.C., Hippocrates wrote about "health" as meaning the harmonious balance of mind and body and "disease" as being disharmony and lack of balance. Later, the French scientist Claude Bernard, who lived from 1813 to 1878, wrote about the stability of the internal landscape and first described the *"milieu interieur* formed by the circulating organic liquid which surrounds and bathes all the tissue elements." While Bernard did not identify this liquid, we now know that it contains acidic wastes and stress that, if triggered on a constant basis as I discussed in Chapter 1, can have harmful effects on the body.

Every one of our 70-plus trillion cells are working and orchestrating the millions of functions day in and day out without letting up in the never-ending process to procure and preserve our health. When the requirements of health are appropriately provided, the self-healing mechanisms of the body attempt to restore and/or optimize health.

Unconditionally cherishing, appreciating, loving, respecting, and nurturing our bodies, no matter what our current shape or level of wellness, is the first step to experiencing vibrant, radiant health. Let your body be your friend; love it with tender, loving care. Remember: **Changes that are loved into being are permanent.** Although your body is only a temporary home for your spiritual being, we must still take care of it daily.

Start today and tune in more to your body. It is an incredible feedback machine. If you listen, you will discover that it actually talks to you. When you get a headache, for instance, your body is trying to tell you something. Maybe you're not getting enough sleep or you are dehydrated; maybe you need to eat more whole foods; or maybe you simply need to carve out some time to just gaze out a window with a cup of your favorite tea while you breathe deeply and count your blessings. The key here is to listen to your body and be willing to deal with its communication.

Our lives are made up of millions of choices. Moment to moment, we are always choosing. What we are consists of the sum of our choices: what we think, what we imagine, how we react, what we eat, what we say, what we feel, and what we expect. Which is why we must each take back the responsibility for our own lives and start using the power that is ours to create what we want—a healthy, fit body and a fulfilling, joyful, peaceful life.

Susan's Top 10 Tips
for a Healthy Nutrition Program

1. Start strong
2. Eat your morning meal
3. Curb your appetite
4. Stop after seven
5. Feel your hunger
6. Go light
7. Eat what you like
8. Slow down
9. Don't give up
10. Reward yourself

---

1. Start strong. Pick a day to begin your new program and make the start date a special date. If you're near the end of the month, wait until the beginning of the next month or the beginning of the next week. I sometimes pick the new moon or the first day of a new season or the beginning of a month. Just as the first 40 minutes of each day set the tone for the day, so we want to make them relaxed, peaceful and positive, the first day of your new program sets the tone the next few months.

The days before your program starts, mentally, emotionally, and spiritually prepare. Do whatever you need to do to clean out your kitchen of unhealthy products, get your workout clothes and shoes in order, and create a monthly calendar you can place on your refrigerator door where each day you will list your physical activities and all the other ways you've loved yourself. For example, you might write that you walked for 30 minutes, lifted weights for 20 minutes, meditated for 15 minutes, ate 3 pieces of fruit, and put a rejuvenation mask on your face before going to bed. Seeing the squares filled in provides you with a mirror of how well you're taking care of yourself and brings a feeling of empowerment.

2. *Eat your morning meal.* Within one hour of getting up in the morning, make sure you have a healthy breakfast. Embracing each day with a strong, positive start makes it easier to make healthier choices throughout the day and also stokes your metabolism. People who eat a healthy breakfast generally feel less hungry throughout the day.

3. *Curb your appetite.* Drink a large glass of water about 15 minutes before a meal. Water does wonders for detoxifying and rejuvenating your body and helps to prevent overeating by making you feel full.

4. *Stop after seven.* If you want to see changes in your body shape fast, establish a habit of not eating after 7 P.M. If you can swing it, I'd say it's even better to stop after 6 P.M. This is what Tina Turner does. If you want to drop some weight quickly, you might even stop eating after 3 P.M., with the exception of fresh fruit or fresh vegetable juice.

5. *Feel your hunger.* Try to snack only when you're hungry, not when you're bored or depressed or tired or anything but hungry.

6. *Go light.* When your tummy really wants food and you don't have much time, opt for low-calorie bites that are quick and nourishing, such as carrot and celery sticks or other fresh vegetables or fresh fruit. If you crave more substance, add a few raw seeds or nuts, but no more than one ounce if you have more than ten pounds to lose.

7. *Eat what you like.* There are so many delicious healthy foods to choose from, there's simply no reason to eat foods you don't like. And nothing makes a food program more difficult than forcing yourself to eat foods you don't care for. So make wise, healthy choices from the foods you really like.

8. *Slow down.* Eat slowly enough to give your body time to release the enzymes that tell your brain when you've had all you need. Inhaling food instead of eating consciously and deliberately causes indigestion and gas. Also, chew your foods well. Half of digestion takes place in your mouth.

9. *Don't give up.* Falling off your health program once or twice does not mean the effort is hopeless. Simply acknowledge that you didn't eat wisely and get back on the program.

10. Reward yourself. Treat yourself with a massage, a movie, a new piece of clothing, or a delicious meal at your favorite restaurant for each week that you maintain your health program, achieve goals, or maintain weight.

(For numerous techniques on creating a new self-image through behavior modification, check out Victoria Moran's *Lit from Within: Tending Your Soul for Lifelong Beauty.)*

Let's explore more closely the importance of your day-to-day choices and the need to reprogram and retrain your senses to release self-limiting beliefs and habits.

Your primary goal on this aliveness eating program is to get to the point where you are eating a reasonable amount of the highest quality foods. Euripides said, "Enough is abundance to the wise."

Although it's important to choose healthy foods, don't become a fanatic about what you eat. It's what you choose to eat on a daily basis that makes the difference, not the occasional lapse. Worrying about every little piece of food that goes into your mouth is far more harmful in the long run than infrequent splurges.

Learn to think in terms of whole foods. Here are those words again. WHOLE FOODS. It's when you begin cutting, cooking, and processing foods that your system gets into trouble. Whenever you are able, eat your foods whole, just the way nature made them, complete with vitamins, minerals, enzymes, amino acids, natural sugars, fibers, and water, in the right proportions for efficient use by your body. Fresh fruits and vegetables, whole grains, legumes, nuts, and seeds carefully selected and prepared to suit your particular needs and desires are ideal foods for the vibrantly alive body.

You may feel that it's too difficult to switch all at once to a new nutritional program. That's a common reaction and that's okay. You can break in gradually if you wish, switching first to the foods that appeal to you the most and gradually adding the others. In fact it may take a while for your digestive system to become accustomed to handling these new live foods.

Your mind may have some negative programming about your eating habits that will trip you up if you aren't careful. The mind will always choose immediate gratification over long-term satisfaction. The mind doesn't care if you achieve your long-term goal for a fit, lean, healthy body. The mind wants you to feel good right now. It's important to realize that the mind isn't necessarily your friend. You must sometimes detach from it to achieve your long-term goals (see Chapter 1 for more information on how meditation can help you to detach.)

Whether for food or something else, the difficulty in resisting sensory desire comes from the force of conditioning. Every time we are negatively conditioned, we lose a little of our freedom and our capacity to choose. So begin by becoming aware of what you are eating. Eating at the table, at mealtimes, and only when you are hungry helps, because you can more fully focus your attention on your food. When our attention is divided, we eat compulsively rather than from hunger. Automatic eating occurs frequently in front of the television set, or at a movie theater, parties, or sports events.

The entire process of eating needs to be given your full attention to get the maximum benefits. Be conscious of the hunger you feel before you eat; how the food looks and smells as you prepare it, serve it, and eat it; how the table setting looks; how the food tastes; the texture of the food; your chewing; your breathing; and how you feel while you are eating. Finally, after all this, be aware of and grateful for the feelings of lightness and high energy derived from the meal and the easy elimination of the food after it's digested. It's embracing this attitude about meals that enables you to appreciate simple, wholesome foods, and to eat less, feeling completely satisfied. Paying attention helps to develop the capacity to enjoy the simplest foods and to be truly healthy.

Stop eating just before you feel really full. In this way you are reprogramming your subconscious and are taking control rather than letting your habits control you. Stopping short of satiety helps you savor your food and helps you to be free and in charge of your choices.

Begin the retraining of your senses by eliminating things that injure the body. None of us would drive into a service station and fill the gas tank with oil. For the car to run efficiently, we must use a particular type of gas, lubricant, coolant, and so on. Yet, when it comes to our bodies, we are often not so careful. We put in all kinds of things that nutritionists and plain common sense tell us impair the body's smooth functioning, just because they taste pleasant. We need to reestablish that the determinant of what we eat should be our body's needs, not merely the appeal of the senses. I have found that meditating for a few minutes before each meal is a powerful tool that fosters choosing foods that promote health and harmony.

Pythagorus said, "Choose what is best; habit will soon render it agreeable and easy." It does seem that our taste buds change and adapt when we alter our eating habits, and the whole wheat bread that tasted heavy and grainy a few months ago may taste chewy and flavorful this month. Feeling better and looking marvelous will soon compensate for the loss of dubious taste thrills of the past, such as fried chicken, white bread, ice cream, candy, and potato chips. You'll find yourself looking forward to more healthful pleasures—the taste of ripe papaya, luscious strawberries, blueberries, ripe pineapple, sweet juicy grapes, a crisp garden salad, brown rice or quinoa with steamed vegetables, and sweet potatoes smothered in sautéed onions, broccoli, and mushrooms.

Your Thoughts Create Your Reality

All this talk about food has probably gotten you hungry, so before we continue, you might want to get a healthy snack. As you're eating, review your thoughts of the day. Do you generally think positive or negative thoughts? Do you think that you have many thoughts? Do you think that you are in control of your thoughts? Many of us are not even aware of how much we think and how negative our thoughts are. When you wake up, are you excited about the new day? Do you say, "Thank you God for this new day filled with opportunity and blessings," or do you say, "Good God, it's morning, another stress-filled day"? Do your thoughts center around the discordant alarm, no time for breakfast, too much traffic on the way to work, and unhappiness with your job? These thought processes go on and on during the day. If you believe that positive thinking doesn't really matter because, "Hey, how many thoughts can a person actually have during a day, anyway?"—well, give it another thought!

According to the National Science Foundation, we each think thousands of thoughts everyday—in fact, about 1,000 an hour. The ordinary human being thinks about 12,000 thoughts a day. A deeper thinker (all of you reading this book, of course) according to this report, puts forth about 50,000 thoughts. So imagine that 50% of the time you are positive in your thinking.

Ralph Waldo Emerson, in all his sagacity, has this to say about thought: "A man is what he thinks about all day long." That's right. What we believe to be true and what we think about consistently—our mental atmosphere—is mirrored back to us in our surroundings. This is not merely my theory but is supported by scientists, psychologists, psychiatrists, hypnotherapists, metaphysicians, and others in the healing profession. So those 25,000 negative thoughts you are thinking each day are making a significant contribution to your reality.

Inevitably, your beliefs and thoughts create your reality. Let's look at an all-too-common example of how this concept works: fat control. Let's assume that you've always had difficulty controlling your weight. You've tried all kinds of diets and they've never worked (diets never bring long-term success!), so you have negative beliefs about diets. You've tried to limit the amount of food you eat without much success, so you don't have much faith in your self-control. And you get on the scale every morning and the figures on the scales usually serve to reinforce your view of yourself as overweight. It really is a vicious cycle. In order to better understand why you keep repeating the same patterns, let's think about the way the mind works.

Reminder: Your beliefs and thoughts create your reality.

Your Mind Can Be Programmed for Positive Results

Brain researchers see the mind as composed of two primary parts: the conscious mind and the subconscious mind. A window to the world, your conscious mind runs your daily waking activities, such as making decisions, relating to others, and so on. Your subconscious mind, however, carries memories of all your experiences. It is the storage center for all the information your conscious mind sends it, based on your daily experiences. Your subconscious mind is a computer that is fed the data of your every thought and experience.

Relating this to the example of weight control: if you get up every morning and worry about what clothes will fit, if you dread getting on your scale, if you dislike being seen in public, if you think about going on a diet but doubt that it will work, **you are programming your subconscious computer in a negative way.**

So you have some excess pounds of fat on you. Rather than getting down on yourself, simply own the fact that you've deposited some extra fat on your body. You don't have to continue repeating the past. You can choose to manifest a different result—being trim and fit. Create new beliefs, thoughts, visualization, and actions. You can reprogram yourself to create what you desire and deserve.

Your mind creates reality according to its programming. If you think of yourself as fat, as having little self-control, as being unable to change, you will see those beliefs reflected in your life.

The same is true for every other area of your life. Your beliefs and thoughts about yourself, your relationships with others, your money, your material possessions, and so on, will be faithfully recreated in your life. Now you may be reading this and thinking, "That isn't true for me. I know that I really want to lose weight and tone up my body (or make more money or get involved in a relationship) but I'm not experiencing that in my life." To that I would say that there is a difference between wanting something on a conscious level and wanting it on a subconscious level.

Reminder: Your beliefs and thoughts about yourself, your relationships with others, your money, your material possessions, and so on, will be faithfully recreated in your life.

You Must Be What You Desire

The conscious mind and the subconscious mind are often in conflict. Consciously you may want something, yet subconsciously you create mediocrity or failure. That's why positive thinking, as it is commonly perceived, doesn't work. It doesn't do much good to force yourself to think positive thoughts on a conscious level while your subconscious still harbors many negative beliefs. What you need to do in order to break the vicious cycle of negative beliefs that is creating a negative reality is to reprogram your subconscious mind through methods and tips we will examine in this section. In addition, you must make some behavior changes on a conscious level that will contribute to new beliefs.

In other words, you must be what you desire. To be it, you must first capture the feeling of whatever it is you desire, whether it's being happy, loving, prosperous, or fit and healthy. Then you'll start acting that way and finally become it. The essential tip here in the process is to capture the feeling, because when you do that, you've captured the ability to internalize it. Then it's only a matter of time.

If you see your world only according to what surrounds you right now, you are judging by appearances and limiting what you are going to have. Instead of thinking, "I'll believe it when I see it," think "I'll see it when I believe it." Trust in the Universe, the power within, regardless of appearances. For as the spiritual teacher Paramahansa Yogananda said, we must trust in the invisible, for it's the sole cause of that which is visible.

As we change our consciousness, we change our lives. Because thoughts create form, the very thing you believe becomes reality for you *because* you believe in it. Richard Bach, in *Jonathan Livingston Seagull*, wrote, "Don't believe what your eyes are telling you. All they show is limitation. Look with your understanding, find out what you already know and you'll see the way to fly."

At the beginning of the twentieth century, William James, founder of one of the first psychological laboratories in the United States, said that belief can be embodied in consciousness through "the path of emotions" and "the path of will." Regarding the emotions, he wrote that the idea must be one that excites our interest. The interest will then stimulate the emotions, particularly feelings of love, and when the feeling reaches the stage of passion it will then be recorded as a belief in the mind: "Gradually our will can lead us to the same results by a very simple method. We need only *act* as if the thing in question was real, and keep acting as if it were real, and it will infallibly end by growing into such a connection with our life that it will become real. It will become so knit with habit and emotion that our interests in it will be those which characterize belief.… If you only care enough for a result, you will almost certainly attain it. If you wish to be rich, you will be rich. If you wish to be learned, you will be learned. If you wish to be good, you will be good. Only you must really wish these things and wish them exclusively and not wish at the same time 100 other incompatible things as strongly."

So first, you must say what it is you desire, and you must be specific. You must put in mind that which you choose to bring into your life. You must direct the power within to create what you want. The creative principle works according to the seeds that you plant. Therefore it's imperative that you plant the seeds that you desire to grow. When you plant seeds that you don't want to grow, it's out of a lack of understanding. If you plant love you get back love. If you plant scarcity, you get back scarcity. So, say what you want, be specific, and act "as if," that is, act as if what you want were already true.

> *Reminder:* If you plant love you get back love. If you plant scarcity, you get back scarcity. So, say what you want, be specific, and act "as if," that is, act as if what you want were already true.

Your Feelings Are the Power that Creates

It's important to understand the role of feelings in being the radiantly healthy, fit person you want to become. Your feelings are the power that creates. Just to simply visualize something without deep, passionate feeling will do little good. From the extensive research I have done in the field of manifestation over the past 25 years, I have come to appreciate the role of feelings. I like to describe feelings as an electromagnetic force field that is so strong it sends up a vibration that pulls like vibrations to itself. Another way of saying this is: **What you think about with feeling expands and grows in your life.** Strong, passionate feelings are like magnets for similar energy particles. The result: more of those situations that produced the feeling to begin with. For example, human behavior specialists know that success begets success and failure begets failure. After interviewing countless highly intelligent, successful people with diverse backgrounds and vast experience, the conclusion I came to was that how you feel about things can be a determining factor in the way your life works out. **And any feeling we want we can have by simply being it.** It's this powerful force of feeling that acts as the generator to bring into creation that which we desire. Negative feelings will bring negative results. Positive feelings will bring positive results.

As I give workshops and do counseling and consulting around the country, I often hear statements such as this: "I continually affirm, visualize, meditate, and believe in my highest good, but I rarely see results." Most of the time this is because we are not really believing in ourselves because we have never forgiven ourselves for our past failures. By practicing forgiveness toward ourselves and others, we unlock the gate to healing and health, prosperity and abundance, joy and happiness, and inner peace. When you don't forgive another person, you give away your power and create a highly charged, emotionally active connection. But when you forgive, you take back your power and are no longer controlled by the other person. And when we don't forgive ourselves and others, the emotions of guilt, fear, worry, and anger take away our power, disconnect us from our Spirit, color our words and actions, and ultimately—because what we think about expands and grows in our lives—negatively affects our lives. These negative emotions are energy—time-wasters. Learn from your feelings and then release anything and everything that you don't want more of in your life. For a simple exercise, try this: In your mind's eye, visualize yourself and the person you wish to forgive seated facing each other. Surround yourselves in a circle of golden or white light. Create a scenario in which you share your feelings in a comfortable, supportive manner. Say everything you need to say. Release, and let go. Take a deep breath and bring your awareness back to the here and now. Go about your business knowing that your heart has changed. Trust that everything will unfold for your greatest good as you allow love to be your guide. (For a more in-depth look at these topics, refer to my book *Choose to Live Peacefully*.)

Reminder: What you think about with feeling expands and grows in your life.

Generating & Igniting Your Inner Power

Now let's take a look at some external, conscious changes you can make. For example, if you feel that your beliefs about money are creating negative results in your life, examine the behaviors that support those negative beliefs. Maybe you are frugal in your grocery shopping; you always buy the cheapest brands and skip the luxuries. Although that frugality might be wise in light of your current financial situation, you should be aware that it also tends to reinforce your belief that you have very little money. One way to attack this belief would be to substitute a new behavior for an old one. In other words, the next time you're in a grocery store, allow yourself to indulge in a little luxury; purchase those beautiful, but more expensive oranges, yellow and purple sweet bell peppers, or the Belgian endive, or the juicer or sprouting kit to help you create more healthy meals.

If your problem is loneliness, make it a point to smile at one stranger every day, just as if you had plenty of friends and an abundance of love to share.

If you are heavier than you'd like to be, buy yourself something appealing that you would normally have denied yourself because of your present weight.

The more time you spend acting "as if" and imagining yourself as already having achieved a given goal, the more likely you will be able to achieve that goal.

Reminder: The more time you spend acting "as if" and imagining yourself as already having achieved a given goal, the more likely you will be able to achieve that goal.

Choose to Reprogram Your Subconscious Mind

Another way to move toward the achievement of your goals is through reprogramming your subconscious mind. There are many methods available: Creative visualization, affirmations, meditation, hypnosis, and biofeedback techniques are just a few. The idea is to alter your state of consciousness so you can temporarily set aside the conscious mind and focus your concentration specifically on your subconscious. According to brain researchers, suggestions given to your subconscious while in an altered state of consciousness, whether they are images or affirmations, will be at least 20 times as effective as suggestions given in a normal state of consciousness. I've seen this validated time and time again in my counseling when I do creative visualization with clients. If you're interested in reading about this further, I suggest Wayne Dyer's book *Manifest Your Destiny*.

Although altering your state of consciousness may sound difficult, it's really easy. In fact, you change your state of consciousness at least twice a day without realizing it: when you wake up in the morning and when you fall asleep at night. That's because you pass through different states of consciousness, or brain wave levels, as you pass into and out of sleep. Brain research tells us that four brain wave levels characterize your state of consciousness: Beta is waking consciousness. As your body becomes relaxed you move into alpha, a state of consciousness in which you are still fully aware of your environment but are probably untroubled by it. Still closer to sleep is theta. While in theta you may still maintain some conscious awareness of your environment, but your mind will be totally concentrating on the relaxed feeling in your body. Delta is the sleep state. While in delta you are completely unconscious and have no sense of your surroundings.

For reprogramming purposes you need only be concerned with the alpha and theta levels of your mind. This is where you can speak directly to your subconscious while still maintaining conscious control of the programming you are supplying.

Before we go any further into actual techniques you can use to reprogram your subconscious, I want to emphasize the importance of recognizing how your beliefs create your reality. What you are at this very moment is the culmination of all that you have ever dreamed, desired, or thought. Remember, if things aren't just the way you would like them to be and you desire some changes in your life, first you must change your beliefs, thoughts, and the words you speak.

> *The greatest force in the human body is the natural drive of the body to heal itself—but that force is not independent of the belief system, which can translate expectations into physiological change. Nothing is more wondrous about the fifteen billion neurons in the human brain than their ability to convert thoughts, hopes, ideas and attitudes into chemical substances. Everything begins, therefore, with belief. What we believe is the most powerful option of all.*
>
> —Norman Cousins

Your beliefs about yourself are based entirely on your past experiences. All of your experiences program your subconscious, and the result is the person you are today.

That is not to say that all you will ever be is the sum of your experiences. Unless you take **conscious** control and **choose** the kind of programming you are feeding into your subconscious computer, however, you are destined to repeat your past experiences. Have you ever noticed that your life experiences are all very similar—it's just the people who keep changing?

The subconscious is programmed; it doesn't reason. When you understand this concept and integrate this knowledge into your life, you will be able to create a healthier, happier life than you ever imagined possible. The subconscious works to create reality according to the programming it has been fed. Although this is normally accomplished by thoughts and through your life experiences, brain researchers have found that the subconscious is incapable of telling the difference between reality and fantasy, between the real experience and the imagined experience.

There have been numerous classic studies in which a person in a hypnotic trance (altered state of consciousness) is touched by an object, such as a piece of ice, that is represented as a piece of hot metal. Almost invariably, a blister will develop at the point of contact. What this demonstrates is that it is not reality that counts, but belief—the direct, unquestioned communication to your nervous system. The brain does what it is told. Or with the placebo effect, you take a pill believed to make you feel happy and energetic, and you do, even though you're unaware that it's only a sugar pill.

Visualize & Affirm Your Goals as Already Achieved

Taking time each day to visualize your goals can have a profound effect on your life. Albert Einstein conceived the theory of relativity by visualizing "what it must look like to be riding on the end of a light beam."

Henry David Thoreau advised: "If you advance confidently in the direction of your dreams and endeavor to live the life which you have imagined, you will meet with success unexpected in common hours." I love that. It always works, but it takes getting out there and advancing confidently in the direction of your dreams. So ask yourself. What are your dreams? What is your vision? What do you expect to achieve in life? An important part of the process is expectation. Always expect to achieve your highest good, the best life has to offer, and live so that the best may become a part of your experience.

This moment, and always, choose consciously to take your attention off those things that you don't want in your life, and think about and visualize what you do want. In addition, you must have faith in yourself. And yes, faith means sometimes having to believe in things that common sense doesn't seem to support. Faith also means living beyond what you can see with your eyes. Don't judge by appearances.

Never allow anyone or anything to cause you to doubt your power and ability to live your vision—to manifest your goals and dreams. Be very clear about what you want to create and then set some goals for yourself. Goals are an important part of living your vision, and goals give you something constructive to think about. So many of us spend our waking hours thinking about all the negative elements around us or about how others should change to meet our expectations. Goals give our thoughts positive direction and purpose and keep us focused on our own thoughts and behavior, which we can control, rather than other people, who we can't control. Remember, what we think about consistently, we get.

Remember, when you use creative visualization, ***see your desire as an already accomplished fact.*** Dwell in perfect confidence, peace, and certainty, never looking for results, never wondering or becoming anxious or hurried. Above all, don't worry. Worry leads to fear and fear is crippling. Know that there is a power greater than yourself within you, guiding you in the right direction. So there's no need to worry. It was Mark Twain who said, "I'm an old man and have many troubles, most of which never happened."

If, for example, you want to lose weight and you are clear on this goal, here's what you might do. Create a mental movie (visualization) in which you see yourself walking into a clothing store and trying on a dress or suit two sizes smaller than the size you are now wearing. Imagine yourself looking in the mirror, and then experience delight when it fits. Then imagine that a sales clerk comments on how well you wear your clothes. When you take the outfit home, imagine your mate or a friend being pleased and surprised by how much weight you've lost. Then in another mental movie you might imagine yourself getting on the scale/monitor in the morning and seeing that you've achieved your desired weight and percentage of body fat. ***Emotion and feeling have more power in your subconscious than reasoning.*** Two affirmations for a fat loss goal might be: "Every day in every way I am becoming more slender and fit" and "I weigh ___ pounds easily and effortlessly, my body is fit and beautifully shaped, and I feel healthier and look more youthful than ever before."

There is power in what you say. Although it is sometimes difficult to control your thoughts, you can always control your words. Be aware of everything you say. Always affirm what you want in life. Words can be a blessing or a curse. Each word is just like a rock that we throw into a lake—the ripples fan out and spread across a large area. Every word we speak is an act of creating, just like our thoughts. There is an unwritten law that we attract to ourselves the equivalent of that which we express by our thoughts and words. That means that every time we bless or praise something we actually bring a blessing to ourselves. The opposite is also true. The old proverb "sticks and stones may break my bones but words can never hurt me" couldn't be more untrue. Words have amazing power.

Now I'm not saying that all you have to do is put different pictures in your head and say a few positive words and immediately your life will turn around. I am saying that **in order to change, you must start with your images, thoughts, and words.** They will then get stored in your subconscious as reality. Then you will start acting on that new reality. I use visualization for everything from healing relationships, to increasing my fitness level, to bringing more peace into my life.

After setting goals for your weight, health, vitality, and every area of your life, write some affirmations supporting these goals. An affirmation is a strong, positive statement that something is already so. It is a way of making firm what you are desiring and visualizing. By using affirmations you can weed out the limiting and false beliefs you have about yourself and program those goals you wish to achieve. Don't underestimate the power of using affirmations. It is an effective technique that can positively affect your attitude, thoughts, and actions, and transform the quality of your life in a short time.

There are a few points to keep in mind when composing your affirmations.

1. *Make sure they are in the present tense, rather than the future.* Remember, the subconscious has no reasoning power and doesn't understand abstract concepts such as future. So rather than affirming, "I will weigh (your goal) pounds by the end of the

month and my body will be firm, strong, and well-defined," say something like: "I am at my ideal weight of _____ pounds and my body is strong, firm, and filled with vitality." It doesn't matter how far away from your ideal weight you are right now. This practice acknowledges that everything always begins on a mental plane and then manifests itself on the physical plane.

2. *Make sure your affirmations are phrased in a positive way*. In other words, don't say, "I no longer feel tired or lack self-esteem." If you phrase your affirmation in this way, your subconscious may hear only the negative words. Instead, affirm, "I always have an abundance of energy and have high self-esteem."

3. *Make up affirmations that truly have meaning for you*—words that you can feel deep in your heart and elicit emotion. It's not enough to just recite them, you must *feel* them and be *moved* passionately and joyfully by them.

These affirmations can be used alone or with visualizations.

4. *Use your affirmations often*. Say them quietly to yourself or say them out loud. Make a recording of your affirmations and play them several times each week. (In my audiobook *Wired to Meditate* and my 7-tape program *Celebrate Life!* I offer many affirmations that you can repeat with me.)

5. *Write down your affirmations on three-by-five-inch cards and place them around your home and office*. Then take each affirmation and write it 21 times on a piece of paper and say it as you write.

Begin to include your affirmations in your daily conversations. Make strong positive statements about yourself, situations, and people that you want to see in a more positive way. Make an agreement with a friend to support each other in choosing only positive words, and to call each other on the use of negative ones. You will discover that over time speaking positively will become natural for you. Remember: Your reality is simply a manifestation of your thoughts, the words you speak, and your beliefs. So choose them all carefully.

To get the most out of your visualizations and affirmations you should use them throughout the day along with visualizing your goals in their successful state. For this programming to be dramatically effective and to bring results more quickly, set aside at least fifteen minutes each day so you can purposely alter your state of consciousness.

"Imagination is more important than knowledge."
—Albert Einstein

Here's a simple way to alter your state of consciousness. Find a place where you can be alone and undisturbed. Sit comfortably with your back straight or lie down, but don't let yourself fall asleep. Breathe slowly and deeply for a few moments. As you breathe, relax your body, progressively, from your toes to your head. Imagine that a wave of relaxation is entering your feet, relaxing every part as it travels up throughout your body. Then start to vividly visualize your goal or goals. Before finishing, say the affirmations that support the reality you want to create. The entire process might take 15 minutes. Then, as you return to your regular state of consciousness, let go of your mental movie and bring your thoughts back to your environment. Remind yourself that you have the power and ability to create the reality you desire. You really do!

It Takes 21 Days to Change a Habit

Your mind is a powerful tool for creating positive change, but it isn't always your friend. Sometimes it is often a less than willing participant.

Perhaps you've taken up walking/jogging and promised yourself that you're going to get out there at least every other day. For the first week you have a lot of motivation, but your resolve is weakening. It seems that something always comes up that is more important than exercise. Perhaps you need to be in the office early and can't take time for a morning run, or your children might begin complaining about not receiving your undivided attention. Or maybe you just stayed out too late and an extra hour's sleep seems more inviting than 10 laps around the track. Whatever circumstances you create—and they always seem legitimate at the time—be aware that your mind is doing a number on you. It is creating excuses so it won't have to change familiar patterns. According to behavioral psychologists, *it takes 21 days of consistently repeating an activity before your mind accepts the activity as a habit*. There are several steps you can take to ensure you'll stick with your new exercise program.

1. *Choose an exercise program that includes activities you honestly like to do.* Ideally, you will choose a variety of activities, such as jogging, walking, hiking, bicycling, swimming, and weight lifting, to work different muscle groups and give you a change of pace. Most important, though, is to choose an activity that you won't dread doing a minimum of three times a week.

2. *Create an exercise plan that seems easy to accomplish.* You might, for instance, want to make an agreement with yourself that every day you will spend 30 minutes jogging or walking, depending upon the way you feel that day. Or you might agree to spend 15 minutes stretching every morning. Don't create a plan that requires you to be running 10 miles a day, pressing 130 pounds on the leg press, and doing the splits within a month. Your mind and body will rebel against these drastic changes, and you won't succeed with any of them.

3. *Resolve to stay with your agreement every day for 21 days.* If you skip a day, you must begin the 21-day cycle over again. The reasoning behind this is simple. Because it takes 21 days to form a new habit, it will probably take 21 days for your mind and body to stop resisting the new pattern. Twenty-one days isn't a very long time, so if you find your mind coming up with excuses, you can regain control by reminding yourself that you only have to do it for 21 days.

If, at the end of that time, you still don't enjoy the activity or feel you aren't receiving any benefit, you can always reevaluate. What you will almost surely find is that by the end of the 21-day period, you no longer mind doing the exercise. It has become a normal part of your life. At this point you are ready to incorporate a slightly more demanding fitness program, which I describe in Chapters 4 and 5.

This 21-day process can be used in any area you choose, including changing your eating habits, establishing a meditation program, or drinking more water.

Discipline & Commitment Bring Freedom & Success

What you're probably seeing by now is that discipline is an important part of this. Discipline is a choice. If we are to achieve our highest potential, we must practice self-discipline in every aspect of our lives. Success and fulfillment are available only to those who learn to control their body, mind, and emotions.

Discipline, to me, means **the ability to carry out a resolution long after the mood has left you.** It also means doing what you say you are going to do, and doing it with eagerness and enthusiasm. If your attitude is positive, you will get positive results. There is no way to get 100% success without putting in 100% effort.

With discipline comes freedom and peace of mind. A disciplined person is not at the mercy of external circumstances. Whereas an undisciplined person is usually lazy, undirected and unhappy or depressed, a disciplined person is in control of what she thinks, feels, says, and does. A disciplined mind creates a disciplined body. And from a disciplined body comes an exhilarated mind. It's a powerful cycle.

Discipline ignites the power within you and helps create miracles in your life. Breakthroughs and miracles occur when people are willing to live out their vision and commitment and to honor their decisions. When you're committed, you allow nothing to deter you from reaching your goal. Discipline keeps you going even when you are not feeling motivated. You get past your excuses so you follow through and do what you said you are going to do.

Make your word count. Be responsible and accountable. **How do you ever expect someone to make a commitment to you or think you will follow through on a commitment to them unless you first show a commitment to yourself?**

I welcome friendships where commitment, discipline, follow-through, and taking risks is a way of living and being. When I'm with those friends, I feel empowered, inspired, motivated, and energized. I have very little patience or respect for people who don't honor their commitments. In fact, I have weeded out several such friends over the past few years. These people are very energy draining.

If you are ready for commitment—if you are ready to create a healthy lifestyle—you will arrange your personal circumstances so that your lifestyle totally supports your commitment. You will do whatever it takes, whatever you need to do to order your life, let go of excess baggage and the superfluous non-essentials, and consciously focus on what is important.

Self mastery begins by recognizing our power and using it to bring our vision to life. Some years ago, I made a conscious choice to stop allowing myself to go where life pushed and pulled me. Instead, I began to acknowledge that I could choose my responses and master my life. Since then I've begun to use the power that I had previously been giving away to self-limiting beliefs.

This moment—right now—can be a new beginning. You no longer need to repeat the past, worry about the future, or struggle through life as a victim of circumstance. Here are the key tips I use in my life and with my clients to help boost self-esteem and make life more of a celebration filled with success.

1. *Take loving care of your body.* Eat healthy foods and exercise regularly. Think of your body as more than pounds of flesh and tissue. Treat your body as the miracle it is and honor it with love and respect.

2. *Be grateful and count your blessings.* Gratitude is a dynamic spiritual energy that allows you to exert a powerful influence on your body and life. Plato wrote, "A grateful mind is a great mind—it eventually attracts to itself every great thing."

Buy or create your own special gratitude journal. Every day, write down at least three things for which you are grateful. Remember, **whatever you put your attention on, expands and grows in your life.**

Look at all the positive aspects about your body and life and write them down so you can see them all the time. Make a list of all the things for which you are grateful: your eyes, which show you beauty; your hands, which let you touch; your children; your spouse and friends; the flowers in your yard; or the park down the street (see the Self-Realization Fellowship in the Resource Directory).

3. *Be patient and trust.* Everything happens in its proper time. Trust that unscheduled events in your life are your own form of spiritual direction and that everything will unfold for your highest good. Be patient with yourself and choose to live one day at a time.

4. *Let go of all criticism and judgments.* Be loving and kind towards yourself and release all criticism and judgments. Harboring critical and judgmental thoughts affect your body and health. When you let go of your self-criticisms and judgments of others, and instead choose to practice living with unconditional love and forgiveness, the extra padding of fat that you've used to armor your body and protect your self falls away and your authentic, beautiful self then reveals itself. So when you catch yourself being judgmental and critical, stop and think of something positive. Say your affirmations. Count your blessings. And at least once a day, look in your mirror and take one minute to praise and support yourself. You deserve it.

5. Be of service to others.   One of the fastest ways to feel better about yourself is to do something nice for another person. It could be as simple as giving someone a hug, cooking a meal for a sick neighbor, watching a friend's child so she or he can have some quality time to themselves, or sending a card saying "thank you." In giving to others, we give to ourselves. Find ways to volunteer. A ten-year study of 1,300 Michigan men found that those who were active in organizations outside the home lived longer, healthier lives than those who were not. Some scientists even speculate that volunteering produces a "helper's high," an exhilaration caused by the release of endorphins, the brain's own mood-elevating chemicals.

6. Live in the presence of love.   There is nothing that will transform your life more quickly than living with a consistent feeling of love in your heart. For the next twenty-four hours maintain a consistent feeling of love; your entire life will change for the better and will be enriched. It's not very easy. Keep practicing and see how long you can go.

Loving, Positive Thoughts Transform Lives

I could hear the frustration in her voice the moment I picked up the telephone. My friend Rose called me because she was on the verge of quitting her job, even though she loved her work. Rose is a very talented window dresser for a popular store on Rodeo Drive in Beverly Hills, in charge of changing the window every couple of weeks. Rose's talents are so well-known that people come from miles around just to see what she has created in the window. She loves what she does, but she had been having a very difficult time with her boss. During our conversation, she described how she was convinced that she was unjustly criticized by her supervisor and felt that some of her best work was being rejected and unappreciated. She also felt he was deliberately rude and unfair to her. On top of that, in the six months since she was hired, she had gained almost fifteen pounds, felt stressed out, and exhausted.

Because I believe that we always attract to ourselves the equivalent of what we think, feel, and believe, I lovingly suggested to my friend that maybe she, rather than her boss, was the one in need of a new attitude. I asked her how she felt about him.

Rose confessed to me she felt critical and unkind toward this man and that she rarely felt positive in his presence because every day she anticipated the way he would treat her as she walked to work. I explained that he was merely bearing witness to her concept of him.

When Rose realized what she had been doing, she agreed to change her attitude and only think of him in a loving, kind way. I recommended to her that, before drifting off to sleep at night, she visualize her boss congratulating her on her fine designs and creativity and that she, in turn, see herself thanking him for his praise and kindness.

To her delight, after only seven days of practicing her visualization, the behavior of her employer miraculously reversed itself. Rose realized that her own attitude was the cause of the problem. She proved the power of imagination and kindness. Rose's persistent desire to change her attitude changed his behavior and his attitude toward her. He even admitted that he was bearing down on her unfairly and inexorably. It is always the same—as within, so without.

Two months after starting her new positive attitude, she lost the fifteen pounds along with another five extra pounds that she needed to lose without even trying. It just came off as she elected to let her love light shine on herself and another. **When you invite and allow love to be the guiding force of your life, you become empowered and this reconnection with your inner power creates miracles in your body, your life, and in the lives of others. And changes that are loved into being are permanent.**

We are powerful spiritual beings meant to create good on the earth. This good isn't usually accomplished in bold actions, but in singular small acts of love and kindness between people. The amount of love and good feelings we have at the end of our lives is equal to the love and good feelings we put out during our lives.

So start now and choose to live life the way you have imagined, without interfering with anyone else's right to do the same. When you advance confidently and boldly, with an excitement and enthusiasm about what you are doing—be it your health and fitness program, your job, or hobbies—then success is inevitable. You will start living your vision when you get out there and act "as if." Advance confidently in the direction of your dreams.

Man is made or unmade by himself . . . in the armory of thought he forges the weapons by which he destroys himself; he also fashions the tools with which he builds for himself heavenly mansions of joy and strength and peace. By the right choice and true application of thought, man ascends to the Divine Perfection; by the abuse and wrong application of thought, he descends below the level of the beast. Between these two extremes are all the grades of character, and man is their maker and master.

—James Allen, *As a Man Thinketh*

Things turnout best for the people who make the best out of how things turn out.

—John Wooden

SUCCESS

Chapter 3

CHOOSE THE OPTIMUM DIET

Nothing will benefit human health and increase the chances for survival of life on earth as much as the evolution to a vegetarian diet.
—Albert Einstein

Last year a man came to see me. He was (and still is) the president of a major corporation. I could tell from our first meeting that he was an impatient, aggressive, sometimes hostile man who was completely unaware of how to make choices to support his well-being. He told me that he routinely put in six or seven fourteen-hour pressure-packed days a week at his office or traveling. He always had to be first, always had to be right, and always had to be busy with work to feel worthwhile. As a fancier of rich foods, he regularly put away vast quantities of cheese, ice cream, steak, butter, processed foods, and cream sauces. His favorite breakfast consisted of a sausage composed of port, liver, white rice, and hot spices, served with eggs, ham, white bread and butter, and two cups of coffee. Despite all the cholesterol and fat, he figured he didn't need to worry because, according to the scale, he wasn't overweight. His only regular exercise was shifting gears in one of his expensive sports cars.

Although he was always tired, he thought a soak in the hot tub and a drink or two each night were all he needed to relax. But eventually he began to sink into a depression. He began to experience bouts of dizziness and was unable to stay focused. His wife encouraged him to have a medical checkup, his first in more than five years. Then came the shocker (to him, not me). This forty-year-old man discovered he had high blood pressure and hardening of the arteries. He was told that if he didn't make some lifestyle changes immediately, he was headed for a heart attack within six months. It was also suggested that he have quadruple heart bypass surgery.

As providence would have it, the following day a friend of his who had heard about the doctor's prognosis recommended that he follow the program outlined in my tape albums and books, which is how we met and worked together on his "Wellness Lifestyle" makeover. He has been a great inspiration to me for the past year because I had never worked with anyone so stressed, so unhealthy, and who led such an unhealthy way of life. During our first visit he made the choice to make the commitment to changing his life. Today, both he and his family are the picture of health. Recently, the family participated together in a 10K run and left the following day for a two-week health and fitness vacation. Oh, by the way, his new wellness program precluded him needing to go through with the bypass surgery.

Of course becoming healthy and fit is more than merely choosing to eat wholesome, nutritious foods, but it's a good place to start.

Diets don't work. Americans spend billions of dollars each year on diet-related products and services, yet obesity is a national epidemic. The only way any diet or weight-loss-fitness program can work permanently is if it is something you can live with for the rest of your life.

Some of the high-protein diets that are rich in animal products and low in fruits and unrefined carbohydrates certainly appeal to those looking to maintain their addiction to a high-fat, nutrient-inadequate diet. Most are downright dangerous. Don't follow any weight-loss plan, no matter how effective it might be in making you lose inches and pounds rapidly, if it places you at risk for serious illness. Remember, any diet program worth following should improve your health, not sacrifice it.

My nutrition program is based on a variety of unrefined plant-based, whole foods. It will not only help you shed any unwanted pounds of fat, but it will also maximize your fat-burning potential, "switch off" carb cravings, help stabilize your mood, supercharge your metabolism, and prevent and alleviate degenerative diseases. But this program also goes beyond just the physical benefits.

Day by day, you'll see and feel the changes taking place in your body, mind, and spirit and you'll begin to blossom with a renewed sense of control over your life, boosting your sense of self-esteem and confidence. You'll feel a restored sense of vitality and will be able to get your weight—and your health in general—under control. I know that's promising a lot but I've been using this program with clients for decades and it's backed by years of scientific research and empirical evidence. It's also important for you to know that I've been eating this way for 30 years, and I can tell you it works! So can the hundreds of people each year who send me letters after attending my workshops or reading my books.

Before we get specific about the foods to eat and avoid and the best tips for guaranteeing success, let's take a brief look at your miraculous body engine and how to assist it in working most efficiently.

Your body is composed of over 70 trillion cells. Think of each cell as a little engine, some of which work in unison, some of which work independently, and they all work 24/7. Like any engine, it requires specific fuels to run right. The wrong fuel blend, or a poor grade fuel, will cause the engine to sputter and hesitate, creating a loss of power. If the engine is given no fuel, it will simply stop.

Much of the fuel for our cells comes directly from the things we eat, which contain nutrients in the form of vitamins, minerals, water, carbohydrates, fats, proteins, and enzymes. Just as a car requires different forms of energy for the brakes, transmission, and battery to run smoothly, the cells of the body require different amounts and types of nutrients depending on their location and function in the body. These nutrients allow us to sustain life by providing our body's cells with needed basic materials.

Each nutrient differs in form and function but each one is vital. Nutrients are involved in every body process, from combating infection to repairing tissue to thinking. To eat is one of the most basic and powerful of human drives. Although eating has been woven into many cultural and religious practices, essentially we eat to survive.

The problem is that most of us simply do not get what we need from our modern diet. **Even if you are not sick, you may not necessarily by healthy. It simply may be that you are not yet exhibiting any overt symptoms of illness.** Unlike a car engine that immediately malfunctions if you put water into the gasoline tank, the human body has tremendous resilience and often camouflages the repercussions of unhealthy fuel choices.

It doesn't help that we are surrounded by bad influences when it comes to what we eat. Fast food is probably the biggest culprit. We have come to believe that any combination of heated, treated, processed, chemicalized 'foods' will meet our nutritional needs so long as we take plenty of vitamin pills, heartburn medicine, headache pills, laxatives, and other remedies.

"Call it science. Call it the state of the art of medicine. I now believe," writes Dr. Lendon H. Smith in his book, *Feed Your Body Right,* "what I learned in medical school in the early 1940s was a calculated effort by the pharmaceutical industry to get fledgling medical doctors to use drugs, their drugs. We were taught to make a diagnosis, clear and simple. Once a label was attached to the patient, a drug was attached to the disease label. It was neat and clean. If we could not remember the name of the drug, the pharmaceutical representative who came to our offices once or twice a month reminded us. Ads in the medical journals kept the name alive in our memory storage banks." And now drug pushers are coming into our living rooms day and night with television commercials for prescription medications!

Heart–Healthy Lifestyles Pay Off

If you read the paper or watch television, you might begin to think that your health is something preordained or beyond your control. Hardly a day goes by without a new article being published about some genetic predisposition for diseases and conditions that are factors that we often can't do anything about. That's why a major study published in the *British Medical Journal* about a major Finnish study is so redeeming.

In the early 1970s, middle-aged Finnish men had the highest mortality rates from cardiovascular disease in the world. They also consumed some of the highest amounts per capita of full-fat dairy products.

Early on, government officials took action, instituting health education programs and tracking the results of various preventive measures. The researchers recruited a random sample of close to 30,000 Finnish men and women ages 30 to 59. In surveys conducted every five years from 1972 to 1992, they kept close track of their medical history, current health, socioeconomic factors, and lifestyle habits. Specially trained nurses measured height, weight, and blood pressure and took blood specimens to determine cholesterol concentrations. Nonsmokers were defined as those who had never smoked regularly as well as those who had smoked regularly but had quit at least six months before the start of the survey.

During this same two-decade period, the rate of heart disease in Finland began to drop dramatically. The researchers concluded that the reductions in mortality rates from heart disease in Finland, which were 55% in men and 60% in women, over the past two decades were brought about primarily by changes in three main coronary risk factors: cholesterol levels, blood pressure, and smoking.

Atherosclerotic vascular disease is a buildup of fat in the blood vessels. The associated heart attacks and strokes caused by this fat buildup prematurely cause half of all deaths each year. Cancer of the breast, colon, prostate, lung, and other organs cause another 25% of deaths each year. Diabetes, cirrhosis of the liver, obesity, and emphysema also kill many people prematurely.

All these conditions have one thing in common: They are caused or greatly influenced by what we put or don't put into our mouths. Of all the things human beings put in their mouths, says Dr. Alan Goldhamer, co-director of the TrueNorth Health Center in Penngrove, California, tobacco, alcohol, caffeine, and recreational and prescription drugs are perhaps the most harmful.

The Impact of Animal Protein

Perhaps the second most destructive habit Dr. Goldhamer sees is the consumption of animal products. In their search for evidence on how food affects health, researchers have often considered Asian populations because, statistically, their longevity surpasses other groups. While they do not have a perfect diet, they do have a much lower risk of cancer, heart disease, and many other serious conditions.

One of the most ambitious nutrition research projects ever undertaken is the China Oxford Cornell Project (called the Grand Prix of epidemiology). Conducted by Dr. Colin Campbell of Cornell University and his colleagues, Drs. Chen Junshi and Li Junyao of Beijing, China, and Dr. Richard Peto of Oxford University, the project looked in detail at China as a natural laboratory. Diets vary significantly from one part of the country to another, yet studying China has the added advantage that people in China tend to stay in the same place all their lives, allowing observable relationships between diet and health to emerge. Beginning in 1983, the team collected information about the typical foods of 65 Chinese provinces. They studied records of health and illness, took blood samples, and made other tests. In 1991, they published an 896-page monograph filled with data from this and subsequent and even larger studies, which they continue to analyze.

The project's hypothesis was that diet substantially enriched with good quality plant foods prevents a variety of chronic degenerative diseases, and that the more the diet contains plant-source foods, the lower the disease risk. "In a sense," explains Dr. Campbell, "one might say that we are testing whether a diet which contains no animal products and is low in fat, is better than, say, an average vegetarian diet which usually contains dairy and egg products and nutrient compositions which are not too different from nonvegetarian diets. Our study suggests that the closer one approaches a total plant food diet, the greater the health benefit."

Their first finding was that, overall, Chinese diets are extraordinarily healthy by Western standards. Rice and other grains, vegetables, and legumes are consumed in much greater quantity than in the United States. While Americans get around 40% of their calories from fat, the Chinese get much less—ranging from 6% to 24%—and their overall health is much better.

The emphasis of the study was on protein (how much and what kinds) and its influence on heart disease, cancer, and other diseases. On average, Americans derive 70% of their protein from animal sources. In China, only 7% is from animal sources. But in spite of these low levels of animal protein intake, those Chinese who add just a little bit of animal protein to their diet register increases in cholesterol levels, heart disease, and cancer. This suggests that it doesn't take much animal protein to start changing cholesterol levels and consequently increase the risk of heart disease and cancer.

"There is strong evidence in the scientific literature that when a reduction in fat is compared to a reduction in protein intake, the protein effect on blood cholesterol is more significant than the effect of saturated fat," explains Campbell. Animal protein is a hypercholesterolemic (cholesterol-increasing) agent. Campbell adds, "We can reduce cholesterol levels either by reducing animal protein intake or exchanging it for plant protein. Some of the plant proteins, particularly soy, have an impressive ability to reduce cholesterol. I really think that protein—both the kind and the amount—is more significant as far as cholesterol levels are concerned than is saturated fat, and certainly more significant than dietary cholesterol itself."

Animal protein is about as well correlated with overall cancer rates across different countries as is total fat. Of course, animal protein is tightly coupled with the intake of saturated fat, so a lot of these associations between saturated fat and various cancers could just as easily be accounted for by animal protein. According to Campbell, "The consumption of animal protein has a profound effect on enzymes that are involved in the metabolism of cholesterol and related chemicals and this occurs very quickly—within an hour after the consumption of the meal."

Protein is so highly regarded by everyone, including most investigators, that there is a tremendous bias against considering its implication in disease. "It is easy to see that fat is greasy and nasty," says Campbell, "so most people more readily accept the idea that fat might have something to do with the emergence of disease. They do not want to imagine that animal protein does the same things as excess fat intake. But it turns out that animal protein, when consumed, exhibits a variety of undesirable health effects. Whether it is the immune system, various enzyme systems, the uptake of carcinogens into the cells, or hormonal activities, animal protein generally only causes mischief. High fat intake still can be a problem, and we should not be consuming such high fat diets. But I suggest that animal protein is more problematic in this whole diet/disease relationship than is total fat."

Perhaps you have switched from beef to skinless chicken breasts and other animal-based foods, to reduce your intake of fat. The evidence suggests that this makes little or no sense. You may reduce fat intake a bit, but even lean cuts of meat or poultry still contain around 20% to 40% of total calories as fat, or even more. This is not going to get us very far. We might get our fat intake down a bit, but our protein intake is not going to change; if anything, the already high level may go even higher. As Campbell says, "One really has to change the total diet." This project also revealed that those people eating the most plant foods rarely had weight problems.

In my opinion, if you want to see big changes in your health, you really must switch to a vegan (no animal product) diet. If you are accustomed to a high salt, high fat, high animal protein diet, you might not like the taste of healthier foods at first. The strong flavors of animal products—meat, cheese, etc.—often mask the cleaner, more subtle flavors of grains, vegetables, seeds, nuts, etc. But after just two or three months or so, you will adapt to these new flavors and even grow to love them.

Since heart disease is the leading cause of death in this country, it is appropriate to also describe a landmark study in heart disease: the Lifestyle Heart Trial, conceived by Dr. Dean Ornish of the University of California, San Francisco. This interventional study, conducted on patients with documented coronary artery disease, split participants into two groups, a control group and an intervention group. All of the patients in the study had cardiac tests before beginning the study. These tests were repeated a year later to document the effect of the intervention.

The control group was placed on the American Heart Association recommended diet, which is similar to the diet recommended by the American Diabetic Association for Diabetics. This diet includes limited red meat, chicken, fish, and substitutes margarine for butter, resulting in a reduction from the American norm of about 40% of calories from fat down to 30%, and reducing cholesterol to less than 300 mg daily (the norm is higher). These patients were also advised to exercise and to stop smoking. To the surprise of many, the majority of participants in this control group that were following the American Heart Association recommendations showed *worsening* of their cardiac status on the one-year follow up.

The intervention group did dramatically better. These patients were placed on a low-fat vegetarian diet, with less than 10% of calories from fat. To achieve this, they ate—without restriction in quantity—unrefined plant foods, such as fresh fruits, vegetables, legumes, and whole grains, with a limited amount of egg whites and nonfat milk or yogurt. They also engaged in light exercise and stress management. After one year, researchers found reversal in atherosclerotic plaque in 82% of this intervention group, all of whom were coronary disease patients. Not only that but those participants who wanted to lose weight found that it came off easily on the whole foods, plant-based diet and ***while eating more food*** than they had before.

In addition to bacterial infestation, carcinogenic agents, toxic poisons, and parasites, animal products all suffer from the problem of biological concentration. Animals consume large quantities of grain, grass, and other foods that are, to a greater or lesser extent, contaminated with herbicides, pesticides, and other agents. In addition, animals are often fed antibiotics and treated with other drugs and toxic agents that concentrate in the fat of the animal and are present in the animal's milk and flesh. This biological concentration of poisons poses significant threats to the health of humans who consume animal products.

In spite of the millions of dollars the meat and dairy industries spend on advertising to try to make us believe otherwise, it is excess protein, not inadequate protein, that is the threat to health. Animal products are extremely high in protein. Excess protein, especially the high sulfur-containing amino acids found in animal products, has been strongly implicated as a causal agent in many disease processes, including kidney disease, various forms of cancer, a host of autoimmune and hypersensitivity disease processes, obesity, and osteoporosis.

Osteoporosis is a condition common to post-menopausal women whose bones have become weak and fracture easily. Campbell found in his study that osteoporosis is not caused by calcium deficiency, and calcium supplementation does not prevent it. In osteoporosis there is a loss of the bone matrix that holds calcium. He found that a diet high in animal protein can cause osteoporosis by creating toxic, acidic nitrogenous wastes that must be neutralized by calcium drawn from the body's reserves, creating a negative calcium balance where more calcium is lost in the urine than is taken in. Thus, for someone eating a diet high in animal protein, no matter how much calcium is taken, the calcium balance will remain negative. To prevent osteoporosis, a low- or no animal–protein diet and regular weight-bearing exercises are essential in addition to eating lots of fresh fruits and vegetables daily.

Researchers at the University of Surrey evaluated 62 healthy women aged 45 to 55. Each woman underwent a bone mineral density screening and completed detailed diet questionnaires about the foods she had consumed in the past 12 months as well as in childhood. The women who ate the highest amounts of fruits and vegetables had higher bone density scores and less evidence of bone loss.

Lead investigator, Dr. Susan A. New, notes that although most studies on osteoporosis have focused on calcium, "intakes of nutrients found in an abundance of fruits and vegetables—namely potassium, beta-carotene, vitamin C, and magnesium—were positively associated with bone health." Researchers believe that potassium slows the excretion of calcium, while it and vitamin C increase rate of bone formation. *So it's a misconception that you have to eat dairy products to prevent osteoporosis.*

Dairy products are also implicated in many other diseases, including autoimmune disorders, heart disease, arthritis, obesity, and cancer.

Dairy Is "Udder" Nonsense

I choose not to eat any dairy products. When I announce this at my workshops, hands inevitably go up and ask why and also what I use in place of milk. Excellent substitutes for milk include nut milks like almond, oat milk, rice milk, and, most popular, soy milk. All of these are available in natural foods stores and they come in plain, vanilla, chocolate, low and nonfat, and organic. I prefer organic, whenever possible. Try to find your favorites. I have included some recipes in Chapter 8 for making your own nut and seed milks. You can also make or purchase soy yogurt, soy cheese, soy cream cheese, and soy sour cream, so you won't miss your dairy. (Be patient. As I mentioned earlier, it might take a couple of months to adjust to the new flavors and textures in your wholesome diet.) And besides, soy has the added benefit of being a phytoestrogen.

Phytoestrogens are the gentle estrogens found in plants such as soy, dong quai, licorice root, black cohosh, and many others. Their power comes from their apparent ability to match up with estrogen receptor sites throughout the body. There they seem to offer protection from the stronger, potentially more dangerous forms of estrogen. And phytoestrogens have a positive effect on the bones, heart, and cells. Numerous studies have confirmed the fact that women who eat foods rich in phytoestrogens seem to have fewer symptoms of PMS and menopause.

Why have researchers become so concerned about dairy products?

1. *Milk is the leading cause of iron-deficiency anemia in children because milk is deficient in iron.* Milk also binds with the iron in

other foods and prevents its absorption. Even so renowned an authority on children as the late Dr. Benjamin Spock changed his recommendations in his later years and discouraged giving children milk. Milk allergies are very common in children and can cause sinus problems, diarrhea, constipation, and fatigue. They are the leading cause of the chronic ear infections that plague up to 40% of all children under the age of six. Milk allergies are also linked to behavior problems in children and to the disturbing rise in childhood asthma. (Milk allergies are equally common in adults and produce similar symptoms.)

2. *Dairy products have no dietary fiber.* Diets low in fiber contribute to constipation and other related diseases (varicose veins, hemorrhoids, and hiatal hernia).

3. *There is evidence that immune system reactions to dairy proteins may cause and/or aggravate rheumatoid arthritis (RA) in some people.* Some studies have shown that eliminating dairy products can help reduce symptoms in people with RA.

4. *Milk may contribute to heart disease.* There's a clear link between dairy products and osteoporosis, obesity, cancer, allergies, and diabetes, and there is now some evidence that we can add heart disease to the group. While we know that high-fat dairy products, such as whole milk and cheese, are significant contributors to high cholesterol levels and heart disease, William B. Grant, Ph.D., summarizes the mounting evidence that nonfat milk is also a major player in bringing on heart disease. Writing in *Alternative Medicine Review*, Dr. Grant points out that nonfat milk, which contains substantial amounts of dairy protein, is very low in B vitamins. The metabolism of all this protein in the absence of B vitamins contributes to the buildup of homocysteine, a marker for heart disease. The protein in dairy products may damage arteries through an immune cross-reaction. High levels of antibodies from milk proteins have been found in severally atherosclerotic subjects. Even low-fat or fat-free dairy products may be culprits.

5. *There is some evidence that cow's milk proteins may trigger type 1 diabetes through a cross-reaction to the protein.* Worldwide, the incidence of type 1 diabetes correlates to the amount of dairy products consumed.

6. *High levels of IGF-1 may be related to an increased risk for certain cancers.* In 1994, the FDA approved the use of recombinant bovine somatotropin (rBST), a genetically engineered hormone made by Monsanto, that increases milk production in cows by 10% to 25%. It is also referred to as BHT. Milk from cows treated with rBST contains elevated levels of insulin-like growth factor-1 (IGF-1), one of the most powerful growth factors ever identified. Recent studies have found a seven-fold increase in the risk of breast cancer in women with the highest IGF-1 levels, and a four-fold increase in prostate cancer in men with the highest levels. In his must-read book, *Milk, the Deadly Poison*, author Robert Cohen, a tenacious investigative reporter, describes a level of corruption between Monsanto, the FDA, and the Department of Agriculture that will have your hair standing on end. This book documents how the public has been misled regarding rBST, its effects on our health, and the amounts of this hormone present in milk. I highly recommend this book for anyone who thinks dairy products are healthful and beneficial. The fact that the dairy industry, the FDA, and Monsanto have chosen to ignore the studies and use BHT is evidence enough that profits are more important to them than your health. If you don't give up dairy, at least, for the sake of your health and life, look for an organic brand.

7. Most African Americans (70%), Asian Americans (95%), Native Americans (74%), and Hispanic Americans (53%) are lactose intolerant. However, milk is touted as "Nature's perfect food."

8. *Beef cattle are routinely injected with estrogen pellets to fatten them up for market.* According to John R. Lee, M.D., in his fantastic book *What Your Doctor May Not Tell You About Menopause*, this estrogen is still present when the beef gets to your table in the form of meat and dairy. It may be present in small amounts but, as he explains, it only takes a very small amount of estrogen to throw your hormones out of balance and cause "estrogen-dominance." This condition brings with it a list of symptoms including acceleration of the aging process, decreased sex drive, depression, fatigue, irritability, decreased metabolism, water retention and bloating, and fat gain, especially around the abdomen, hips, and thighs, just to name a few. Are you sure you want to continue eating dairy products?

For a majority of my clients who come to me with weight issues and want to lose fat, I suggest giving up dairy. Across the board, those who do have a much easier time losing weight than those who don't. Most even say that the weight came off easily and effortlessly when they gave up dairy as well as all animal products.

Don't take chances with your health! The health risks associated with milk and dairy products, from clogging arteries to allergies, to weight gain, and difficulty in losing weight, are well documented. If these products still play a role in your diet, start cutting back. Check at your natural food store for more healthful substitutes.

It's ironic that the chief argument used to promote the use of animal and dairy products—the purported need for large quantities of protein—is one of the greatest reasons for avoiding them. If animal and dairy products are included in the diet in significant quantities, it is virtually impossible to design a healthful, slimming diet. So, to speed weight loss and increase vitality:

The 3 Greatest Weight Loss & Vitality Secrets of all Time

1. Eat a diet derived from whole, natural, plant-based foods— fresh fruits, vegetables, legumes, whole grains, and the variable addition of a few raw nuts and seeds. I'm often asked, "If I have to avoid drugs (including alcohol, coffee, cola, and tobacco) and animal products (including meat, fish, fowl, eggs, and dairy products) and refined carbohydrates (sweets, white sugar, and white flour products), what's left?" The answer is (and this is the first secret to slimming down and maintaining your natural weight easily): a diet derived from whole, natural, plant-based foods. *These foods are high in nutrients in proportion to their caloric content.*

Calories come only from carbohydrates, fats, or proteins. The non-caloric portion of the food is comprised of all the other dietary components including vitamins, minerals, enzymes, phytochemicals, antioxidants, and fiber, and unrefined plant-based foods are rich in all these components. A food is good or not-so-good for you based on how much of these health-providing components and other unnamed or undiscovered nutrients it contains in proportion to its calories. Based on this simple fact, the nutrient/calorie ratio, you can grade food quality, construct menus, and make food choices to support excellent health. Once you know which foods have the highest nutrient density, you will become an expert in nutrition and weight loss. It's that simple. You can then begin to lose weight in a healthful manner. Judging from the experiences of hundreds of clients I've worked with over the past three decades, you can expect to lose between 20 and 30 pounds in just three months and, if you continue with your healthy lifestyle, you will be able to keep it off. **What's more, if you consume a diet that contains 90%-100% nutrient-dense food, you can practically disease-proof your body, as well.**

Nutrient dense foods—fresh fruits, vegetables, whole grains, and beans—are rich in fiber and nutrients, while processed foods are nutrient-deficient. Interestingly, one food has shown a strong positive association with increased longevity—raw leafy greens, normally referred to as salad. Leafy greens, such as romaine lettuce, kale, spinach, collards, Swiss chard, red leaf, arugula, and all kinds of sprouts, are the healthiest foods you can eat. **The more you eat of these foods, the more weight you will lose!**

Strive to eat 7 to 12 servings of fruits and vegetables each day, emphasizing the vegetables. Here are some tips to help you get more fruits and vegetables into your health program.

1. Drink vegetable juice instead of soda.

2. Add extra vegetables to your favorite entrées.

3. Try making some all-vegetable-based meals (see recipes).

4. Try one new fruit or vegetable each week. Experiment!

5. Eat fruit for breakfast or add it to whole grain cereal.

6. Double your normal serving sizes of fruits and vegetables.

7. Eat two salads daily and use a variety of chopped vegetables.

8. Add extra fruit to a smoothie.

9. Eat fruit instead of candy for snacks.

10. Take one to two pieces of fruit to work each day.

11. Take fresh fruit with you when you go to the movies or sporting events.

12. Make frozen fruit kabobs and serve as a refreshing treat.

13. Make frozen fruit sorbets or ice creams for dessert or snacks.

14. Keep zip-top bags of vegetables with you when you're running errands or plan on being in the car for awhile.

2. Eat at least 50% of your diet raw. The old saying "You are what you eat" is only half true. We are actually no more than we can digest. We must effectively assimilate what we eat through good digestion. Optimal digestion depends on more than just eating the right foods. The key to good digestion is the class of complex chemical substances known as enzymes.

Three types of enzymes have been identified: digestive enzymes that diminish as we age (which digest our food), food enzymes (available only in fresh, live food), and metabolic enzymes made by the body in a fixed amount (which science has discovered no means of replenishing). When we eat cooked food over a period of many years, we eventually deplete our digestive enzymes and have to rob our pool of metabolic enzymes to assist the digestion process. As the metabolic enzymes are depleted, deterioration of the body sets in. The aging process begins.

Food enzymes are necessary in order to break large food components into smaller ones that the body can absorb. Each enzyme has a specific job and can only break down certain components. The three main components that we consume are fats, proteins, and carbohydrates.

Most nutritionally aware people take care to get a daily ration of fruit and vegetables, grains and legumes. But they may not be absorbing the nutrients effectively. And herein lies the second greatest weight loss and vitality secret of all time: Eat as much raw (unrefined, plant-based, natural) food as possible, at least 50% of your daily diet. If you know your meal is going to be cooked, start with something raw first, such as a few carrot or celery sticks to help your digestion. Also, devote one or two days each week, such as Monday and Thursday, to eating only raw foods. If that seems too extreme, try eating only raw foods during the day and then eat a big, raw salad with dinner. This simple practice alone will be a great bonanza to your health.

Once a piece of food is cooked, whether steamed, baked, fried, boiled, broiled, barbecued, toasted, roasted, sautéed, poached, grilled, or microwaved, it is really as good as dead. Its 'life force,' its vital energy, is lost. If you take a handful of raw sunflower seeds, bury them in the earth and water them, chances are good they will sprout. If boiled first, they will rot in the ground. The difference between raw and cooked is the difference between life and death.

The reason a cooked seed won't sprout is that the enzymes have been destroyed by the heat of cooking. "Enzymes are substances that make life possible," explains one of the world's leading experts in enzyme research, Dr. Edward Howell in *Enzyme Nutrition, The Food Enzyme Concept.* "They are needed for every chemical reaction that takes place in the human body. No mineral, vitamin, or hormone can do any work without enzymes.

"Our bodies, all of our organs, tissues, and cells, are run by metabolic enzymes. They are the manual workers that build the body from proteins, carbohydrates, and fat, just as construction workers build our homes. You have all the raw materials with which to build, but without the workers (enzymes) you cannot even begin," he says.

Among many important enzymes so far identified, three start out as major league players in the assimilation of food. The body needs **protease** for the digestion of proteins, **amylase** for breaking down carbohydrates and starch, and **lipase** for digesting fats. These and other enzymes can be gotten from raw foods, in which naturally present enzymes tend to correlate with the nutritional factors of the food itself. Raw fatty foods such as oils and nuts, for example, contain lipase. But if these same fatty foods are cooked, the lipase and other enzymes are destroyed, placing extra demands on the body (especially the pancreas) to produce more enzymes in order to facilitate digestion. This is why, as you'll see in the recipe section, when a dish calls for any oil at all (and many of mine don't), I recommend only cold-pressed oils, such as olive oil. The term "extra virgin" means that it is the first, and purest, pressing.

The human body produces its own enzymes, but only in a limited quantity over the course of a lifetime. When the enzyme potential is depleted beyond a certain point, according to research documented in Howell's book, a given life is effectively over. Researchers in Chicago have found that enzyme levels in the saliva of young adults are thirty times higher than in persons over 69 years of age. Research in Germany has found that the urine of young people contains nearly twice the amount of the starch-digesting enzymes amylase than the urine of older people. An individual's enzyme potential, maintains Howell, not only determines the length of that person's life but is directly related to good health and resistance to disease.

According to Humbart Santillo, ND, author of the excellent book, *Food Enzymes: The Missing Link to Radiant Health,* a diet of mostly cooked foods is a disservice to the body. The pancreas must borrow enzymes from other parts of the body to properly digest cooked food. Inadequately digested food can putrefy the intestines, creating gas and toxins and further impede nutrient assimilation. For these reasons, whether you are young or old, and especially if you include cooked food in your diet, I suggest supplementing your diet with enzymes. The ones I use and recommend are called Living Enzymes. You can find out more about them in Living Food in the Resource Directory.

Finally, and perhaps the most important reason to eat a diet of mostly live foods, is the effect it has on your spiritual life. Over the years I have observed in myself and in many of my clients that eating a live food diet helps us become more sensitive to the sacred in our lives. When you're more sensitive to the sacred, you're more sensitive to the divine unfolding in your own life and that, in itself, helps you have a brighter attitude. One of my favorite books on the subject of a live foods diet is *Conscious Eating* by Gabriel Cousen, M.D. A respected medical doctor, Cousen doesn't just validate the importance of live foods diet, he lives it. His book is another must-read for anyone desiring healing, radiant health, and vitality. He's founder of the Tree of Life Center in Patagonia, Arizona, where you can go for a retreat to fast and/or learn how to live a physically and spiritually rich lifestyle.

3. Include a well-rounded exercise program into your daily regime. As we will discuss in Chapters 4 and 5, the best way to guarantee fat loss is through proper exercise. You must exercise often, combining the triangle of cardio, weight lifting, and flexibility training to help burn fat, increase muscle and metabolism, reduce bone loss, and keep energy levels revved. As we age, we lose muscle, strength, bone density, and energy. The best way to counteract this is with exercise, as described in detail in Chapters 4 and 5.

Changing to a Healthy Diet

When changing from an animal-based diet to a natural plant-based diet, you may experience headaches, indigestion, and other uncomfortable symptoms. Have no fear—what you are experiencing is actually a good sign! Your body is going through transition, much like the withdrawal from caffeine or tobacco. Most people who initially experience such symptoms find that they resolve within the first two weeks, and from that point on, they feel better and more energetic than they have in years.

1. *You may experience some uncomfortable symptoms.* Headaches, in particular, are a natural part of your body's recovery process. During the transition time, you might experience diarrhea, bloating, gas, or other digestive discomforts. The increase in fiber and water in your new diet means a change in stool. Your new stools will be heavier, allowing them to pass through the digestive tract at a faster rate. The peristaltic waves that propel the food have to adjust to this. It can take two weeks or longer for this adjustment to take place.

2. *You may slow down.* It's not uncommon at first to feel enervated and lethargic when you switch to a lower protein, low-fat diet, because the body starts to eliminate retained proteinaceous wastes, fat cells also are broken down, and the toxins stored in the fat cells are released into the bloodstream. This is the body 'cleaning house,' but it can temporarily leave you feeling sluggish. These symptoms are the result of detoxification. Don't let temporary discomfort lead you to abandoning your new eating habits. You cannot accomplish healing overnight. Try eating slowly and chewing everything thoroughly, or just eat a few leaves of lettuce with each meal rather than one big raw salad at dinner. If you are experiencing indigestion and cramping, do not eat asparagus or the cruciferous vegetables (cabbage, cauliflower, broccoli, or Brussels sprouts) for the first two weeks, as they may produce bloating and gas. Fruit juices and other sweet drinks also can increase gas, so these should be avoided temporarily if you are experiencing this problem.

3. *Be informed.* Educate yourself as much as you can on nutrition and an optimum diet. There are numerous excellent books and maga-

zines available to give you support, inspiration, motivation, and delicious, nutritious recipes. Here is a list of my favorites.

Becoming Vegan: The Complete Guide to Adopting a Healthy Plant-Based Diet by Brenda Davis, R.D., and Vesanto Melina, R.D.

Conscious Eating by Gabriel Cousens, M.D.

Do No Harm by Yoshitaka Ohno, M.D., Ph.D.

Eating in the Light by Doreen Virtue, Ph.D., and Becky Perlitz, R.D.

Everyday Cooking with Dr. Dean Ornish* by Dean Ornish, M.D.

Fasting and Eating for Health and *Discover the Health Equation* by Joel Fuhrman, M.D.

Fight Fat After Forty by Pamela Peeke, M.D.

Flax for Life* by Jade Beutler

Foods That Fight Pain and *Turn Off the Fat Genes** by Neal Barnard, M.D.

The Food Revolution by John Robbins

Healing with Whole Foods by Paul Pitchford

The HRT Solution by John M. Kells and Marla Ahlgrimm, RPH

Juice Fasting & Detoxification by Steve Meyerowitz

Love Yourself Thin, Get the Fat Out, and *Fit from Within* by Victoria Moran

Milk, the Deadly Poison by Robert Cohen

Natural Beauty & Health Magazine

The New Whole Foods Encyclopedia by Rebecca Wood

The Pritikin Principle: The Calorie Density Solution by Robert Pritikin

Raw: The UNcook Book* by Juliano

Sea Salt's Hidden Powers by Jacques de Langre, Ph.D.

Thin Through the Power of Spirit by Lucia Capodilupo

Tired of Being Tired by Jesse Lynn Hanley, M.D.

Vegetarian Magic* by John Nowakowski

Warming Up to Living Foods* by Elysa Markowitz

What Color Is Your Diet? by David Heber, M.D., Ph.D.

What Your Doctor May Not Tell You About Menopause by John R. Lee, M.D.

What Your Doctor May Not Tell You About Premenopause by John R. Lee, M.D., and Jesse Hanley, M.D.

Your Body's Many Cries for Water by F. Batmanghelidj, M.D.

And for children

Dr. Attwood's Low Fat Prescription for Kids by Charles Attwood, M.D.

How to Get Kids to Eat Great and Love It! by Christine Wood, M.D.

Pregnancy, Children, and the Vegan Diet by Michael Klaper, M.D.

Vegetable Soup/The Fruit Bowl by Dianne Warren and Susan Smith Jones

*cookbooks or includes recipes

The long-term rewards of improvement in your diet—increased vitality, improved sleep, more energy, regular and soft bowel movements, lower cholesterol and a healthy heart, lower cancer risk, stronger bones, and a life without ever having to battle the bulge again—are well worth any temporary discomfort. But to eat well, we have to understand the factors that drive us to eat unhealthfully.

Very often we eat for the wrong reasons. One reason is genetics— we are programmed to eat concentrated foods when they are available, which is an important survival trait. In a natural setting, there are no ice cream cone trees, hot dog vines, or candy bushes. But today, surrounded by unlimited access to concentrated foods, we must overcome instincts with our intellect and create alternatives for ourselves other than reaching for a candy bar, a beer, or a bucket of fried chicken when we are stressed out.

If you eat when you are emotionally distraught, try taking a walk, listening to relaxing music, or doing some deep breathing.

If you feel tired and eat for stimulation, try taking a nap or going to bed earlier.

Fear of being different may drive you to make poor food choices. Friends can create a lot of pressure with comments like, "You're no fun anymore," "You're so thin," "Don't you think you're carrying this food thing a bit too far," "I made it just for you," or "A little won't hurt." Thank them for their concern and stay committed to your health program. Often a short explanation is all that is necessary. **You don't need to justify yourself or your health habits.**

Your body is a wonderful feedback machine. It is continually giving you messages about what's working and what's not, so pay attention to the signs and symptoms it gives you. I really like what Dr. Lendon H. Smith has to say about this in his book *Feed Your Body Right*. "The more we investigate the origin of symptoms, signs, and diseases the more we find that nutrition is at the bottom of what ails us. The triggering event that precipitates an actual disease may be an emotional upset or a physical injury. Something has stressed our body chemistry beyond its ability to compensate; our ability to buffer the changes accompanying stressors has been compromised by our lifestyle, which includes diet. We are all at risk—some more, some less."

Set Point Theory

Each of us has a biologically predetermined set point for body weight that controls how much we eat and at what rate we burn calories. Dieting and fasting often will raise the body's set point. Prolonged or drastic reduction in calorie intake tricks the body into thinking it is starving so the body's natural defense is to slow down the rate at which it burns up food.

A truly permanent weight loss program must involve resetting the set point to a lower level. This can be accomplished by making the following lifestyle changes:

1. *Avoid total daily calorie restriction.* Less than 1,200 calories a day triggers a starvation response by the body and raises the set point.

2. *Eat smaller but more frequent meals during the day* as opposed to one or two larger meals.

3. *Decrease dietary fat* to around 15% of your total calories.

4. *Avoid refined carbohydrates* (sugar), soft drinks, and other fluids containing calories. Excessive sugar releases insulin, which decreases blood sugar, creating the strong urge to eat.

5. *Increase consumption of grains, legumes, and vegetables, especially leafy greens.*

6. *Exercise at least five times a week.* Physical activity increases the metabolic rate, builds muscle mass and strength, causes an increased demand for fuel, and adds enzymes that stimulate fat burning (as you'll read more about in Chapter 5).

Susan's Top 20 Tips for Accelerating Fat Loss

1. Drink lots of water.   We often turn to food when we're really just thirsty. Water makes you feel fuller. Drink a large glass of water

15 minutes before your meal on an empty stomach and drink lots of water throughout the day (I recommend 80 ounces for the average, active person). Your urine should be clear, light-colored, and plentiful. Drink even more in hot weather, low humidity, high altitude, when you're ill or stressed, when you want to accelerate fat loss, or if you're pregnant.

2. Eat frequently.   Three meals a day, along with two or three low-calorie, nutrient-dense snacks between meals, will control hunger. Eat breakfast within one hour of rising to help rev up your metabolism.

3. Avoid foods that contain a significant amount of fat, which is the most calorically dense substance in the food supply. Fat has 9 calories per gram while both protein and carbs have about 4 calories per gram.

4. Eat unlimited quantities of raw vegetables, including raw starches, such as carrots. Raw foods have high transit times; they fill you up and will encourage weight loss. You can't overeat them. Eat as much salad and lettuce as possible. Every lunch and every dinner should begin with a salad and some raw vegetables. I also encourage you to eat close to a head of romaine or other similar lettuce daily. The more of these foods you eat, the quicker you will lose fat.

5. Sequence your food selection during meals.   First eat those foods that have the lowest caloric and highest nutrient density. Salads (without tons of dressing, of course) are the best choice, not to mention that it's also important to make your first few bites of food from raw foods to aid digestion. Other good foods to consume early in the meal would be steamed vegetables and broth-based soups. All these will help fill you up and leave less room in your stomach for higher-calorie-dense foods. The feeling of fullness is created largely by the volume of your food, rather than its calorie content.

6. Don't drink your calories; eat them, with the exception of freshly-made, healthy fruit and vegetable juices and smoothies. Processed juices, sugar-sweetened sodas, and alcoholic beverages contribute calories without affecting your sense of fullness.

7. Eat as many fresh fruits as you want.   Avoid processed fruit juices and, if you have a lot of weight to lose or want to see an acceleration in fat loss quickly, even avoid fresh fruit juices. Avoid all refined sugary foods; satisfy your sweet tooth with fruits.

8. *Eat steamed green vegetables* with each dinner, unless going all raw, (as I'll describe in the Retreats, Chapters 19 and 20), such as broccoli, green beans, collards, kale, Swiss chard, and spinach.

9. *Limit cooked, starchy foods* to about one cup a day if you want a more rapid weight loss. This would include one ear of corn, one baked potato, or one sweet potato. Don't feel that you'll go hungry. You can still eat as much low-starch plant food as you want and as many raw vegetables as you want.

10. *Eat legumes daily.* They absorb most of the water they're cooked in and they're rich in fiber. They fill you up, have staying power, and offer a high nutrient-per-calorie profile that helps prevent food cravings.

11. *Stay clear of more refined foods* until you've reached your weight loss goal. This would include bread, rolls, bagels, croissants, crackers, pretzels, pasta, and other flour products. In other words, focus more on those foods with the highest water content—fruits, vegetables, beans, and whole grains.

12. *Limit nuts and seeds, unless sprouted, to no more than 1 ounce daily* (2 tablespoons), if you desire a more rapid weight loss. The fat in nuts is a heart-healthy unsaturated fat. They're also packed with B vitamins, calcium, fiber, vitamin E, and hard-to-find minerals like magnesium and phosphorous. Make sure they are unsalted and raw and as fresh as possible. Always store nuts and seeds in the refrigerator or they'll go rancid.

13. *Include Barlean's Organic Flax Oil in your diet daily.* The omega-3's in the flax may help protect against cancer, boost immunity, and help with fat loss. Also, grind fresh flax meal on some foods each day. (See recipes for suggestions.) Stay away from other oil except extra virgin, cold-pressed olive oil in small amounts.

14. *Eat slowly.* Chopsticks help in slowing you down. It takes a while for your brain to register that your stomach is filled up with food and you're no longer hungry. If you eat really fast, you're going to overeat before it registers. To help keep you from wolfing down your food, here are three tips: Use chopsticks, put down your fork (or chopsticks) after every bite, and eat your meals with other people, conversing between nibbles rather than gobbling. Chew well so digestion will get off to a favorable start in your mouth.

15. Stay away from dairy and all other animal products. If you're in a transition period on the way to a plant-based diet, adjust using animal products as condiments, to no more than 12 ounces a week. If in transition, have only plant-based foods four days a week and limit animal-as-condiment foods to the other three, alternating back and forth.

16. Find ways to add fruits and vegetables to everything. Put fruits in smoothies; add banana, diced apple, or berries to oatmeal; toss asparagus or lightly steamed broccoli in salads; mix salsa with nonfat bean dip to use as a topping on potatoes. You'll feel full sooner, with fewer calories. (Supplement with Barlean's Greens.)

17. Make whole, natural plant-based foods—fruits, vegetables, legumes, and whole grains—the mainstay of your diet, as raw as possible.

18. Stay away from desserts except fresh fruit, or fresh fruit sorbets or ice creams (see Chapter 18 for healthy dessert ideas).

19. Eat moderate amounts of "good" fats. Research has shown that including monosaturated fat in the diet increases good cholesterol level, possibly protecting against heart disease. Monosaturated fat is found in avocados, and nuts, such as almonds, and seeds, such as sunflower and flax. But because all fat is high in calories, it's still a good idea to exercise moderation with these foods—or you may find it more difficult to lose fat.

20. Make mealtime pleasant in conversation and beautiful to the eye. Don't save your good china, silver, and crystal for special occasions. *You deserve the best all the time*. Use nice linens or placemats, have a lovely centerpiece of fresh flowers or fresh fruit, and don't forget to always give thanks for the food you're about to eat that will nourish your body, mind, and spirit.

Is a Calorie a Calorie?

For each pound of fat you want to lose, you have to create a "caloric deficit" of about 3,500 calories. Researchers have looked at several popular diets—Dr. Atkins, The Zone, Protein Power, and others—randomly assigning people to eat either a test diet or a control diet and making sure that each has the same number of calories. Dozens of these studies have found that if you cut any calories—from fat, protein, or carbs—you'll lose the same amount of weight. "Any differences in how well calories are used by the body are trivial," says Susan Roberts, head of the Energy Metabolism Laboratory at the Jean Mayer U.S. Department of Agriculture Human Nutrition Research Center on Aging at Tufts University in Boston. So, it just makes sense to me to cut calories by restricting animal products and refined carbs so that you'll lose fat while you improve health.

But if you want to lose weight, you do need to decrease your calorie consumption. (Be careful not to cut calories too severely. Nature has programmed the human body to protect you from starving in times of famine. If you limit food intake too drastically, nature's safety net kicks in and slows your metabolism.) Many studies corroborate this important tip: **If you eat as many vegetables, fresh fruits, whole grains, and legumes as you want, you will eat about half the number of calories that you would by choosing from sugars, meats, cheese, and fried foods.** Part of the reason for this is that high-fiber foods tend to be very filling and have fewer calories than other foods. Also, keep in mind the second greatest secret for weight loss and vitality of all time—raw foods. **You simply can't, and won't, overeat raw foods.** And the more you eat, the faster you will lose fat, reshape your body, and restore vitality.

While we're at it, let's clear up some misconceptions about the latest fad diets. In the high protein diet, where you sharply reduce carbohydrates and consume mostly protein and fat, those pounds that seem to drop so miraculously are mostly water lost through dehydration. These diets are unhealthy, potentially creating loads of acidic wastes, elevating lipid levels, which can cause cardio problems, taxing the kidneys, leaching essential minerals from your bones and body, clogging the arteries, increasing blood pressure, giving you bad breath, and causing dizziness and extreme fatigue, just to name a few.

We hear a lot these days about insulin resistance and about carbs making you fat. First off, carbs don't make you fat, and insulin doesn't make you fat, as many of the latest books claim. **Calories make you fat.** It's like a bank book, as Gerald Reaven, M.D., so aptly describes in his informative book, *Syndrome X: Overcoming the Silent Killer that Can Give You a Heart Attack.* Reaven was the director of the Division of Endocrinology and Metabolism and the Division of Gerontology at Stanford University School of Medicine and is now professor of medicine at Stanford. As he so clearly states, it's a matter of how much you put in and how much you take out. The more you eat and the fewer calories you burn up, the heavier you'll get. "The law of thermodynamics, to the best of my knowledge, hasn't been repealed recently," says Reaven.

He explains the process of insulin very simply. In a normal person, the rise in blood glucose after a meal stimulates the pancreas to secrete insulin. Insulin attaches to the insulin receptors on the cell surface and enables glucose to enter the muscle and fat cells, where it is stored or burned for energy. In an insulin resistant person, as in type 2 diabetes (in type 1 diabetes, the pancreas stops secreting insulin), the pancreas secretes sufficient insulin, but the body is resistant to the insulin. To compensate, the pancreas secretes more and more. The excess insulin manages to keep blood glucose levels within the normal range—though usually at the upper end of that range—so diabetes doesn't occur. However, the high insulin levels lead to high triglyceride levels, low HDL ("good") cholesterol, high blood pressure, and/or other signs of Syndrome X, which raise the risk of heart attack. To compensate for insulin resistance, the body secretes more and more, but it can't keep up. Because glucose has trouble getting to the cells, blood glucose levels rise, and the person is diagnosed with diabetes.

In his book, Reaven cites numerous studies showing that insulin resistance does not cause obesity as many diet books claim. "Years ago, we put people with different degrees of insulin resistance on dramatically different diets—in one study, carbohydrates were either 85% or 17% of calories. The only thing that affected their weight was how many calories they ate. More recently, we've published long-term studies showing that weight gain is unrelated to how insulin resistant people were when the studies began. And weight loss with low-calories is also unrelated to the degree of insulin resistance. So there's not one shred of evidence that insulin resistance causes obesity. He says the most important lifestyle changes you can make are how much you weigh and how fit you are. If you're insulin-resistant and overweight and you lose weight, you become less insulin resistant. And you stay that way as long as you keep the weight off. The average overweight person, says Reaven, would benefit by losing only 10 to 15 pounds.

Finally, what about carbohydrates? First, let's be clear: All carbs are not the same. "If you take a grain of whole wheat and process it into white flour to make white bread or pasta," writes Joel Fuhrman, M.D., in his book *Discover the Health Equation*, "more than 90% of the fiber and vitamin E is lost and about 75% of the minerals are lost. The body breaks the carbohydrate down into simple sugars and the physiologic response is not much different than if we consume cotton candy." Pasta and bread are just like sugar; because their fiber has been removed, they will be absorbed too rapidly, shoot up glucose and insulin levels in our blood, and raise triglyceride levels. Refined grains are undesirable and will sabotage your weight loss goals, explains Fuhrman.

All refined sweets are rapidly absorbed and are low in nutrients and fiber. Not only sugar, but also honey, corn syrup, molasses, corn sweeteners, and even commercial fruit juice has an unfavorable nutrient density. Many studies detailed in his book offer evidence that the consumption of these sweets and white flour products is an important cause of obesity, as well as diabetes, heart disease, and even cancer.

"White flour products and sweets cause a dramatic increase in the production of fat-storing hormones. The overall effect is that your body will raise what it believes to be its ideal weight, known as the **set point.** There are many other negative side effects to eating refined and fatty foods, such as insulin surges which serve to promote fat storage, and appetite stimulation, to name a few," writes Fuhrman.

In a six-year study of 65,000 women, those whose diets were high in refined carbohydrates from white bread, white rice, and pasta had two and a half times the incidence of type 2 diabetes, compared to those who ate high-fiber foods—vegetables, beans/legumes, whole grains, and fresh fruit. Diabetes is no lightweight problem; it is the fourth leading cause of death by disease in America, and growing.

Walter Willet, a professor of epidemiology and nutrition at the Harvard School of Public Health and a co-author of the study, finds the results of this and other research so convincing that he'd like our government to change the Food Guide Pyramid, which recommends six to eleven servings of any kind of carbohydrate. He says, "They should move refined grains like white bread up to the sweets category because metabolically they're basically the same."

Every time you eat a processed food, you exclude from your diet not only the important nutrients that we are aware of, but hundreds of other undiscovered or newly discovered phytonutrients that are essential for normal human function. It is precisely this outer portion of the wheat kernel, the part removed in the refining process, that contains the trace minerals, phytoestrogens, lignins, indoles, phenolic compounds, and other phytochemicals, as well as all the vitamin E naturally found in wheat. And so, removing the most important part of the food by refining it significantly increases your cancer risk.

The brain reads the fiber content and nutrient content of every morsel of food we digest. **When our diet is deficient in nutrients and fiber, the brain will signal us to eat more.** These refined grains, because they lack the fiber and nutrient density to turn down our appetite, contribute to obesity in yet another way. A recent 9-year study reported in the *American Journal of Clinical Nutrition* in 1998, involving 34,492 women aged 55 to 69, showed a two-thirds increased risk of death from heart disease in those eating refined grains. Summarizing 15 epidemiological studies, researchers found that diets containing refined grains and refined sweets were consistently linked to stomach and colon cancer, and at least 12 breast cancer studies connect low-fiber diets with increased risk.

As Fuhrman says in his book, "Pasta is not a health food, it is a hurt food." As far as the human body is concerned, low-fiber carbohydrates such as pasta might as well be white sugar. Unrefined carbohydrates, by contrast, supply us with energy and are naturally low in fat and calories. They are good for us and can satisfy our hunger far longer than sugary processed foods. Whole grains stabilize blood sugar and are the only food, along with legumes, that contain all the major nutrient groups in balance needed by the body: carbs, protein, fats, vitamins, minerals, and fiber.

Colors Galore & Flavonoids

Dark green leafy or yellow, orange, and red vegetables (such as spinach, squash, carrots, and peppers) and some fruits (such as apricots, cantaloupe, mangos, and papayas) are good sources of beta carotene. Fresh citrus fruits and some vegetables (such as peppers, tomatoes, collard greens, and broccoli) are rich in vitamin C. Green leafy vegetables, nuts, and wheat germ contain vitamin E.

What we're seeing here is that nature has provided us with important clues in the colors of the foods we eat. By eating from the whole palette of nature's food colors, we can help prevent diseases like cancer, heart disease, and other illnesses. Blackberries, blueberries, strawberries, plums, squash, pumpkin, apples, oranges, grapefruit, tomatoes, and other fruits and vegetables colored purple, blue, red, orange, or yellow are nearly all rich sources of carotenoids and flavonoids, maintains David Heber, M.D. in *What Color Is Your Diet?*

You may have heard of citrus flavonoids, including rutin and hesperidin. Biochemical dictionaries say there are 3,000 or more naturally occurring flavonoids, of which only several hundred are colored. However, even colorless flavonoids often contribute to plant coloration by interaction with other flavonoids. As some of the specific effects of individual bioflavonoids are researched and documented, a few of the better known—including quercetin and pycnogenol—have joined rutin on the health food store shelves.

A 1994 report in the prestigious medical journal *Lancet,* states that "Flavonoids in regularly consumed foods may reduce the risk of death from coronary heart disease in older men." In this study, 805 men, ages 65 to 84 years, were studied over a five-year period for flavonoid intake and incidence of heart attacks. The highest risk of heart attacks was found in those with the lowest flavonoid intake. Conversely, those men who consumed the most flavonoids had the lowest risk of heart attacks. It was also reported that flavonoids also interfere with cancer growth and development.

Eat at the Bottom of the Food Chain

The pesticides and herbicides used in conventional growing are among the most toxic chemicals known to science. After all, they are designed to kill living creatures. Along with other industrial metals and chemicals, pesticides run off into our lakes, rivers, and oceans, polluting both water supplies and marine animals. All of these toxins become more concentrated as they move up the food chain. From phytoplankton to zooplankton to small fish to larger fish, the metals and chemicals concentrate as they move up. That's why a large fish like tuna has more mercury than a smaller fish like cod; tuna is further up the food chain.

Livestock animals also concentrate toxic chemicals in their fat and livers. This toxic concentration as we move up the food chain has been confirmed in tests. Compared to the average pesticide residues found in plant foods, dairy foods have about three times as much; meat, fish, and poultry have about six times as much.

If you want to lower your ingestion of harmful toxins, eat organic produce, and stay low on the food chain (plant-based foods). The closer we come to being vegans (vegetarians who eat no animal products, including dairy or eggs), the fewer harmful metals and chemicals we take in. The lower you eat on the food chain the less energy it requires to produce food and the less damage it does to the environment. And it's more economical, too. Eating a plant-based diet is a safe, simple way of reestablishing a relationship with nature.

Unrefined Living Sea Salt, Baby/Kid's Weight, Mouth–to–Hips Gain & Aspartame

Finally, a few words about four subjects I'm asked about constantly:

Salt

I never recommended using salt until a few years ago, when I found out about Celtic Sea Salt®. Harvested by hand in Brittany in the northwest of France, this living salt hasn't been artificially heated—it's naturally sun-dried—thus it revitalizes the body with an exquisite flavor enhanced by more than 80 naturally balanced minerals from the ocean. Unlike table or refined sea salt, Celtic Sea Salt contains no added chemicals. The traditional method of harvesting salt maintains all the rich nutrients of the ocean while producing a salt that transforms dining experiences. Lower in sodium than regular refined table salt (sodium chloride) and rich in minerals, it is certified pure, clean, and free from pesticides and herbicides. (See the Grain and Salt Society in the Resource Directory for more information.)

Baby/Kid Weight

Not only are American adults fatter than ever, but so are American children. We need to get the whole family up and moving and eating a healthier diet. We develop fat cells between the ages of 12 and 18 months and again during puberty. After that point, our 25 to 35 billion (yes billion!) fat cells respond to weight gain by growing up to twice their size. But if all of your fat cells have already doubled in size and you continue to gain weight, your body starts making new ones. So if you gained more than 30 or 40 pounds since your teens, you could have more fat cells than someone who has gained less.

Mouth-to-Hips Gain

Finally, I'm often asked how fast one can gain weight. If you've eaten a big dinner and splurged on a rich dessert, the next day the scale might say you've gained two pounds. Don't believe it. True weight gain—or loss—is gradual. That two-pound gain is *not* fat. To gain just one pound you need to consume 3,500 *extra* calories. If you normally eat and burn off around 2,000 calories daily, you'd need to eat 5,500 calories in one day to gain a pound and 9,000 calories to gain two. Most of your two-pound "gain" comes from a combination of yet-to-be-excreted food and fluid retention caused by unusually high sodium and carbohydrate intakes. (Carbohydrates as well as sodium can make you retain water. And when you eat more than usual, the effect of both is increased.) As long as you return to your normal eating and exercise habits and drink lots of water, most of the extra pounds will disappear.

Aspartame

Aspartame is the chemical sweetener and sugar substitute in NutraSweet and is found in more than 5,000 different products, especially many convenience foods. Since the 1970s, the FDA has known about independent studies on aspartame in lab mice that document brain seizures, holes in the brains, dead and deformed fetuses, etc.

Researchers for the NutraSweet Corporation say that aspartame is safe for public consumption. That's all the FDA needed for its approval. Since aspartame's approval, over 5,000 complaints have been registered with the FDA, including vomiting, diarrhea, hives, dizziness, and four deaths. In over 100 years of saccharin use, for instance, there have been six complaints. (I'm not recommending saccharin or any artificial sweetener but I mention this for comparison.) Aspartame was originally intended as an ulcer drug whose sweet taste was discovered by accident. Did you know that 10% of aspartame is methyl alcohol which, if heated to 86 degrees, produces formaldehyde, an embalming fluid?

In my holistic health counseling, one of the first things I ask clients when doing their medical history and food diary is if they are consuming any foods containing aspartame. If so, I encourage them to eschew those products immediately. I tell them it's found in coffee, diet sodas, ice cream, gum, cookies, candies, breath mints, yogurt, many baked goods, vitamins, over-the-counter drugs, and prescription medicines, just to name a few. I show them a list, put out by the FDA in 1995, of over 25 symptoms from aspartame, ranging from sleep problems, memory loss, fatigue, edema, weight gain, changes in vision and sexual function, and cramps to hallucinations, seizures, shortness of breath, difficulties with pregnancy, developmental retardation in children, cancer, and even death.

Then, if they are still not convinced to give it up, I highly recommend they read the compelling book *Sweet Poison: How the World's Most Popular Artificial Sweetener Is Killing Us—My Story* by Janet Starr Hull. This is the true story of an average woman who wanted to lose weight after having three children. She did what most people would do: participate in regular workouts, eat low-fat frozen food, and drink diet cola. After a short while, she suffered blinding migraine headaches and night sweats, her hair fell out in clumps, and her heart raced to over 180 beats per minute. In the hospital, she was diagnosed with Graves' disease, told her thyroid gland would have to be destroyed, and she would have to take expensive thyroid medicine for the rest of her life. Hull had the presence of mind to conduct her own investigation. Searching through countless medical texts and journals, following up clues and reports, as well as conducting personal interviews, she discovered the true source of her illness—aspartame poisoning.

One of the most stunning revelations of all was Hull's unearthing of evidence of a cover-up by several high-ranking government officials. Hull's true, courageous, and multilayered story reveals the deadly truth about aspartame poisoning, and the greed of the individuals and corporate entities who put personal profits before the public's safety. Needless to say, if you or anyone you know is hooked on aspartame-laden products, this is the book to read.

As mentioned throughout this chapter, here is another reminder—one of the most alarming ones—that we must get back to the basics. Choose from a variety of whole, fresh foods and, by all means, stay away from aspartame.

Above all, I want to say this: Enjoy your food, but remember, food is fuel. ***Eat to live, don't live to eat.*** There is more to life than food. Honor yourself by selecting foods that support your body and promote optimum health.

SUCCESS

Chapter 4

CREATE A TONED, FIT BODY— FITNESS FOR LIFE!

Even the best diet combined with the most potent vitamins will never tune up your muscles the way good exercise will.
—Covert Bailey

I live in Los Angeles, the fitness capital of the world. People are so body conscious here, the first thing you might be asked when you meet someone is, "Have you got a good trainer and gym?" I wouldn't be surprised to start seeing ads in the personal columns that read: "Fit, trim, female weightlifter who bench presses 150 pounds and has a cholesterol level of 150 looking for a tan, strong, toned man who has completed at least a dozen triathlons and has a triglyceride level of 75."

Of course there are many reasons to stay in good shape beyond the fact that it's fashionable. Fitness is the key to enjoying life—it can unlock the energy, stamina, and positive outlook that make each day a pleasure. Along with good eating habits, adequate rest and relaxation, enough sleep, and a positive attitude about yourself and life, exercise is an important facet of a total program for well-being. It is one of the common sense ways to take responsibility for your own health and life.

In this chapter I want to get you excited about all the reasons you should start or upgrade your fitness program, then guide you on ways to stay motivated, suggesting exercises that tone, strengthen, lengthen, and reshape the body, and encourage you to make that commitment and make exercise a top priority in your life from today forward.

Exercise Your Way to Vitality

Let's take a closer look at the latest research on all the beneficial effects of exercise on your health—physically, emotionally, and spiritually.

HORMONAL BALANCE and ENRICHMENT: Exercise sweeps excess cortisol (stress hormones) from the bloodstream. (As I wrote about in Chapter 1, stress hormones favor fat uptake in the body and increase insulin.) That's why a good workout feels so soothing after a stressful day. Also, when you exercise, your body makes chemicals called endorphins, which are natural painkillers and mood enhancers.

MENTAL HEALTH: Exercise physiologists and medical researchers are now discovering that our sense of happiness and well-being is greatly influenced by the presence of certain chemicals and hormones in the bloodstream. Vigorous exercise stimulates the production of two chemicals that are known to lift the spirit: norepinephrine and enkephalin.

A British medical team headed by Dr. Malcolm Carruthers spent four years studying the effect of norepinephrine on 200 people. Their conclusion: "We believe that most people could ban the blues with a simple, vigorous ten-minute exercise session three times a week. Ten minutes of exercise will double the body's level of this essential neurotransmitter, and the effect is long-lasting. Norepinephrine would seem from our research to be the chemical key to happiness."

FATIGUE: Inactivity actually leads to fatigue. According to Dr. Lawrence Lamb, consultant to the President's Council on Physical Fitness and Sports, part of the reason for this has to do with the way we store adrenaline. Lamb reports, "Activity uses up adrenaline. If it isn't used, adrenaline saps energy and decreases the efficiency of the heart." The downward spiral of energy you feel at the end of a workday will only be worsened if you come home and collapse in an easy chair. "Exercise will get the metabolic machinery out of inertia," says Lamb, "and you'll be refreshed and ready to go."

STRESS: According to the medical profession, 80% to 90% of today's illnesses are stress-related. But stress does not need to be a way of life. We can choose to live productive, energetic lives, based on an inner strength and calmness. One of the most effective ways of reducing stress and tension is through physical exercise. It has even been shown that among persons with symptoms of anxiety and tension, a single dose of exercise is a more effective muscle relaxant than tranquilizers, without the undesirable side effects (see Chapter 1).

HEART HEALTH: Regular exercise is also an important partner in helping reduce the risk of heart attack. Exercise improves blood circulation throughout the body, allowing the lungs, heart, other organs, and muscles to work together more effectively. Exercise also improves your body's ability to use oxygen and provide the energy needed for physical activity.

Exercise raises HDL (the so-called "good" cholesterol, a lipoprotein associated with decreased probability of developing atherosclerosis) and, in some people, also lowers both LDL (the so-called "bad" cholesterol, a lipoprotein associated with increased probability of developing atherosclerosis) and triglycerides.

In a Harvard-based Nurses Health Study published in the June 2000 issue of *JAMA (Journal of the American Medical Association),* involving 72,000 women, ages 30 to 65, it was found that daily 30-minute brisk walks (brisk is walking 1 mile in at least 20 minutes) reduced the risk of stroke by 30% compared to sedentary women. If you walk briskly for 45 to 60 minutes, you reduce the risk of stroke by up to 40%. They also discovered brisk walking helpful in reducing the risk of heart disease, adult onset diabetes, hypertension (high blood pressure), osteoporosis, and even cancer. Because it's so beneficial and easy to do, I'll give you some tips on enhancing your walking program later in this chapter.

OSTEOPOROSIS: This is a condition characterized by decreased bone density. It is never too early or too late to build bone mass. Strength training may be the best exercise for cutting the risk of osteoporosis. Researchers indicate that after the mid-thirties, 1% of our bone mineral mass dissolves each year.

Strength training (weightlifting) workouts tug on the bones, exerting pressure—much more pressure—than nonweight-bearing exercises such as cycling or swimming or even moderate weight-bearing exercises like walking or jogging. That tugging action triggers bone mineralization, stimulating the flow of bone-hardening calcium into the skeleton. Studies reveal that **40 minutes of weight training, 2 times a week** strengthens the body and can reverse or prevent osteoporosis, even in menopausal women.

CANCER: Investigations during the past decade at the Harvard School of Public Health and Center for Population Studies showed that the risk of cancer was lower in athletic women. Regular, long-term, vigorous exercise established a lifestyle that lowered the risk of breast cancer and cancers of the reproductive system. The study of several thousand women, both athletic and sedentary, found that the less-active women were nearly twice as likely to suffer from breast cancer and almost three times as likely to suffer from cancer of the reproductive system. The incidence of benign tumors of the breast and reproductive system was also significantly lower in athletic women.

The study points out the importance of starting vigorous exercise at an early age. The great majority of the active women in the study started exercising in high school or earlier. Prevention is clearly a long-term effect. Lead investigator, Rose E. Frisch, Ph.D., said the best time to start exercising is about the age of nine, and to keep it up. Those who began exercising young also avoided fatty foods in favor of those foods that supported their activities, namely fresh fruits and vegetables.

Research shows that women who do not exercise tend to become obese, with increased levels of toxic forms of estrogen. After menopause, this condition is an established breast-cancer risk factor. Studies at the Norris Comprehensive Cancer Center of the University of Southern California showed that women under age forty who exercised at least four hours a week could cut their risk of the disease up to 60%. That's remarkable! Those under forty who exercised one to three hours a week lessened their risk by up to 30%.

STRENGTH and ENDURANCE: Even into the ages of 80 and 90, resistance training (weights) can help or prevent deterioration of muscles and bones and increase energy and strength. Not long ago, Dr. Maria Fiatarone of Penn State and Dr. William Evans at the Tufts USDA Nutrition Research Center on Aging engaged ten nursing home residents, all between the ages of 86 and 96, and asked them to sit on exercise benches and lift weights, extending one leg at a time, three times a week. At the end of just 8 weeks (!) the men and women had tripled their muscle strength. The amount of absolute weight they could lift increased from about 15 pounds on each leg to 43 pounds. The researchers found similar results with a 12-week program of resistance training for 60- to 70-year-old men. Muscle strength of all the men doubled and tripled. Muscle mass grew by 10% to 15%.

Recently, Dr. Fiatarone and associates were able to show just how important these muscle-building efforts were for enjoyment of everyday living. The scientists recruited 100 frail nursing home residents between the ages of 72 and 98 and placed 50 of them in a strength-training program; the other 50, the control group, remained sedentary. Over a 10-week period, muscle strength among the 50 exercisers more than doubled, which resulted, the researchers discovered, in a 30% increase in spontaneous physical activity. "The exercise intervention," wrote the researchers, "significantly improved habitual gait velocity (speed of walking), stair climbing ability, and the overall level of physical activity." As reported in the *New England Journal of Medicine,* several participants who had been limited to using a walker graduated to the use of only a cane.

According to studies conducted at Tufts University, **from age 20 to age 80 we lose up to one-third of our muscle mass and gain fat if we don't stay physically active.** This results in decreased metabolism (and osteoporosis).

WEIGHT CONTROL: While I've covered this in other chapters, I'll briefly summarize it here. Increased muscle mass from strength training raises your body's energy requirements. That means more calories are expended all day long, every day. **Food fuels the furnace of metabolism and exercise fans its fire.** Exercise that causes sweating and heavy breathing is sugar-burning exercise. However, overweight people need fat-burning exercise, which requires slow, sustained activity such as brisk walking. Thirty to sixty minutes of vigorous walking every day will help people lose fat. In addition, **lifting weights helps increase lean muscle mass. Sufficient muscle mass is desirable because it burns calories, whereas fat stores calories. The idea that fat turns to muscle isn't true, but if you have more muscle, you burn more fat. As a person loses muscle due to inactivity, she or he loses the ability to use calories effectively and usually gains fat and weight even when eating fewer calories.** The lack of consistent exercise (both aerobics and weight training) may be the most important factor in explaining why more than 50% of the U.S. population is overweight.

DIABETES: Obesity and a sedentary lifestyle are major risk factors for several diseases. Type 2 diabetes, also known as non-insulin dependent diabetes, is strongly associated with obesity. Losing weight is usually the first step in treating the disease. People don't usually associate diabetes with lack of exercise. However, a study reported in the October 1999 issue of *Journal of the American Medical Association,* found a clear relationship between exercise and diabetes risk. Responses to questions about the intensity and duration of physical activity provided by approximately 70,000 women participating in the Nurses Health Study were evaluated. The women were free of heart disease, diabetes, and cancer at the time they answered the questions (1986). During the 8 years of follow-up, 1,419 women developed diabetes. After taking into account known risk factors for diabetes, a relationship between physical activity and the risk of type 2 diabetes emerged.

"Increasing physical activity substantially reduced the risk of type 2 diabetes," said Dr. Frank B. Hu of the Harvard School of Public Health, who led the study. "What is particularly interesting," he said, "is that the risk reduction for moderate intensity activity, such as walking, is the same as that for more vigorous forms of activity, such as running or jogging, if the energy expenditure is the same. Total energy expenditure is the most important factor." The study found that just an hour of brisk walking every day can cut the risk of developing type 2 diabetes in half, as much as more vigorous exercise does. Physical activity can help reduce the risk of type 2 diabetes by assisting in fat reduction and by helping the body use insulin more efficiently.

No more excuses! Get out there and walk whenever possible.

LONGEVITY and VITALITY: A recent study suggests that baby boomers may not have to rely on injections of human growth hormone to compensate for age-related declines in their later years. Researchers found that people in their 60s who had exercised regularly for most of their lives had higher levels of the muscle-building, skin-toning hormone (human growth hormone) than sedentary people in their 20s. For more information on staying youthful and strong, I recommend the book *Strong Women Stay Young* by Miriam E. Nelson, Ph.D.

There is no guarantee that exercise will add years to your life, but there's compelling evidence that it might. A study done by Dr. Ralph

Paffenbarger, a noted medical researcher at Stanford University, showed that those participants who expended 2,000 calories a week in vigorous exercise such as brisk walking and cross-country skiing lived 2 years longer than those who did not.

WOMEN'S HEALTH: We now have ample evidence that menstrual cramps and PMS are soothed by a good workout. Exercise can also alleviate some of the undesirable symptoms of menopause. Two recent studies have documented a reduction in hot flash severity in women who work out (one study involved runners; the other, women were in an aerobic conditioning program). Exercise increases endorphin levels, which ultimately works to counteract, at least in part, the decreasing levels of estrogen and progesterone hormones, that can cause hot flashes and other symptoms in menopausal women.

Exercise, by improving mood and relieving stress, also alleviates fatigue, depression, tension, insomnia, weight gain, and irritability that may accompany the change of life.

SEX and LIBIDO: If none of the above interests you, maybe this one will. Exercise makes you sexy. A physically fit body is brimming with sex appeal, and exercise unleashes the libido. A recent comprehensive survey showed that exercise increased the sexual confidence of most women; a third of them made love more often, and nearly half of them had an enhanced capacity to be sexually aroused. There's no doubt about it: Women who exercise have more satisfying sex lives. I've heard this from hundreds of women I've counseled over the years. Studies also show that exercise is a potent stimulus to hormone production in both men and women, chemically increasing desire by stepping up the levels of such hormones as testosterone and prolactin. It is a scientific fact that exercise can dramatically improve your sex life, at any age.

SPIRITUAL HEALTH: Exercise is also very important for spiritual health. A well-exercised and fit body can relax and meditate better. I know my meditations are deeper when I exercise every day.

OTHER BENEFITS:

Immunity is boosted after each exercise session, so a regular exercise program means better resistance against infectious diseases. Sleep quality improves on the days you workout. Exercise causes an increase in the body's natural antioxidant defenses. Exercise is a natural appetite suppressant when you exercise no more than one hour a day, and a good way to ease cravings. If you exercise longer, you might eat more but it will be burned up from the increased metabolism, especially when you eat healthy foods.

With all these benefits to the whole body—physically, mentally, spiritually—you really have no excuses left not to make exercise a top priority in your daily health regime, do you?

Susan's Top 10 Tips to Walk Your Way to Radiant Health

I love to walk. Next to hiking, it's my favorite aerobic activity. We now know that a regular walking program affords many aerobic benefits, such as lowered blood pressure, reduced cholesterol, improved cardiovascular endurance and circulation, a higher metabolism that burns more calories, reduced stress and a more positive state of mind, a better skin complexion, and an increased energy level. WOW! At this point, you're probably eager to get out and walk before reading any further. First let me give you a few tips to help you along.

1. Wear bright, reflective clothing when walking in the dark, and especially at dusk and dawn when visibility is poor. Wear comfortable shoes with good support and replace them at least every six months. Make sure they are suitable for the type and amount of walking you will be doing. To avoid blisters, wear quality walking socks, padded at the toe and heel.

2. Carry identification, change for a pay phone, and tissue or a bandana. In warmer weather or on walks over an hour, bring a water bottle. I put a few supplements (Emer'gen-C and AlkaLife) in my water for workouts (see Resource Directory).

3. If you walk near traffic, use sidewalks or walk on the left side of the road facing traffic. Make eye contact with drivers or assume they don't see you.

4. Bring your dog along for company and/or protection, but if your dog stops at every rose bush and visits with other dogs, it's best to leave her at home as she'll slow your walking progress and you won't be able to keep a nonstop, brisk pace.

5. *Don't run from a threatening dog.* Calmly face the accosting canine, speak in a low, clear, and authoritative voice and tell him to go home. Then back away if necessary.

6. If you walk where you pass by friends and acquaintances, ***don't stop to chat en route.*** Tell any friends you see you're not being anti-social, but your walk is most effective if done continuously.

7. When you have a busy day with little walking time available, ***don't skip your walk.*** A short walk provides a physical and emotional boost and helps you maintain your everyday walking commitment.

8. *If it's a cold windy day, dress warmly in layers and walk into the wind first.* You'll get the hard work out of the way and avoid the problem of getting a chill while working up a sweat with the wind at your back.

9. *Drink at least eight to ten 8-oz glasses of water a day.* Also, drink a large glass of water about 15 minutes before you start your walk.

10. *Have fun!*

A Few Helpful Techniques

1. *Be aware of your posture.* Make sure your shoulders are directly over your hips and your hips are moving front to back, not side to side.

2. *Keep your head up* and your chin parallel to the ground.

3. *Bend your arms* at a 90° angle to help propel you forward.

4. *Keep up a good pace* by rotating your hips front to back while pushing off with one foot and pulling the other forward.

5. *Warm up slowly* and establish a pace that is brisk, but not exhausting or painful.

6. *Be light on your feet.* Make sure your weight rolls though your entire foot, from your heel through to your toes.

7. *Easy does it.* Start by walking 15 to 20 minutes a day if you're a beginner and progressively increase the time.

8. Increase your workload by walking uphill, in sand, or against the wind. Hand weights probably won't help your walk.

A Few Motivating Facts

1. The faster you walk, the more calories you'll burn. If you walk for a half hour at 3 miles per hour, you can expect to expend 120 calories. If you walk for the same amount of time at 4 miles per hour, you'll burn closer to 170 calories.

2. The more you weigh, the more calories you burn, so with weight-bearing exercise, such as walking, you'll burn more calories than someone who weighs less than you.

3. Caloric expenditure increases when you increase intensity, such as walking uphill. For every 3% grade, your body uses as much energy as it would to go a mile per hour faster. This is one of the reasons I love to hike so much: lots of hills and the scenery is so beautiful, I hardly notice that I'm working out harder. Instead of saying I'll push harder to the end of the block as I might if jogging in my neighborhood, I say that I'll push harder to the top of the hill from where I can see the entire Santa Monica Bay sprawled out in all its glory.

4. The harder you work during your aerobic workout, the longer the "afterburn," the length of time after exercise that your body continue to use more energy than it does at rest (see Chapter 5 for more on this).

Finding Your Target Heart Rate

How do you know if you're exercising at the proper level to reap all the aerobic benefits?

Two formulas are used to compute the percentage of maximum heart rate at which you should work to improve aerobic capacity. One method involves multiplying your estimated maximum heart rate (obtained by subtracting your age from 220) times a percentage (from around 60% to 80%) that's related to your fitness goals and condition. For example, if you're thirty years old, your estimated maximum heart rate would be 190 beats per minute (220-30=190). Multiplying 190 by 60% (or 0.6) equals 114; 190 times 80% (0.9) equals 171.

The older, less conditioned, or more obese you are, the better it is to start off easier. Work at the low end of your target heart range and keep up the activity for longer periods. As your condition improves, you can up the intensity so that you're working harder, perhaps 70% to 80% (0.7 to 0.8 times maximum heart rate, which would be 133 to 152 beats per minute).

How do you know what your exercise heart rate is? To take your heart rate, place your index and middle finger just to the side of your windpipe with a slight pressure toward the back of your neck until you feel the pulse in your carotid artery. Count the beats over a 10-second period and multiply by 6 (or you can count for 6 seconds and multiply by 10—or simply add a 0—or count for 15 seconds and multiply by 4) to get your heart rate for 1 minute. Take it about 5 to 7 minutes into your exercise and every 10 to 15 minutes thereafter until you learn what the appropriate intensity feels like.

Constantly trying to increase your exercise intensity will help burn more calories as well as increase your aerobic power, but what matters in the long run is consistency. When in doubt, always be conservative and go easier than harder. The real key is to work at activities that you like and at a pace or intensity that you're comfortable with. You should finish each exercise session feeling exhilarated—not exhausted—and looking forward to your next session.

As an alternative to measuring your exercise heart rate (I recommend that you do so for safety, effectiveness, and to enhance your body awareness), you can use the talk test. If you're breathing harder yet can still carry on a conversation without significant difficulty—gasping for air—while exercising aerobically, you're working at a level that's well within your capacity.

If all this is too complicated for you, consider using a heart monitor. This electronic device—typically consisting of an electrode-studded strap that's worn around the chest and a wristwatch-like digital display—gives a continuous reading of your heart rate. With a heart monitor, there's no need to stop exercising to take your pulse.

See the following chart to help you locate your target heart rate easily and quickly.

As I said before, I love to walk/jog for exercise and, whenever possible, I find beautiful places in nature to hike. I live a couple of minutes from the magnificent Santa Monica mountains and hike

Monitoring Your Pulse

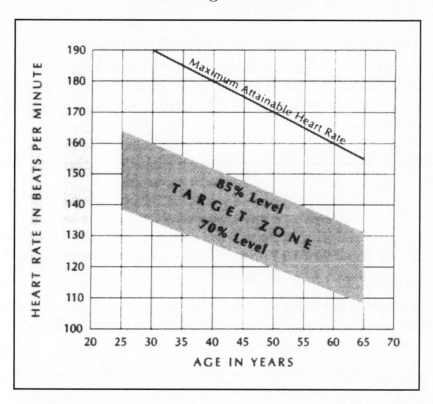

several times each week. I get a great workout for my body, mind, and spirit.

Although I enjoy working out at the gym and do so a few times weekly, I think many people get into a rut of only working out indoors. We can feed our bodies and souls more effectively by getting outside into local parks, school tracks, golf courses, and public gardens. Walt Whitman wrote, "Now I know the secret of making the best persons. It is to grow in the open air and sleep and eat with the earth."

Outdoor activities you might want to consider are the following: Jogging on the beach, rock climbing, white-water rafting, kayaking, rowing a boat, tossing a Frisbee, beach volleyball, windsurfing, sailing, surfing, tennis, or speed golf. Speed golf is the type A personality's answer to traditional golf. After putting, you literally run to the next hole. The person with the lowest score—the total of your running time and golf score—wins. Combining different activities (cross-training) assures I'll never get bored and helps me to stay motivated to exercise regularly.

Susan's Top 10 Tips for Staying Motivated

Every person who exercises regularly, whether an athlete or not, will have to cope with lack of motivation, boredom, or burnout at one time or another. Here are some helpful tips that can keep you motivated to stick to your routine

1. Make a commitment. Once you decide to make exercise a part of your life, take precautions that will keep you on the right track.

- Arrange your personal circumstances so your lifestyle supports your commitment.
- Make time for exercise.
- Seek the support of others, but realize the prime reason to exercise must come from within yourself.

2. Define your fitness goals. Write down realistic short-term and long-term goals. Your goals provide a path for a specific direction and let you know how you are doing.

3. Repetition. Repetition is the key to mastery. Remember: It takes 21 days for the mind and body to create a new habit. During this time, remind yourself that for at least 21 consecutive days you'll stick to your new exercise program. It also helps to share your goals with a trusted friend.

4. Reaffirm your fitness goals daily. Post your goals and your plans for achieving them where you can see them every day.

5. Visualize your fitness goals. Visualizing your fitness goals as already completed will increase your motivation, keep you on course, and hasten your success.

6. Keep track of your daily progress. Plan your workouts in advance and keep track of your progress in a diary or on a calendar. Seeing your daily accomplishments is encouraging and increases self-esteem.

7. Be realistic. Don't set yourself up to fail. If you've just started a walking program and are now up to 2 miles nonstop, don't make it one of your goals to run a marathon at the end of the month.

8. Exercise with someone else. Working out is easier when you have someone to do it with. Many times I've been grateful for friends who got me through a workout I might have skipped if I were working out alone.

9. Use affirmations. Affirmations greatly enhance motivation. They can be mental, verbal, written, or recorded on a cassette. Keep affirmations positive and in the present.

10. Reward yourself. You've kept your agreement, you've worked out hard, you've been consistent, and you're seeing positive results. Reward yourself. Rewards increase motivation and create positive associations toward your exercise program.

Be More Active Throughout the Day

1. Get creative. If you're exercising primarily as a way to lose weight, you may have read that 30 minutes of exercise 3 to 5 times a week is all that's needed. Not true. A study recently published in the *Journal of the American Medical Association* suggests that a total of at least 40 minutes—and preferably 60—is needed *each* day of the week to lose weight and keep it off. An hour a day might be daunting, but that's mainly because few of us exercise as effectively—or as creatively—as we could. The study revealed that so-called lifestyle exercisers (people who regularly took the stairs, walked instead of drove, cleaned the house, etc.) lost almost as much weight and body fat as those who exercised in a more structured way (in health clubs, for instance).

The key to weight control, especially when time is too limited to be able to carve out structured time to work out, is to become more active in general. Check out the following chart for the calorie burn of everyday actions. If you're not working out regularly (and I do recommend you *create* time to do this especially if your goal is to accelerate fat), aim for at least 30 to 40 minutes of unstructured activity every day.

Activity	Calories burned in 10 Minutes
Dancing to a song on the radio	27–54
Ping-Pong	35
Horseplay with the kids	40
Vigorous housework	40
Walking up stairs	70
Walking down stairs	25
Gardening (hoeing, raking, weeding)	50
Shoveling snow	65

2. Exercise early in the day. Morning workouts burn no more calories than workouts late in the day, but they do give you more options if your schedule changes. I find that if unforeseen circumstances force me to cancel a workout that I've scheduled for the morning, I still have the rest of the day to break a sweat. If I'm forced to cancel the evening workout, I've lost the chance for the entire day.

3. Put exercise on your calendar. If you want to be the best you can be and be radiantly healthy, you must give exercise the same priority as you would a business meeting or lunch with a friend or time spent going to a movie or shopping. So write it down! Mark your workout days and times on your calendar to make it a priority.

4. Exercise to music. Most people exercise more vigorously to fast-tempo music than they do without it. They also tend to keep at it longer.

NO MORE EXCUSES! If there's any concern that weather or darkness might keep you from working out, invest in a X-ISER™ (see Resource Directory). Recent research suggests that it's the most effective machine for fat loss and increased metabolism, strength, and energy. It takes only a few minutes, depending on the program you use, and it takes up just a few inches of floor space, so you can easily use it at home or in your office. It's like a stair climber without the top part, but it's so much more than that and it does produce fast results! I've seen it in all my clients and friends who have one. Most importantly, it's fun to use.

Attaining Optimum Flexibility

Take time to stretch or do yoga every day. A flexible body, especially for an active person, greatly reduces the risk of injury because muscles that restrict the natural range of motion in the joints are susceptible to pulls, tears, and stress injuries.

For the less athletic, flexibility can provide relief from everyday muscle tension and stiffness, and is also crucial for proper posture.

When we lack flexibility, our bodies compensate in ways that create poor posture, resulting in mechanical imbalances in the back, hip, and neck. These imbalances pull the body out of line, causing stress, strain, and even worse posture. Inflexible joints and weak muscles in the shoulder and chest can cause rounded shoulders, which can lead to kyphosis (humpbacked spine), a sunken chest, and impaired respiratory capacity.

Tight hip-flexor muscles, hamstrings, and back muscles can rotate the pelvis forward, resulting in excessive curvature of the lower back, chronic lower back pain, and sciatica.

Drooping your head forward may produce dizziness and chronic strain on the muscles along the back of the neck, resulting in neck and shoulder pain.

Yoga

Yoga is a great way to increase flexibility. The most ancient of all fitness systems, yoga has many benefits. Yoga can increase lung capacity and height, aid digestion and circulation, while reducing stress, insomnia, back pain, and asthma attacks. New studies show it can even help to reverse heart disease.

Hatha yoga (physical yoga, as opposed to meditative or devotional) is a system of breathing exercises and postures (asanas). Some poses may look contortionistic, but they can be modified for any body. What's important is content—breathing and inner awareness—more than form.

In yoga, the diaphragm (the floor for the heart and lungs; the ceiling for the liver, stomach, and spleen) is retrained to move vertically, thus massaging the adjacent vital organs and stimulating digestion and circulation. Yoga is also a stress buster, offering a respite in fast-paced American life, a way to quiet down and work on your body from the inside out.

It does require instruction. Check out fitness clubs, dance studios, hospitals, wellness centers, colleges, YMCAs, churches, recreational parks, and back clinics for classes. Find the right teacher for you. You may also consider video programs. There are some great ones available at your video store. Rent first to make sure it's one you'll use often.

Stretching

Another way to increase flexibility is through a stretching program. Again, you can find stretching videos if you need the structure or find a class to attend. Muscles exert force by pulling, not pushing. Most muscles attach to bones and cross over one or more joints. When the muscles contract and shorten, they cause a limb or body part to move in a particular direction. The external opposing force can be applied by gravity, by the contraction of an opposite muscle, or by a stretching partner.

The approach to increasing flexibility in a progressive stretching program is related to the overload principle used to build muscle strength. To increase muscle strength, you must regularly contract the muscle against progressively more resistance with a slightly greater force than that to which it is accustomed. In time the muscle responds to the overload by becoming stronger. Similarly, to increase flexibility, you must regularly stretch the muscle slightly beyond its normal length. It will adapt to this overload by increasing its length, thereby rewarding you with a greater range of joint motion. To increase a muscle's length, you must regularly pull it about 10% beyond its normal length; that is the point where your muscles feel stretched enough to be slightly uncomfortable but not enough to cause pain. Ideally, you should hold this position for 30 seconds while breathing deeply; then relax, and repeat the stretch 2 or 3 times, if time permits. Stretching 3 to 7 days a week is optimal. In one study, 57 men and women with tight hamstrings (back of the thigh) stretched that muscle for different periods over 6 weeks. Groups held stretches either 15, 30, or 60 seconds, or didn't stretch at all. Only when the muscle was stretched for 30 seconds or more did it respond by lengthening, thereby allowing more range of motion. Anything less than that was just going through the motions. As reported in the September 1994 issue of *Physical Therapy,* the surprise was that more wasn't better—the minute-long stretch was only about as effective as the half-minute hold. This was the first study to test which stretch offered the most benefits over a long period of time. Be patient. You will see results if you are consistent.

It's worth adding those 30-second segments of stretching to your walking, cycling, or other exercise routine, says study leader William D. Bandy, Ph.D., PT, associate professor of physical therapy at the University of Central Arkansas. Tight hamstrings may force your quadriceps muscles (front of the thigh) to work harder, and that may set you up for knee problems. In addition, tight muscles can be injured by sudden overstretching.

I really enjoy doing some type of stretching every day. My rule of thumb is to stretch half the time I've engaged in an aerobic or weight workout. For example, if I hike, bike, jog, or do a weight workout for 30 minutes, I would devote 15 minutes to stretching. It's best to stretch before *and* after a workout. But if you only have time for one stretch session, make it after. Stretching increases your joints' range of motion, and warm muscles respond better than cold muscles. Warm up with enough light activity to break a sweat, then hit the stretching mats before your workout, if time permits. Follow up with a post-sweat stretch, when your muscles are at their most flexible. I usually do 5 minutes of stretching before the aerobic workout and the remainder after the workout. When lifting weights, I stretch before, during the workout—in between sets—and after the workout is over. Besides elongating your muscles and increasing flexibility, stretching is also a wonderful way to breathe deeply and just relax.

So make it a short-term goal to incorporate stretching into your daily life. The best time to stretch is whenever you're really going to do it. I teach fitness clients and students to stretch during commercials on television. If I were to ask them to warm up, run, and come back and stretch, I don't think they'd do it. But you can easily fit in at least a few 30-second stretches during your average commercial break.

If you'd like to start stretching today, here are five important stretches:

GENERAL FLEXIBILITY and UPPER THIGHS: Sit on the floor with the soles of the feet together, grasp your ankles and pull toward the groin area. Then place hands on the inside of your knees and push them out and down toward floor until you feel a stretch. Hold seconds and repeat.

QUADRICEPS: While standing, bend one knee and grasp the ankle behind you. Pull the ankle toward buttocks until you feel a stretch. Hold on to something if you need to. Hold for 30 seconds. Repeat. Alternate legs. Variations: Use a towel to help you stretch if you cannot easily reach your feet. You can also do this one lying on your side on the floor. Bend your top knee and pull your foot toward your buttocks with your top hand.

HAMSTRING: Sit on the floor with one leg straight, the other leg bent with the heel against upper part of the other inner thigh. Lean over the straight leg and grasp your calf or ankle, wherever your extended arms reach, pulling your chin towards your knee. Keep your knee straight and soft (don't lock the knee). Hold for 30 seconds. Repeat. Alternate legs.

CALF: Stand facing a wall. Using your hands against the wall for balance, take a step back and lean toward the wall until you feel a stretch in your lower calf. You can do one calf or both at the same time. Hold for 30 seconds, relax. Repeat. Alternate legs.

LOWER BACK: Lie on your back. Raise one knee to your chest, keeping the opposite leg slightly bent. Grasp your knee with your hands and pull in towards your chest, while keeping your lower back pressed flat on the floor. Hold the stretch for 30 to 60 seconds. Relax and repeat with the opposite leg, then both legs together. End by curling your head up toward your knees.

I also use my BodySlant for adding variety to my stretching. It's like a slant board and improves circulation, increases energy and relaxation, and helps relieve back, shoulder, and neck strain or pain. (Refer to the Resource Directory for more information.)

If time is really limited—say I have 15 minutes to workout and stretch—I'll do my quick jumping jack/stretch routine. I'll start with 3 minutes of stretching on the floor and follow that with 7 minutes of jumping jacks to work up a light sweat, and then end with 5 more minutes of stretching. While it's not a very intense or complete work-out, at least it's something and I don't need any equipment. I can do this just about anywhere, including hotel rooms. Also, the X-iser (see Resource Directory) is a great way to get a quick intense workout in only minutes.

SAFE JUMPING JACKS: Although jumping jacks were com-mon during the early days of aerobics, they disappeared when low-impact aerobics, step, and spinning came into vogue. But the emer-gence of boot camp, kick boxing, Tae-Bo, and athletic-style fitness classes has brought them back in a big way. Jumping jacks boost workout intensity, so they're a great calorie burner. And you don't have to worry about the pounding forces of jumping if you have good form. Stance: First, when jumping out, keep your feet hip- to shoul-der-width apart, and avoid opening them too far. Jump: To absorb impact, soften your knees when you land, and make sure that both heels contact the ground after every jump. Upper Body: Lift rib cage and contract abs throughout the move. Arms: Avoid shoulder strain: Don't raise arms above shoulder level.

How to Develop Strong, Toned, Impressive Abdominals

As a fitness instructor to students, staff, and faculty at UCLA for over 30 years and a personal fitness trainer for more than 25 years, I get asked lots of questions about fitness. One of the most-asked ques-tions is, "Why aren't my sit-ups helping me lose fat around my waist?" Some people mistakenly think they can burn fat around their waists by doing exercises involving muscles in that area, such as sit-ups and side bends. Unfortunately, sit-ups will not reduce observable fat around the waist. *Exercises aimed at any single muscle group do not burn enough calories to noticeably reduce fat in that area. In other words, spot reducing doesn't work!*

You cannot work a specific muscle with the idea that the fat on top of the muscle will be burned off. Like blood, fat belongs to the entire body. The fat around your waist and tummy is not tummy fat—it's body fat. For example, when you're hiking, your body doesn't say, "Oh, she's hiking, so let's use her leg fat." It says, "Send me some fat from anywhere in the body to fuel her activity."

To burn the most amount of fat from all over the body, you must exercise large sets of muscles like you do when you use your thighs and buttocks—the very muscles used in all aerobic exercise. If you exercise only one muscle or a small set, like the abdominals or biceps, you don't burn many calories or use much fat. Leg raises and abdominal exercises, while not effective for burning fat, are still great for spot *building*. They will enhance the shape of your body by emphasizing a particular area, thus making the surrounding areas appear slimmer. And when you lose your extra body fat, those toned muscles underneath the fat, such as the abdominals (abs), will look awesome. So do your floor exercises, as I do often, but know that you're not spot reducing, you're spot building.

Like other muscles, your abs thrive on variety and change. And in terms of toning and tightening, they seem to respond best when constantly thrown new stresses.

Have you ever heard someone complain that they've been doing 200 crunches every day for the past six months with no results? Or have your noticed how a new ab routine you could barely finish the first time became pretty easy after a few sessions? That's because muscles adapt to the stress placed upon them rather quickly. In the case of your abs, since you're only lifting your body weight, you can't really increase the load. Once this happens, they aren't being challenged anymore and you stop making improvements in strength and tone. So what do you do? Get out of the rut. Change your routine. Sneak up on your abs and they'll respond. With your abdominals in a perpetual state of surprise, they'll be exerting more effort and if you work the muscles in your torso from a variety of angles, you will recruit different muscle fibers from each of the abdominal muscles.

The following exercises for ab strengthening are among the best. They will not place any stress on your back. You should do them in the order listed so you work your lower abdominal muscles before the uppers. If you tire the upper abs first, fatigue will limit the amount of lower abdominal work you can do. Do them to your favorite music so you can coordinate the movements with the music's beat. Nothing helps motivate and energize better than great music with a strong beat.

KNEE LIFT REVERSE CRUNCH: Lie on your back, feet up in the air and knees bent at a 90-degree angle so they're directly over your hips. Place your hands behind your head in the basic position. (Don't lace your fingers together or pull on your neck; instead, put your thumbs behind your ears, fingertips just touching. Lengthen your neck. You should be able to see your elbows out of the corners of your eyes.) Keeping your upper body still and flat on the floor, contract your abs and lift your buttocks upward 1 to 2 inches, allow your knees to move slightly toward your chest while lifting your upper torso at the same time until your shoulder blades clear the floor. Hold a moment, return to the start, and repeat to fatigue. (By fatigue I mean until your muscles are exhausted and it's difficult to do another repetition. A specific muscle fatigue is a different fatigue from a general over-all body fatigue or tiredness.) Your hands function as a cradle to prevent your lower back from arching. Your lower back should remain flat against the floor throughout the exercise with your abdominals pulled in and tight.

BASIC CRUNCH: Lie on your back, knees bent, feet on the floor, with your heels a comfortable distance from your buttocks. Align your spine in the neutral position. (Rotate your hips backward and pull your abs inward so your lower back is in contact with the floor. Not only will this neutral position protect your lower back, but it will make the exercises more challenging and effective.) Place your hands behind your head in the basic position. Curl your upper body upward in one smooth movement until your shoulder blades clear the floor, exhaling as you lift. Hold a moment, return to the start, and continue until fatigued.

ROTATION CRUNCH: Lie as in the basic crunch. Bend your right leg and place the heel on your left thigh (your right knee will point out to the side). Put your left hand behind your head and your right arm at your side on the floor. Curl your upper body upward and then, leading with your left shoulder, rotate your torso toward your right knee. Return to the start and do several reps until fatigued, then change sides.

CONTINUOUS ROTATION CRUNCH: Lie on your back as you did in the basic crunch and keep your lower back flat against the floor with your abs pulled in during the entire exercise. Curl your upper body up until your shoulder blades are off the floor and then, leading with your right shoulder, rotate your torso toward your left knee. Without rolling down, rotate your torso toward your right knee, leading with your left shoulder. Continue your reps without stopping or rolling down until fatigued. (One rotation left and right equals one repetition.)

DOUBLE ARM CRUNCH: Lie on your back with feet in the air, knees bent directly above hips so that your calves are parallel to the floor. Extend both arms straight behind your head close to your ear, fingers interlaced. Lift your arms, head, neck, and shoulders up and off the floor in a smooth motion. Hold a moment at the top, lower to the start and do several reps.

OPEN KNEE CRUNCH: Lie on your back with your feet in the air, knees bent directly over hips. Place your hands behind your head in the basic position. Cross your ankles and turn your knees out to the sides. Curl your upper body upward and forward until your shoulder blades clear the floor. Hold a moment, lower to the start and repeat to complete reps.

When doing these abdominal exercises, exhale when you lift, inhale as you lower. Don't just go through the motions. Always work your abs slowly and with control. Don't bounce up off the floor between repetitions. You're moving at the right speed if you feel a contraction through your abs on the way up *and* on the way down. Also, when you exercise, be sure to wear comfortable clothing that allows you freedom of movement as well as evaporation of perspiration. Think about what you're doing! Research has shown that if you visualize each contraction you may actually use more muscle fibers.

Individualize Your Exercise Program

Consider the following factors when setting up an exercise program in which your time is used efficiently and for maximum results.

Aerobic Exercise

FREQUENCY: This means how often you should work out. If fat loss is your goal, and you want to see fast results, do some type of aerobic activity 6 times a week and leave 1 day just for extra stretching and/or yoga, an ab workout, some pushups, and maybe an easy walk out in nature. If you just want to tone up, strengthen, and reshape your body, shoot for at least 3 to 4 times a week for aerobic activity.

INTENSITY: This refers to how hard you work, that is, how much your heart rate increases (refer back to the monitoring heart rate section and chart) or how quickly you burn calories. Exercise in your target zone and, if you're not a beginner, intensify your workouts at least twice a week. This means to push harder a few times during the workout for 30 to 60 seconds and then fall back into your target heart rate zone (refer to Chapter 5 for more detailed information). Space these higher intensity periods out, such as Tuesday, Thursday, and Saturday, 3 to 6 times in your workout. If you're a beginner, wait for about 4 weeks before adding intensifying your workouts. It's not the intensity of the sprint (faster walk, jog, hike, steep hill, etc.) that makes your body burn calories. It's the intensity of the recovery (see section below on weightlifting). You must force your body to recuperate while it is under stress. In other words, you are still working out and recovering in your target heart rate zone after the higher intensity interval.

DURATION: This refers to the length of each workout. For beginners, start with 15 to 20 minutes and progressively build up to 45 minutes to 1 hour. If you're not a beginner, shoot for at least 20 minutes, preferably 45 minutes or more. If you want to accelerate fat loss, go for an hour a day, with 3 days of higher intensity intervals, and 1 day a week with an easier aerobic workout than usual.

METHOD: Any aerobic activity using the large muscle groups (legs, buttocks, and back) performed continuously in a rhythmic manner is suitable. Fast walking is highly recommended for people of all ages since walking provides all the benefits of aerobic training with a minimum of impact stress on weight-bearing joints like hips, knees, and ankles. Combine indoor and outdoor activities so you won't get bored. And remember to breathe. It may be hard to believe but lots of people have an unhealthy habit of holding their breath, especially when increasing intensity. During weightlifting, in particular, holding your breath can cause a sharp rise in blood pressure. Focus on the muscle group being used and have fun!

Weight lifting

Contrary to popular belief, weight lifting (or strength training as it's also called) is not aerobic. Even though you may be breathing deeply when you're lifting heavier weights, you'll never supply enough oxygen to the muscles to make it aerobic because the demand is simply too intense. But weight lifting is essential if you want to perform aerobic activity more intensely without becoming anaerobic, burn more fat even while sleeping, build more fat-burning enzymes, reshape your body, and restore and maintain youthful vitality.

You don't burn fat during a weight workout but you burn lots of fat during the recovery period as your body strives to replace the sugar that was used by the sugar-burning enzymes during the workout. *If you feel the burn, then your muscles are using sugar for fuel, not fat.* In other words, our bodies break down fat supplies to build up the sugar supplies. And restoring sugar requires a lot of energy, which means that lots of calories are burned. And *all* of this energy must be supplied by the fat-burning enzymes. Now you can see how important it is to include weight lifting in your program if you want to increase lean muscle mass and stimulate metabolism, lose fat, and reshape your body.

Whether with cables, barbells, dumbbells, or machines, or even free-hand movements such as push-ups and sit-ups, this type of training is an essential accompaniment to aerobic and flexibility activities.

In more than 25 years of fitness training and teaching, I've seen that you need at least 2 sessions a week in which the major muscle groups of the body are exercised with weights. For those of you who are beginners to weight lifting and don't know what to do, here's a sample program on the opposite page:

You should weight train at least 2, or better yet 3, times a week. Allow at least 1 day between sessions. An ideal system would be to take 2 days off between training sessions. I do 2 days on, 1 day off. A typical week of weight training for me might look like this: Monday I focus on back, legs, and biceps. Tuesday I work out chest, shoulders, and triceps. Wednesday I'll take off and then repeat Monday and Tuesday routines on Thursday and Friday. With this routine, I'm lifting weights 4 times a week and still getting 48 hours of recovery between the muscles I worked out. Muscles need to repair after weight lifting. If you don't give your muscles time to recover, you won't get the beneficial metabolic effects. Sometimes I'll spend 2 hours just on my legs or back/chest. I add cardio by hiking 3 times a

Exercise	Sets	Rep
Leg Press or Squat	1-3	10-15
Lat Pull-Down	1-3	10-12
Chest Press	1-3	10-12
Bent-Over or Machine Row	1-3	10-12
Overhead Shoulder Press	1-3	10-12
Biceps Curl	1-2	10-12
Triceps Extension	1-2	10-12
Abdominal Curl	1-3	15-20
Calf Raise	1-2	15-20

week in addition to incorporating some of the other aerobic activities I mentioned above. On a rest day, I frequently include a walking meditation (Chapter 19) as part of my 3-Day De-Stress Retreat.

If all this seems too complicated, consult a fitness trainer to help you set up a program geared to your specific needs.

Perform at least 1 set (which consists of a series of continuous repetitions) of each exercise and work up to 3 sets, time and energy permitting. (If you're a beginner, start with just 1 set.) When you've finished the set, it should be difficult to perform more repetitions. If it isn't, you need to go up in weight until you find the correct amount to lift. You should be able to do only, say 10 to 12 reps before fatigue. Rest for 2 or 3 minutes between sets. I usually use this time to stretch or, if I'm working out with a partner, I'll spot them in what they're doing with the weights. One of the great things about lifting weights is that you can see your strength improving, which will keep you motivated to continue.

Always remember to breathe when you're lifting weights. It's not so important when you should inhale or exhale as you might consciously do with yoga positions; just breathe comfortably and remind yourself to do it.

Remember, as with aerobic exercise, the goal is to enjoy yourself, not kill yourself. Try to make progress in the amount of weight you lift, but remember that the most important thing is to **be consistent.** Listen to your body and keep the weights and pace within comfortable limits. Learn as much as you can about strength training and body building from your trainer and fitness magazines. And don't forget to always use good exercise form. You will progress if you just stick to it and don't overdo it.

For Better & Faster Results

Make sure you change your workout routine every 6 weeks. One way is by simply switching the order of what you do—if you usually do weights and then cardio, flip them. Or substitute new moves for old ones in your weight routine and try a brand new cardio activity or video program to challenge your muscles and force your body to work harder and avoid the dreaded plateau. When Tae-Bo and spinning started, people raved about their huge body changes. But it wasn't that these workouts were so much better than other kinds of exercise—it was just that people were using their bodies in a totally new way.

And finally, take a look at what you eat—your exercise efforts won't trim you down if you eat a high-fat, high-calorie diet. Adopting a healthy, nutritious plan will help you reach your weight-loss goal in record-breaking time.

Exercises You Can Do at Home/Hotel/Office That Really Work!

Arms

This is great for the triceps (the back of the arm) and will help make heads turn when you wear something sleeveless.

DIP: Sit on the very edge of a chair with arms straight, hands gripping the seat, knees bent, feet flat. Scoot your rear off the chair, and slowly lower your bottom until your arms are bent at a 90–degree angle. Raise yourself. Use your legs to make this easier, if you need to. The farther your feet are from the chair, the harder the exercise. Beginners, start with your feet under your knees. Intermediate and advanced, straighten out your legs when you do the dip.

ADVANCED DIP: Since one leg is off the floor on this one, the upper body has more weight to support. The longer you stretch the leg, the greater the effort. Sit on the floor with one knee bent at 90 degrees and one leg extended. Place hands behind you about a shoulder-width apart, palms down, and fingers facing your body. Keeping your bent leg still, use your arms to push the rest of your body off the floor until your elbows are slightly bent.

With your outstretched leg straight and parallel to the floor, slowly lower your body until your elbows are bent 90 degrees. Hold, then push back to the start position. Work up to 3 sets of 8 to 12 reps, alternating legs.

Chest & Shoulders

PUSH-AWAYS: Beginners can start with a push-away, from the wall. Start with your feet about 24 inches from the wall and with your hands flat on the wall. (To increase difficulty, move farther away.) Bend your elbows so your body falls toward the wall, then slowly straighten your arms, pushing your body away from the wall.

PUSH-UPS: As you get stronger, move on to these. Push-ups work out your arms, as well as your chest and shoulders. Get down on your hands and knees on the floor. Place your hands a little wider apart than shoulders, knees bent, and back flat, not arched. Keep arms bent slightly for starting position, never locked. Slowly lower yourself to the floor and then push back up. Moving hands closer together or farther apart works different muscles, so do a few sets and vary the hand position.

For a more advanced push-up, straighten your legs, and do the same movement as above, from your toes curled under rather than from your knees.

Very advanced: the higher your feet, the more of your body you're lifting with your arms and the more the push-up resembles a bench press with a barbell. So you can put your feet up on a chair and do the same movement of slowly lowering yourself to the ground and push back up.

CHAIR LIFT: This is great for your shoulders and arms. Sit back in a chair, your spine straight. Firmly grasp the ends of the chair's arms. Steadily lift yourself using your shoulders and arms. Assist as needed with your legs. Lower. Do 8 to 10 reps. Rest. Repeat for 3 sets.

Back

Here's a strengthening pose for your back. Kneeling on all fours, extend your right leg and left arm parallel to the floor. Hold for a breath, relax, then do the other side. Repeat 8 to 10 times on each side.

Legs & Butt

WALL SIT: Back up to a wall, your feet a shoulder-width apart and your heels 12 to 16 inches from the wall. Slowly slide down the wall until your legs are almost at a 90 degree angle. Hold for a breath, 4 to 8 seconds, then rise. Do this a few times until you are fatigued

KNEELING LEG CURL: This zeros in on the back of the thigh. Start on your elbows and knees, hands and forearms flat on the floor in front of you. Extend your left leg straight back, toe pointing down. Raise your left foot until your leg forms a 90 degree angle. Your neck should be still and shoulders relaxed. Hold for a breath, 4 to 8 seconds, then lower your foot. After a set of 8 to 10, switch legs.

For a more advanced move, place a 3- to 10-pound weight behind your knee. Hold the weight by squeezing calf to thigh. Lift your knee until your thigh is parallel to the floor, foot flexed. Lower to the floor. Do three sets of 10 with each leg. For another variation, in the lifted position, slightly pulse your thigh in an upward movement a few inches only, while tightening thigh and glutes.

HEEL RAISES: This one gets the calf area. Place your heels shoulder-width apart, toes pointed in. Slowly rise up on your toes, then lower. Then set your heels shoulder-width apart, this time pointing your toes out. Slowly lift heels, then lower.

PLIÉ: This is great for sculpting your thighs and butt and can be done anywhere. To make it harder, hold hand weight on your hips. Spread your feet wider than shoulders (a straddle position) to form a box when you lower your hips. Point toes to 10 and 2 o'clock and shift your body weight to heels. Keep a natural curve in your back by pushing your butt back. Lower your body, keeping knees behind toes. Straighten legs. Repeat until fatigued.

Form is very important here. Even a slight bend can strain your knees if your form is off. If you tilt your pelvis under, you'll increase pressure on both the lower back and knees. Standing with feet close enough that legs form a diamond adds to knee strain, so keep your feet much wider than shoulders.

PLIÉ PRESS: I love this one because it works shoulders, upper back, upper arms, and legs. Stand with your legs in a straddle position with your feet wider than shoulders, toes turned out slightly. Hold hand weights with your elbows at shoulder level and bend to 90 degrees, hand above elbows, palms facing forward. As you exhale, push the weights overhead and simultaneously bend knees and lower hips. Hold a few seconds and return arms to starting position as you straighten legs to stand. Repeat until you get fatigued.

SIDE LEG LIFT: Lie on left side, head resting on your left arm. Bend both knees, positioning them slightly in front of your body. Roll the pelvis forward so hips are stacked. Use an ankle weight or hold a dumbbell on your outer thigh. With foot and knee facing forward, squeeze your glutes (tighten your buttock muscles as though you're holding a coin between then) and raise your right leg sideways as high as you can. Hold, then lower. Repeat several times; then switch sides.

Don't prop your head up in your hand as that can put undue stress on your neck and your wrist. And if you rotate your leg out so that your knee faces up as you lift (rather than facing forward) you'll target the hip flexors instead of the glutes. So practice good form. Tighten your glutes during the entire lifting and lowering phase to increase intensity.

SQUATS: There's no better home exercise for your lower body. Because we're working the biggest muscles here, the buttocks and thighs, you're going to get the same wonderful metabolic aftereffect of weightlifting. If you do them properly, ***in only 3 weeks of daily practice, you'll see a positive difference in your lower body.*** And in 6 weeks, watch out! If you're not using weight, you can do them daily to speed up progress. If you're using weight, especially a heavy weight, do these only on alternate days, 3 to 4 times a week.

Beginners should use a chair for this. Stand about a foot in front of the chair, your back to the chair. Squat in such a way that your butt sticks out and you almost tip over backward. Lower yourself until your glutes just barely touch the chair, then stand up again. Don't let your knees extend in front of your feet. Your knees down to your feet will stay straight up and down. In other words, your knees should be in line with your toes, keeping lower legs vertical. Okay, I know, it's funny looking, but it sure strengthens the lower body. Do several reps. Rest, then repeat. For balance, you might want to reach hands out in front of you. As you feel more confident, do these without a chair.

As you get stronger, add some weight. I usually add a bar on top of my shoulders, behind my head, held in place with my hands. The extra weight makes these squats very effective. Go slowly and *SQUEEZE* your glutes as you move.

SINGLE LEG SQUAT: These are more advanced. Stand with feet at shoulder-width, toes pointed forward. Shift your body weight to the right heel, propping up your left toes to balance. Tighten abs and lean slightly forward. Lower hips until right thigh and calf form a 90-degree angle, your right calf nearly perpendicular to the floor. Squeeze glutes and hamstrings to straighten right leg and stand, then repeat. Switch sides. Repeat until fatigued.

To maximize slouch, I usually interlace my fingers behind my head, open my elbows wide, and press my chest forward. Don't place your hands on your thighs for balance because this shifts your weight forward. Keep your weight shifted back. Letting your body weight shift forward when squatting can stress knee and cause upper body slump, straining the low back. Try this test: If you *can* lift the heel and *can't* wiggle the toes of your supporting leg when squatting, your weight is in your toes.

I urge you to develop a well-rounded fitness program that includes aerobics, strength training, and stretching. This trio (cardio, weight lifting, and flexibility training) will reduce bone loss; accelerate fat loss by increasing fat-burning enzymes, lean muscle, and strength; and keep your energy levels revved. As we age, we lose muscle, strength, bone density, and energy. Exercise is the only way to counteract this trend. Remember these three points: move, lengthen, and strengthen and make your exercise program a top priority in your life.

SUCCESS

Chapter 5

ENHANCE YOUR METABOLISM

Regardless of our body size, self-respect and self-acceptance are the starting points for making peace with our size.
We must know that we have the power to get off the weight treadmill and start enjoying our life, no matter where we are.
—Christiane Northrup, M.D.

In this chapter, we'll look at ways to supertune your metabolism, because you can change your body chemistry to burn more calories more efficiently so you can eat more without worrying about gaining fat. Let's begin with looking at the difference between **overweight** and **overfat** and how extra fat wreaks havoc on all systems in the body.

While millions of people starve to death in many parts of the world, the United States has the dubious honor of being the fattest country on the globe, with 50% of us being obese. Meanwhile, Americans are preoccupied with their waistlines. We spend more than 40 billion dollars a year on diet foods, diet programs, diet pills, and other 'guaranteed' weight-loss regimens and products. Yet according to the National Center of Health Statistics, we're getting fatter all the time.

These unhealthy numbers show no sign of going down. Experts call obesity an American epidemic—one that brings with it major health problems. Heart disease, endometrial (uterine) cancer and possibly breast cancer, high cholesterol, high blood pressure, immune dysfunction, osteoarthritis, stroke, gout, sleep disorders, gallstones, and diabetes are all associated with obesity. Put in a more positive way, *losing even a little weight may significantly*

improve your health and well being. Even if you're only interested in losing 10 or 20 pounds to look better, you'll also benefit in
many other ways.

On the flipside, eating disorders such as anorexia and bulimia are
on the rise, and women's magazines are not helping when they continue to use models who look like waifs. Take Barbie™, a doll that's
part of most little girls' upbringing. This model of good looks and
perfect body is giving the wrong message about what a healthy
woman's body should look like. Were Barbie an actual person, her
body fat would be so low that she probably wouldn't even be able to
menstruate. As little girls treasure Barbie, and teens try to emulate
her, she has one accessory that is consistently missing—food.

Your body has an unlimited capacity for storing fat. Fortunately, it
also has ample capacity to use and reduce it. So how do you know
what's an ideal weight for you?

Until recently, we have usually referred to height and weight tables
provided by Metropolitan Life Insurance Company (MetLife). Yet,
according to Dr. William P. Castelli, medical director of the famed
Framingham Heart Study, these MetLife tables, which were revised
recently to allow for more weight, have become too lenient. In fact, the
American Heart Association has urged people to ignore those guidelines. According to the current MetLife tables, 155 pounds is within
the desirable weight range for a 5'5" woman. That may be fine for a
female bodybuilder with lots of lean muscle tissue, but it's too high for
a normal non-bodybuilder female. These MetLife tables are based on
death rates and vital statistics from millions of insurance holders in
the United States. They don't account for the fact that many thin people with high death rates are cigarette smokers or otherwise ill. If
those people had been eliminated from the current tabulations, says
Dr. Castelli, the desirable weights would be lower. Dr. Castelli and
other experts are exploring better ways to evaluate optimal body
weight based on the latest research on weight-related health risks.

What Your Shape Says About Health Risks

Two approaches, when used together, are emerging as the new 'gold
standard' for weight: Body Mass Index and Waist/Hip Ratio.

Body Mass Index (BMI) is a ratio of height to weight. It's determined by a mathematical formula: first divide your weight (in pounds) by your height (in inches) squared, then multiply the resulting number by 705. You should get a BMI that's somewhere between 10 and 30. For example, let's say you weigh 140 pounds and you are 5'8" tall. You would first figure out your height (68") squared which is 4624. Then take your weight (140) and divide it by 4624, which gives you .030. Multiply this number by 705 and you get 21.

Calculating Body Mass Index (BMI)

HEIGHT   BODY WEIGHT IN POUNDS

Height												
4'10"	91	96	100	105	110	115	119	124	129	134	138	143
4'11"	94	99	104	109	114	119	124	128	133	138	143	148
5'0"	97	102	107	112	118	123	128	133	138	143	148	153
5'1"	100	106	111	116	122	127	132	137	143	148	153	158
5'2"	104	109	115	120	126	131	136	142	147	153	158	164
5'3"	107	113	118	124	130	135	141	146	152	158	163	169
5'4"	110	116	122	128	134	140	145	151	157	163	169	174
5'5"	114	120	126	132	138	144	150	156	162	168	174	180
5'6"	118	124	130	136	142	148	155	161	167	173	179	186
5'7"	121	127	134	140	146	153	159	166	172	178	185	191
5'8"	125	131	138	144	151	158	164	171	177	184	190	197
5'9"	128	135	142	149	155	162	169	176	182	189	196	203
5'10"	132	139	146	153	160	167	174	181	188	195	202	207
5'11"	136	143	150	157	165	172	179	186	193	200	208	215
6'0"	140	147	154	162	169	177	184	191	199	206	213	221
BMI	**19**	**20**	**21**	**22**	**23**	**24**	**25**	**26**	**27**	**28**	**29**	**30**

To find your BMI, locate your height in the left column. (If you've lost inches over the years, use your peak adult height.) Move across the chart (to the right) until you hit your approximate weight, then follow that column down to the corresponding BMI number at the bottom of the chart.

Numerous studies have already been conducted to validate the efficacy of the BMI and weight-related health risks. The conclusion is that 21 to 22 is the optimal body mass index because there are no weight-related health risks at this level.

One large-scale study indicated that a BMI below 22 is ideal for preventing heart disease in women. This Nurses' Health Study, co-directed by Dr. JoAnn E. Manson and conducted at Brigham and Women's Hospital and Harvard Hospital in Boston, followed 115,886 initially healthy American women ages 30 to 55 for 8 years. During that time, 605 of the women experienced coronary-artery disease, of whom 83 died. There was no elevated risk of heart disease among women whose BMI's were under 21; the risk was 30% higher than that of the lean group for women whose BMI was between 21 and 25, 80% higher for a BMI 25 to 29, and 230% higher than the lean group for those with a BMI greater than 29. The researchers concluded that "obesity is a strong risk factor for coronary heart disease in middle-age women." They reported in the March 1990 issue of the *New England Journal of Medicine* that "even mild-to-moderate overweight is associated with substantial elevation in coronary risk."

There's no consensus yet among the experts on how much is too much. Some insist that although a BMI between 23 and 25 isn't ideal, the excess risk for cancer and other weight-related diseases seems to be small. At around 26, these health risks appear to rise, although it's not quite clear to scientists where to draw the line. Jean Pierre Despres, Ph.D., associate director of the Lipid Research Center at Laval University in St. Foy, Quebec, says that between 25 and 27 is a gray zone. "A lot of people in this range are perfectly healthy, but others have a substantially higher risk of developing diabetes and premature coronary disease." Most scientists do agree that a BMI over 27 increases risk for many people. But their risk also depends on other factors, including their waist/hip measurement, notes Dr. Despres.

Although less common than overweight in the United States, excessive thinness can also be a problem. It is linked with osteoporosis and other health problems, even early death, especially if weight loss is sudden. The experts feel that someone with a BMI under 19 should be evaluated. "That doesn't mean everyone low is going to be unhealthy, but it's worth taking a closer look," says James O. Hill, Ph.D., associate director of the Center for Human Nutrition at the University of Colorado Health Sciences Center.

In addition to knowing your BMI number, it's equally important to be aware of your Waist/Hip Ratio (WHR). You get this number by measuring your waist (at the midpoint between your bottom rib and hip bone) and your hips (at their widest point). Then divide the waist measurement by the hip measurement. For example, if your waist is 29 inches and your hips measure 39 inches, then your WHR is 0.76.

Why is this ratio important? In the last few years, researchers have determined that the fat most associated with health risks is on the upper body—the abdomen and above, rather than the thighs and hips. (This pattern of upper-body fat is often called 'central obesity.') "Central obesity is turning out to be the most lethal risk factor associated with excess body weight," says Dr. Castelli. That's because upper-body fat is strongly correlated with visceral fat, which is fat that is packed around the internal organs.

The WHR, though not perfect (it isn't very reliable for women who are very thin, very overweight, or for bodybuilders), can in most cases be used to predict cardiovascular disease risk, especially in women. Researchers at the University of Miami School of Medicine and the University of Minnesota School of Public Health examined data on 32,898 healthy women ages 55 to 69. As reported in the January 1998 issue of *Annals of Epidemiology*, there were nearly 3 times as many heart-disease deaths in a 4-year period among women with the greatest waist/hip ratio (0.86 and over) than those under .80. A high waist-to-hip ratio has also been associated with diabetes, hypertension, stroke, breast and endometial (uterine) cancers, and high cholesterol.

If the ideal BMI is around 21 or 22, let's see what the experts say about the ideal WHR. Most would target 0.80 as desirable. If you're a woman, a number greater than 0.85 indicates higher health risks. If you're a man, health risks are related to a ratio greater than 1.0. Dr. Castelli believes that the WHR measurement is even more important than BMI in predicting risk. "If someone has a healthy BMI but a high WHR, it is important to try to bring that WHR down," he explains. "Someone with a higher BMI but a low WHR might not be quite as bad off."

There's another point to consider. Are you overweight or overfat? Weight tables can classify you as overweight when you actually have average or below average body fat. Athletes are often overweight because of a large frame or muscle development, but they aren't overfat.

Obesity means an excess accumulation of body fat. Usually, obesity and overweight are related. If you're 25 pounds or more overweight by most weight charts, you're probably overfat. At this point, the health risks of obesity surface. And when you are 25 pounds overweight, your heart must pump blood through nearly 5,000 extra miles of blood vessels each day.

So how do you know if you're overweight or overfat? First of all, the term "overweight" is obsolete. Fat can be hidden inside of the body in such a way that you can carry a lot of excess fat without seeming overweight. And I've worked with people who have this ideal number they want to be, weight-wise, on the scale, without realizing that they're supposed to weigh more naturally because they have big bones and/or big muscles. An easy way to judge whether you're overfat is by looking in a mirror. This, along with percentage of body fat, are what I use with my clients to help determine how much fat loss they need to make to create radiant health. If, despite good BMI and WHR numbers, you look flabby in the mirror, you probably are. You'd do well to measure your body fat and to embark on an exercise regimen that burns fat and tones muscles.

Most of us know our blood pressure and cholesterol numbers but few of us know our percentage of body fat. But, in my estimation, it's equally important and simple to monitor. Higher than the average ideal suggests that fat is slowly settling into arteries and putting you at a great risk for future heart attacks, strokes, kidney disease, etc. Fitness expert Covert Bailey, author of *The Ultimate Fit or Fat*, recommends that premenopausal women shoot for no more than 22% fat. If a woman's fat percentage gets a little higher than this, say 26%, she's probably still quite active and living a good life, but she'll have to struggle to keep from gaining weight, being at risk for heart disease, diabetes, and other fat-related problems.

It is true that women have a harder time than men losing weight. The female hormone estrogen increases body fat especially if progesterone is low, and after having a baby, it's even harder for a woman to lose weight. Combined with having less muscle than men on average means a lower capacity to burn fat. Birth control pills raise the fat percentage somewhat, and hormone replacement therapy (for menopausal symptoms) seems to raise it even more, so shoot for about 25% fat if you're in that category.

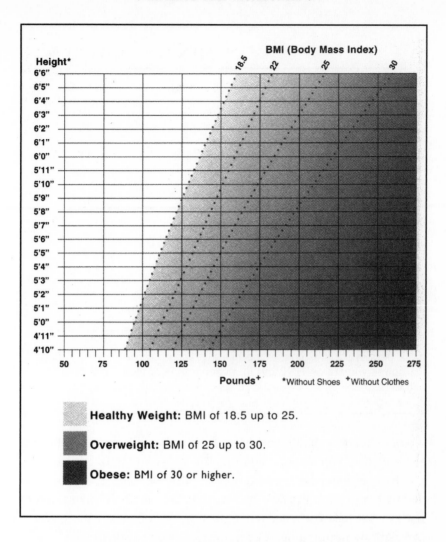

BMI (Body Mass Index)

Healthy Weight: BMI of 18.5 up to 25.

Overweight: BMI of 25 up to 30.

Obese: BMI of 30 or higher.

Men should try to keep their body fat to 15% or less. These numbers of 15% and 22%, while not carved in stone, give you a number to shoot for, like you do with blood pressure 120/80 or cholesterol below 180. Of the thousands of people measured by Covert Bailey and his staff, the average man is 22% fat and the average woman is 32% fat. For comparison, consider the following from Bailey's studies.

There are several ways to determine your body fat. You can get calipers that pinch skin fold or use a special fat monitor/scale. You can use a bioelectric impedance test (running a mild current through the body to measure resistance) or do underwater weighing, which

	MEN %	WOMEN %
Top Athletes	2 to 12	10 to 18
Gymnasts	5	10
Rock Climbers	5	10
Runners	7	14
Body Builders	10	16
Aerobic Dance Instructors	12	18
Cyclists	13	20
Swimmers	14	22
Healthy*	15 max.	22 max.
Average	22	32

* The percentages, 15% for men and 22% for women, are the highest a person should have to be healthy, according to Covert Bailey, unless you are on HRT and in menopause, and then it can be up to 5% higher.

are not widely available and are not always reliable. In fact, all methods only give you a ballpark figure. The older and fatter you are, the less reliable the measurement may be. The method I use personally and with my clients is a fat monitor scale. You stand on it like a weight scale and it tells you your percentage of fat. Whatever method you pick, stick with the same one for a period of a year or so.

I'm often asked if I've thrown away my regular weight scale since it doesn't weigh fat. I use mine to see if I'm a pound or two higher or lower than normal. If I am, I consider my fluid intake, my fatigue, or stress levels, or how much sodium I've eaten. If you've been losing weight consistently without trying, then I'd be concerned about bone loss. So keep your weight scale and use it every so often, but go more by your percentage of fat for a more accurate reading on your health.

Obesity in infancy and childhood can lead to a life battling the bulge. During the first few years of life, new fat cells form rapidly. As the rate of fat storage increases, so does the number of fat cells. In obese children, the number of fat cells is often 3 times that in normal-weight children. As a result, overfeeding children, especially in infancy, can lead to a lifetime of obesity. After adolescence the number of fat cells remains almost constant throughout the rest of life, unless you gain excessive weight.

Although the extra pounds and less than ideal BMI and WHR numbers could be explained by exercise-induced muscle (which, inch for inch, weighs more than fat), unless you're an avid fitness enthusiast or athlete, it's not likely. This culture is still geared toward overeating. If you don't want your eating habits to get the best of you, you should consider raising your basal metabolic rate.

Metabolism & Ways to Increase It

Statistics reveal that most people are not happy with their weight or the shape of their body. Half of the women and a quarter of the men in this country are currently trying to lose weight and reshape their bodies. The sad thing is that a majority of these people are going about it in the wrong way, the hard way—by dieting, which doesn't work! Throw away diet books that tell you that you can lose weight and keep it off without moving a muscle. They're rip-offs. Dieting is not the cure for excess fat. ***After you finish a diet, you may have lost some fat, but you haven't lost your tendency to get fat.*** Rather than constantly worrying about how to lose weight, fat people should ask themselves, "Why do I gain weight so easily?"

The control mechanism for obesity is not diet, it's muscle metabolism. Your basal metabolic rate is the rate at which your body utilizes energy. Put another way, it has to do with how efficiently your body burns calories. Calories are the measuring unit of heat energy. When your metabolism is higher, you burn more fat and have an easier time losing weight (fat) or maintaining your ideal body weight. You can feed your muscles the best food and vitamin supplements in the world, but if they're not tuned up—if they're not exercised—they won't burn up the calories in those foods. As you age, if you don't continue to keep your muscles exercised, your metabolism slows down and you'll gain weight more easily than you did when you were young. If you try to lose weight on a diet, you aren't fixing the slow metabolism that makes you quickly gain weight again. The major ultimate control of metabolism is exercise along with a few minor things you can do to make a big difference.

Statistics reveal that two out of three people who go on a diet will regain their weight in one year or less; 97% will gain the weight back in five years. To make matters worse, a majority of dieters who lose weight will gain back even more fat than they had before they started the diet. They have all violated an important rule in creating and maintaining a healthy, fast metabolism: They lost lean body mass, or muscle. A fat person needs to retrain his or her body so that it burns up ALL the calories it gets, storing none as fat. Yes, she may need a diet at the start to help break bad eating habits, retrain her taste buds, jump-start her metabolism, and lose some excess fat, especially as a motivator. That's one of the reasons I've offered the 3- and 7-Day Rejuvenation Retreats at the end of this book. **But long-term weight control requires a change in body chemistry so you won't get fat all over again. And EXERCISE is the only way to change your metabolism so that your body converts fewer calories to fat.** You need aerobic exercise to burn the fat out of your muscles and then add weight lifting to build up your muscle which, in turn, increases metabolism.

In my workshops around the country, people tell me they get plenty of exercise doing household chores or walking around at work. I emphatically tell them that it's not enough! You need intentional exercise, like fitness walking and lifting weights or hiking, to call yourself anything but sedentary.

Adults who are not active with regular exercise lose about 1% of their muscle every year after about age forty. At the same time, many of those people gain about a pound of fat a year. But the slide to fat really doesn't have to happen if you participate in appropriate physical activity programs that include both aerobic and some strength-training (lifting weights) exercise, and if you select the healthiest foods.

So let's go over some tips for increasing your metabolism, selecting the right exercise and foods, and making healthy choices for creating a fit, lean body. I call this my Aliveness Program. I've used it for over 25 years in my workshops, counseling, and trainings, and it works.

14 Steps to a Fit, Lean Body

1. Increase your muscle mass.

2. Increase your aerobic exercise.

3. Break up your exercise into manageable parts.

4. Add higher intensity bursts to your exercise plan.

5. Graze.

6. Choose whole foods.

7. Eat good fats.

8. Cut your alcohol consumption.

9. Drink at least two quarts of water a day.

10. Start weight lifting.

11. Use common sense for lasting results and success.

12. Be sure your hormones are in balance.

13. Get some sun.

14. Nourish your spirit.

1. Increase your muscle mass. Muscle burns fat. It's that simple. Exercise increases muscle, tones it, alters its chemistry and increases the metabolic rate. When you exercise you actually continue to burn calories even when you're sleeping but you must exercise correctly to get the best results. Before I describe the best exercises to lose fat, burn calories, and increase metabolism, let's briefly explore why lean muscle tissue is so important.

More muscle means a faster metabolism because muscle uses more energy to exist than fat. Because muscle is a highly metabolic tissue, it burns five times as many calories as most other body tissues, pound for pound. In other words, muscle requires more oxygen and more calories to sustain itself than does body fat. When you have more muscle mass, you burn more calories than someone who doesn't, even when you're both sitting still, which is why people who build muscle have an easier time maintaining a healthy weight. They're simply more efficient calorie burners.

Many men can eat more than women without gaining weight because men have more muscle and less fat than women and they don't have the higher estrogen levels that promote fat deposition. Because men have more muscle, they burn 10% to 20% more calories than women at rest.

If you increase muscle mass, you increase the number of calories your body is using every moment of the day, not just during exercise, but also at work, play, and even when sleeping. The addition of 10 pounds of muscle to your body will burn approximately 600 extra calories per day. You would have to run 6 miles a day, 7 days a week to burn the same number of calories. Ten extra pounds of muscle can burn a pound of fat in one week—that's 52 pounds of fat a year.

To increase muscle, you must engage in weight lifting. Please don't skip this if you've never lifted weights before. It can really be fun and you don't necessarily have to go to some intimidating gym to do it. You can lift weights at home (see Chapter 4 for my recommendations). Actually it's not the weight lifting itself, but the physiological effects that take place in the 48 hours AFTER weight lifting during the recovery period, that enhance metabolism. In other words, very little fat is burned during the weight lifting session. But LOTS of fat is burned during the *recovery* from weight lifting.

Weight lifting is not aerobic because the oxygen demand is simply too intense. But lifting weights strengthens your muscles so you can perform your aerobic exercise (such as jogging or hiking) more intensely without becoming anaerobic. When your muscles get stronger through anaerobic weight lifting, it enables you to burn more fat during your aerobic exercise (brisk walking) because you don't get out of breath so quickly.

And now the key reason to lift weights. The recovery phase, the 48 hours after your weight lifting session, has a profound impact on fat burning enzymes. After you've finished your weight training session and you shower, maybe sauna, and are feeling refreshed and relaxed, your fat-burning enzymes are working harder than ever to repair the damage. They must replace the sugar that was used by the sugar-burning enzymes. To build up the sugar supplies (glycogen is stored muscle sugar that's used up during weight lifting), our bodies burn fat. It takes a lot of energy to restore sugar, which means that lots of calories are burned. ALL of this energy must be supplied by the fat-burning enzymes. That's why you *must* make weight lifting a part of your fat loss/vitality program. Let me say this one more way: **Weight lifting stimulates metabolism and fat-burning.**

The best way to increase lean muscle mass is through resistance training, which means weight lifting or resistance machines—barbells, dumbbells or machines, cables, or even 'free-hand' movements such as push-ups, sit-ups (crunches), and dips. All it takes to add 10 pounds of muscle is a regular weight training program involving only 30 to 40 minutes, 3 times a week for about six months. Isn't that fantastic! The wonderful thing about increasing your metabolism through increasing your muscle mass is that you don't have to restrict your caloric intake.

2. Increase your aerobic exercise. Aerobic exercise trains muscles to burn fat and increase metabolism. Aerobic exercise means exercising with oxygen, not being winded or out of breath. These types of exercises, which are fairly gentle and nonstop, change your metabolism and also train your muscles to burn more fat. Here's a key point to keep in mind. **Muscles burn fat ONLY in the presence of oxygen.** For example, if you're jogging with your husband and he's breezing along and singing a song, and you're so out of breath that you can barely put two syllables together, he's burning fat but your fat-burning mechanisms have shut down. Muscles burn two kinds of fuel—sugar (glucose) and fat. Your muscles really do prefer to burn fat because it's a more efficient burning system; there's more of it so it lasts a long time and it produces lots of energy, but oxygen must be present to burn fat.

Does that mean you shouldn't do high-intensity sprints every so often? No, as I'll explain shortly, but you must make aerobic exercise part of your fitness program at least 5 days a week if you want to lose fat and tone up. By using the big muscles of the thighs and buttocks in an activity that is steady and nonstop (such as jogging, hiking, walking, cross-country skiing, bicycling or rowing), and makes you breathe deeply but doesn't make you out of breath, you're supplying oxygen to the muscles, which promotes fat burning in the muscles and makes you burn more food calories.

Let's put this another way. While the best exercise for permanent fat loss is weight lifting because it increases muscle, which burns more calories, low intensity aerobic exercise such as walking is also an excellent way to burn fat efficiently. Cutting 250 calories from your daily diet can help you lose half a pound a week (3,500 calories equals one pound of fat). But add a 30-minute walk 4 days a week, and you can double your rate of weight loss.

Frankly I'd like to suggest that you get out of the habit of thinking which activity burns the most calories in an hour because that's not really what's important. It's much better to find aerobic activities you'll continue on a regular basis because they increase your metabolic rate for hours AFTER exercising.

In a study conducted at the Cooper Aerobic Center, Dr. John Duncan took 102 sedentary women and divided them into 3 groups. Each group walked 3 miles, 5 days a week for 6 months. The first group walked 5 mph, the second group 4 mph, and the third group 3 mph. He found that the slowest group lost the most weight. Any aerobic exercise that raises heart rate above 80% of maximum (220 minus your age times 0.8) will cause you to burn more sugar and less fat. An exercise heart rate kept closer to 60% of maximum (220 minus your age times 0.6), or 108 beats per minute for a 40-year-old person, will burn mostly fat. This is why walking is superior to overzealous running as a fat-burning exercise. Walking is one of the most underrated exercises. The risk of injury is lower than for many other exercises, it's inexpensive, and you can do it just about anywhere. All you need is a good pair of walking shoes.

As you get in better and better shape, which means you can exercise harder without getting out of breath, you'll burn MORE fat. And, most importantly, as you get into better shape by exercising often, you'll be making more fat-burning enzymes, which means that you are slowly changing your body into a fat-burning machine.

What follows are some the best aerobic activities. For your aerobic exercise, I encourage you to get outdoors as much as possible and not get into a rut of only going to your gym.

Machines: treadmill, stair climber, elliptical machine, aerobic rider, X-ISER, step/ladder climber, rowing machine, mini-trampoline, stationary bicycle, and cross-country machine.

Aerobic exercises: hiking, rowing, walking, jogging/running, mountain biking, race walking, bicycling, water aerobics, jumping rope, aerobic classes such as Tae-Bo and Step, cross-country skiing and swimming. (Swimming helps your overall fitness but is poor for losing fat, because in water the body wants to keep its fat. If you love swimming, add it to other aerobic activities.)

In other words, for a rapid fat loss, select weight-bearing and/or whole-body exercises such as hiking, walking, aerobic dance, jogging, rowing, treadmill, cross-country skiing, etc. Swimming, water aerobics, and stationary bicycle, while not conducive to rapid fat loss, are still excellent for overall fitness. Combine indoor and outdoor activities so that you have no excuse to avoid exercise on bad-weather days. And remember, moving your weight around from one spot to another burns fat more quickly than staying in one place sitting on a bicycle, jumping rope, or bouncing on a trampoline.

If fat loss is your goal, make sure to include aerobic activity at least 3 to 4 days a week and weight lifting 2 to 3 days a week until you reach your goal. Non-aerobic exercises—horseback riding, golf, basketball, ice skating, football, soccer, racquetball, baseball, tennis, windsurfing, dancing, field/ice hockey, downhill skiing, in-line skating, water skiing, most yoga, gymnastics, and motorcycle riding—can still be done and, in fact, I encourage you to be as active as possible with all types of activity. You'll get a little aerobic benefit and much enjoyment. The stop-and-go movement in some of these activities helps your proprioception, which is your 'sense of body position' that we tend to lose as we get older if we don't stay active.

3. Break up your exercise. The news from the American College of Sports Medicine and the U.S. Centers for Disease Control and Prevention is that exercise need not necessarily occur in one continuous session (unless you have lots of extra fat to lose, or desire a more rapid fat loss, which might make exercising longer more effective.) The daily training can be broken up—with equivalent fitness benefits—into segments. For example, in lieu of spending one hour doing aerobics at the gym in either a class or on the aerobic equipment, you can take a 15-minute walk in the morning, walk up and down the stairs during the day instead of taking the elevator, take another 15-minute walking during your lunch hour and finish up with a 20-minute walk after dinner. I will say, based on working as a trainer with hundreds of people, that this way of getting in workouts is not quite as effective for rapid fat loss as the higher intensity sessions described below. But it's still a way to get in your workouts, especially when you have a very busy day and can't spare a full hour for exercise.

The key here is to MOVE, MOVE, MOVE. Successful weight control is all about becoming more active. If you're not working out regularly, aim for at least 30 to 40 minutes of unstructured activity every day.

4. Add higher intensity bursts to your exercise plan. I will often work in some high-intensity activity a few times each week. For example, if I'm hiking, I'll spend 30 to 90 seconds going faster than normal on a steeper hill interspersed with more level or declining grades a few times during the workout. (Notice I didn't say "a break-neck run." Just go a little faster than usual.) If you're cycling, pedal faster for several seconds. High intensity bursts of exercise help burn fat. Why? When you force your body to raise the level of intensity for a short burst of "getting winded," you are forcing your body to recover under stress; in other words, while you continue to exercise. This little sprint adds intensity without causing injury. And those fat-burning enzymes are realizing that not only do they need to grow when you're doing regular aerobic activity, but now they must grow even faster. In other words, **a few moments of exercising just a little bit harder than usual will help force you to recover while still exercising, which will burn more fat.** If you're just a beginner and have never exercised before, wait for about one month before adding in these bursts of higher intensity workout.

Case in point: Seventeen exercisers on stationary bikes followed a moderate-exercise training program (30 to 45 minutes, 4 to 5 times per week for 20 weeks). All burned about 300 to 400 calories per session. Ten other exercisers did only about one-third as many sessions of 30-minute bike riding over 15 weeks. They filled the other sessions with short bursts of high-intensity cycling for 30 to 90 seconds and repeated these bursts several times per exercise session. These folks used only about 225 to 250 calories per session, but they lost more fat (according to skin-fold measurements) than did the moderate exercisers (who technically burned more calories). When expressed as calories expended during exercise, their fat loss was 9 times greater than that in subjects performing lower intensity exercise. Muscle biopsies confirmed that the important step of fat oxidation occurred in the cells of the high-intensity exercisers to a greater degree than in the low-intensity exercisers (as reported in the journal *Metabolism*, July 1994).

It seems to be a paradox that less exercise time could result in more fat burning. Standard thinking says that high-intensity exercise burns the available carbohydrates (sugar) as the fuel source before it digs into fat. Researchers think that what happens here may have to do with two things that happen between and after exercise. First, intermittent high-intensity exercise may encourage a higher rate of fuel burning during the recovery periods AND after exercise—and that fuel may come from fat. And second, high-intensity exercise may have an anorectic effect—that is, you may feel more satisfied with fewer calories (and fewer fat calories) in what you eat for a while after your workout.

The high-intensity exercise levels in the above study were equivalent to sprinting. What I recommend is that you go just a little higher intensity than you're used to. Going all out—breakneck sprint—can be done but isn't for everyone, says study leader Angelo Tremblay, Ph.D., professor of physiology and nutrition at Laval University, Quebec. "Something comparable might be vigorous circuit training. Or it could be reasonable—if you are healthy and accustomed to performing vigorous exercises—to briefly increase walking to a level where speaking is not possible. You can do that for 60 to 90 seconds, 3 to 5 times during a walk." Later, he says, you can increase the number of high intensity bouts. Of course, even if this is confirmed in other studies, it's not an excuse to cut your exercise time. Even trained athletes can't sustain day-in/day-out workouts at super-high intensities.

Endurance exercise may have benefits we're just beginning to tap. Another study, for instance, found that 35 to 45 minutes of endurance exercise 3 times a week reduced insulin levels in the blood of 70- to 79-year-old men and women.

So pump up the intensity if your doctor says you can. Just find a way to fit that extra vigor into your regular workout program.

5. *Graze.* Liquid meals, diet pills, and special diet packaged food aren't your answers to increasing metabolism, weight control, or better health. Instead, and in addition to regular exercise, learn how to eat so that your body becomes an efficient fat-burning machine.

The results of four national surveys show that most people try to lose weight by eating 1,000 to 1,500 calories a day. However, cutting calories to under 1,200 (if you're a woman) or 1,400 (if you're a man) doesn't provide enough food to be satisfying in the long term. Eating fewer than 1,200 calories makes it difficult to get adequate amounts of certain nutrients, such as folic acid, magnesium, and zinc. It also promotes temporary loss of fluids rather than permanent loss of fat.

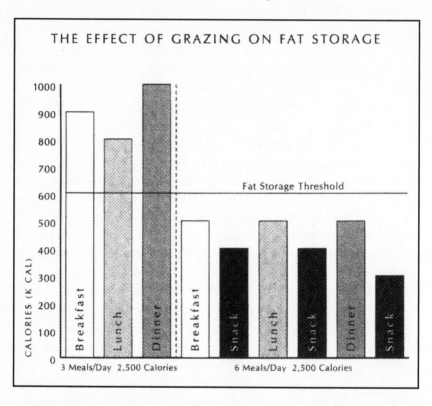

The typical dieter will often skip meals and, as research points out, *the worst meal to skip, if you want to increase your metabolism, is breakfast*. This temporary fasting state sends a signal to the body that food is scarce. As a result, the stress hormones (including cortisol) increase and the body begins 'lightening the load' and shedding its muscle tissue. Decreasing muscle tissue, as you know now, is very metabolically active, and decreases the body's need for food. By the next feeding, the pancreas is sensitized and will sharply increase blood insulin levels, which is the body's signal to make fat. And if you're insulin resistant, as many sedentary people are, you make extra amounts of this hormone (insulin) and make/deposit fat very easily, especially if you eat refined carbohydrates. Have you ever wondered how the Sumo wrestlers get so big! They fast and then gorge themselves with food. As you can see, this approach is absolutely counterproductive if your goal is to lose fat.

If you want to increase your metabolism, it's best to eat several small healthy meals a day (see the chart above). This kind of grazing approach to meals keeps your metabolism stoked. It also keeps you from feeling deprived—one of the chief complaints of everyone who has ever been on a diet.

Because undereating can actually have the effect of slowing your metabolism, you want to be sure you're getting *enough* calories. You should be eating at least 10 calories per pound of your ideal body weight, so if you are aiming for a weight of 150 pounds, your daily menu should contain at least 1,500 calories.

If this information is not enough to motivate you to eat smaller meals (with the exception of salads with lots of leafy greens), maybe the following will be food for thought. One of the best things you can do to retard the aging process is simply to eat smaller amounts of the highest quality foods available. In a landmark 1982 study published in *Science*, Richard Weindruch, Ph.D., and Roy L. Walfor, M.D. (author of *Maximum Life Span* and *Anti-Aging Plan*), reported that when the food of 'middle-aged' mice was gradually restricted over a 1-month period and then kept at that level, they lived an average of 10% longer than the control group. They also had fewer spontaneous cancers than the control mice. Their conclusion and recommendation is to strive for "undernutrition without malnutrition." In other words, limit caloric intake while providing adequate amounts of all the necessary nutrients. It's not absolutely clear how dietary restriction slows down the aging process, but evidence points to its retarding the age-related decline in immune function.

When you eat the diet recommended in this book, with emphasis on plant-based foods, you get all the nutrients your body needs without an overconsumption of food and calories, and if you eat several small meals per day based on my recommendations, you prime your body to burn fat and slow the aging process. This approach to eating results in success.

6. *Choose whole foods.* In the 80s, I had a wonderful opportunity to work as the consultant for the Los Angeles City Fire Department. For 30 weeks I worked with the first group of women recruits. In the areas of motivation, holistic health, and particularly nutrition, I saw many of the concepts and principles discussed in this book come alive.

One female recruit liked a big breakfast, high in animal protein and fat, typically consisting of two eggs, sausage or bacon, toast with butter and jam, milk, and coffee with cream and sugar. Although she didn't have a weight problem, by midmorning she was often tired and had difficulty in the endurance and strength aspects of her training. She also complained of an inability to think clearly for more than short periods. Within 2 weeks of changing her breakfast to more healthy, energy-promoting foods, she experienced an abundance of energy and increased mental clarity, important for participation in the rigorous training program. Her new breakfast typically included fresh fruit and freshly squeezed juice, whole grain cereal like oatmeal or millet, and herb tea.

Another woman ate too many dairy products—lots of cheese, milk, butter, sour cream, cottage cheese, and ice cream. The rest of her diet was healthy, with lots of fresh fruits and vegetables, whole grains, beans, a few seeds and nuts, some broiled fish, and lots of water. When she cut down on her dairy intake, using nondairy substitutes (soymilk products instead of cow's milk), she experienced a noticeable increase in energy. As soon as the third day on her new nutrition program, she was able to perform the endurance events, which included running, continuous stair climbing, and the fire hose pull, more easily.

If you change what you eat, you don't have to be as concerned with how much you eat. By doing this, you can eat whenever you're hungry until you feel satisfied. You'll lose weight without hunger or deprivation and you won't need to count calories. You need information, not willpower.

The healthiest foods are the plant-based foods described in Chapter 3 and used in all my recipes (see Chapters 8 through 18). They are lower in fat than most animal products, are faster burning, and are rich in vitamins and minerals. They are also high in fiber, which means you can feel full on fewer calories. Plant-based foods are nutrient-dense, meaning they offer an abundance of vitamins, minerals, antioxidants, enzymes, phyto-nutrients, and fiber, without an over-abundance of fat, calories, and refined carbohydrates.

At the risk of repeating myself, if I had to offer one dietary recommendation it would be this: **eat a whole foods diets—foods as close to the way Nature made them as possible.** Whole foods, as opposed to refined foods (white flour/sugar products such as bagels, refined pasta, white bread, pastries, donuts, cakes, candy, sweets, other desserts, etc.) usually have a low glycemic index. A low glycemic index means that blood sugar is not rapidly elevated after a meal. High glycemic index foods, such as sugary, refined, and processed foods put your blood sugar on a roller coaster. When blood sugar rises too rapidly, an overabundance of insulin is secreted. This excess insulin stimulates fat production and storage. The superfluous insulin will cause too much sugar to be stored, resulting in low blood sugar. Low blood sugar, in turn, will then cause stress hormone release (which decreases muscle), depression, fatigue, and hunger.

The high fiber in this recommended plant-based diet will actually slow digestion and absorption for a more even blood sugar level. Fiber will also bind with some fat and cholesterol (if you eat animal products) and prevent its absorption. High fiber foods speed up bowel transit time, taking some stress off the liver. The body can then more efficiently metabolize fats. (See Chapter 3 on fiber for more information).

After three decades working with thousands of people, I see a significant connection between toxicity and weight problems. Toxicity in the body causes retention of fluids, called edema. (I write about this in detail in Chapter 7.) The short-term solution to toxicity is to drink more alkaline water. In other words, **dilution is the solution to internal pollution**. When toxins are eliminated, the body no longer needs to retain water, and a significant loss of fluid occurs. Water retention alters the body's energy-production systems and affects metabolism. The long term solution is to eat wholesome foods. A diet emphasizing plant foods doesn't create the toxic overload in your body that unhealthy foods do.

Eating healthy, nutrient-rich foods increases your mitochondrial bioenergetics (energy production, which helps increase metabolism). Such nutritional support includes adequate levels of B vitamins, trace minerals (copper, iron, and chromium), and nutrients necessary for supporting proper detoxification—including molybdenum, selenium, manganese, zinc, the antioxidant vitamins E, C, and bioflavonoids, along with pantothenic acid, biotin, and folic acid. These nutrients, plus a well-designed nutrition program, help reset your body weight to a lower set point by improving your body's heat-producing properties.

Investigators at the Department of Community Health at the University of Oregon published a paper in which they reported on the use of a specific, controlled weight-loss program in moderately overweight women. In this study, reported in the 1994 *Journal of the American College of Nutrition*, 18 sedentary, moderately overweight women followed a 7-week program consisting of a diet of whole food meals and a specific vitamin and mineral-fortified drink, along with a progressive walking program. Mitochondrial energy production was assessed in these women before, during, and after the weight-loss program. The weight loss was principally body fat, not muscle. In fact some women actually gained muscle as they lost fat, causing their bodies to be much leaner at the conclusion of the program.

The bottom line: Eat a wholesome diet with lots of nutrients, drink plenty of water between meals, and exercise regularly.

7. Eat good fats. Sedentary, overfat people tend to eat a higher fat diet than people of normal weight. Fatty foods slow metabolism and the body converts dietary fat into body fat very easily. Gram for gram, fats not only have twice the calories of carbohydrates and proteins (9 compared to 4), they also burn only 2% of their calories to be stored as fat. Protein and carbohydrates, on the other hand, will burn about 25% of their calories to be stored as fat. It is considerably more difficult to convert protein and carbohydrates into body fat: your body actually burns calories doing so. Even when calories are the same, a person eating a high-fat diet tends to store more excess calories as body fat than someone eating a lower-fat diet. The closer you can adhere to a low-fat diet, the less fat will remain on you. Diets that are high in saturated fat and low in carbs go to an extreme, putting the body in a state of ketosis that compromises health. You may lose weight, but it's not a healthy way to go about it. So, if you are currently maintaining your weight on 3,000 calories a day, and then decrease the percentage of fat from 40% to 20%, you can lose 1 pound of fat in about 3 weeks—while at the same time eating 20% more food from complex carbs and protein. The bottom line: *eating too much fat makes you fat.*

But not all fats make you fat. In fact, you can also fight fat with healthy fat. Sounds paradoxical, doesn't it? Omega-3 fatty acids, as I discuss in the next chapter, can actually increase your metabolic rate. They also rid the body of excess fluids and can increase your energy level. The best source of omega-3 (LNA) fatty acids is organic Barlean's Flax Oil or Forti-Flax meal, available in the refrigerator section of health food stores; other sources include flax seeds (which you can grind yourself in a Flax Seed grinder) and fish. Omega-6 (LA) fatty acids (especially gamma linolenic acid or GLA) are also essential to a healthy metabolism but are less likely to be deficient in a healthy diet. Good supplementary sources of GLA and omega-6 fatty acids are borage seed oil, black currant oil, and primrose oil.

8. Cut your alcohol consumption. One of the greatest ways to sabotage your fat loss program is through alcohol consumption. Aside from having 7 calories per gram, alcohol shifts metabolism in favor of fat deposition, burdens the liver, and stimulates your appetite.

9. Drink at least two quarts of water a day—between meals. Water is very important in helping to maintain a healthy metabolic rate. At least 2 quarts a day, between meals, is essential—more if you're physically very active—that's at least 8 glasses of water daily. Water suppresses your appetite naturally. Have a large glass of water about 15 to 20 minutes before each meal or snack. I cannot stress enough how simply drinking purified, alkaline water (see Chapter 7) —between 10 and 14 glasses of water a day, and not changing anything else—not food or exercise—helps with fat loss and reshaping the body.

The liver's main functions are detoxification and regulation of metabolism. The kidneys can get rid of toxins and spare the liver if they have sufficient water, especially supplementing it with AlkaLife drops (see Resource Directory). This allows the liver to metabolize more fat. Adequate water will also decrease bloating and edema caused by fluid accumulation by flushing out sodium, acidic wastes, and other toxins. A high water intake also helps relieve constipation by keeping your stools soft.

10. Start weight lifting to eliminate cellulite. Millions of people, especially women, have cellulite. In fact, about 90% of all women over the age of 18 are plagued with this problem. Cellulite is not a fat problem, it's a skin problem. According to Covert Bailey, author of *The Ultimate Fit or Fat*, cellulite is just plain old fat bulging out under skin that has lost some of its elasticity.

You can have cellulite removed with plastic surgery, but you may be disappointed with the results, because your fat was helping to keep the skin taut. Once the fat is suctioned out, the skin that covered it may be even looser, so it dimples and puckers even more. **The best way to counteract cellulite is through weight lifting.** If you build up the muscles in an area, the skin on top of those muscles may smooth out because fat under the skin looks lumpy, but muscle under the skin looks smooth.

Cellulite, which is a combination of fat, water, and wastes, is the result of habits and lifestyle patterns such as stress, poor posture, improper diet, lack of exercise, poor elimination, and sluggish circulation. A sound anti-cellulite program incorporates exercise—aerobics, weight lifting and stretching/yoga, daily dry skin brushing (see Chapter 7), deep breathing, regular massages, and proper nutrition. Here are the things that have worked with my clients.

- Eat plenty of fresh vegetables and fruits and a variety of whole grains.
- Increase water intake to at least 96 ounces (3 quarts) a day and add 2 drops of AlkaLife in 5 of the glasses of water daily.
- Eliminate salt with the exception of small amounts of Celtic Sea Salt.
- Avoid all sugar, caffeine, alcohol, and saturated fat.
- Eat more unrefined complex carbs: they provide energy and fiber necessary for proper elimination.
- Eliminate red meat. Gradually phase out other animal products and byproducts. If being a vegetarian is not your cup of tea, fish is better than chicken and meat, but limit it to the size of your palm, no more than 4 times a week.

- Avoid preservatives, pesticides, and food additives such as food coloring and flavor.
- Make at least 50% of your diet living foods (not cooked).
- Pick two days a week where you eat all raw foods (or at least until dinner when 50% can be raw), such as Monday and Thursday.

11. *Use common sense for lasting results and success.* Despite the latest wave of research into new and better ways to fight fat, from prescription drugs, to meal replacement drinks and bars, to stimulating herbs, I believe that the most efficient fat busters have never changed: exercise and proper nutrition. But you must be consistent. Starting and then stopping your program doesn't work. Make health and fitness top priorities in your life and make your actions each day support your commitment.

There are some spices you can use to season your food that help raise body temperature, a natural trigger for metabolism. These include cayenne pepper, ginger, mustard, and cinnamon. You'll see that I've used these in many of the recipes.

The thyroid gland's action in the cell is to increase the biosynthesis of enzymes, resulting in heat production, oxygen consumption, and elevated metabolic rate. The thyroid stimulates the release of free fatty acids from adipose (fat) tissue, stimulates the oxidation of fatty acids (energy production), and reduces cholesterol by oxidizing it into bile acids.

If the thyroid gland becomes sluggish and underactive, calories are burned more slowly, weight becomes more difficult to lose, and you feel tired, have little cold tolerance, and thinning hair. Sea vegetables, such as nori, kelp, and dulse, are rich in the mineral iodine, which can help boost and normalize thyroid function. Just the simple addition of sea vegetables into the diet, as I recommend to all my clients who have had a hard time losing fat, can yield positive results.

12. *Be sure your hormones are in balance.* While hormone balance involves a complex harmonious blend of all hormones, there are 2, in particular, that affect the thyroid gland and our ability to lose fat.

First, there is an inseparable connection between fat and estrogen. There's a vicious cycle I see with women. Increased body fat raises estrogen levels, and estrogen increases the tendency to accumulate body fat. In other words, estrogen causes food calories to be stored as fat. Thyroid hormone causes fat calories to be turned into usable energy. Therefore, thyroid hormone and estrogen have opposing actions. The lack of progesterone in a woman still making estrogen or taking estrogen supplements leads to the condition of unopposed estrogen or estrogen-dominance. If you are estrogen-dominant, a term coined by John Lee, M.D., in his wonderful books, *What Your Doctor May Not Tell You About Menopause* and *What Your Doctor May Not Tell You About Premenopause,* you will have a hard time losing fat and keeping it off.

Now here's the key point to keep in mind. Most women 35 and above are estrogen-dominant. The reason, according to Dr. Lee, is an overabundance of estrogen and estrogenic substances in the food we eat and in our modern environment (animal and petroleum-based products). Further, estrogen dominance occurs naturally as you reach perimenopausal and menopausal age and can also occur as a result of a stress-filled life. What woman these days doesn't have lots of stress? Stress hormones, such as cortisol, decrease the metabolically active lean muscle tissue, and also lower your progesterone level. Put another way, when your estrogen levels increase and your progesterone levels are low, you put on weight more easily, have a harder time taking it off, and all this negatively affects your thyroid gland, which further lowers metabolism.

So what can you do? Everyone I work with who desires to lose fat first takes a hormone balance test. (I test my own hormones 2 times each year to make sure everything is in balance). It is a simple at-home saliva collection kit, which is then sent to a lab (see Aeron Life Cycles in the Resource Directory) to monitor hormones and bone density. I usually check 7 different hormones, including a form of estrogen (estradiol) and progesterone.

What is most interesting and enlightening to me is that over half of the women I test are estrogen dominant with low levels of progesterone. They start taking ProgestaCare (my favorite), a natural progesterone cream that you rub on your skin (several brands are recommended in Dr. John Lee's *What Your Doctor May Not Tell You About Menopause).* This transdermal cream will bring up the progesterone levels in your body and may have a positive effect on your ability to lose fat more easily and effortlessly. Most of my clients who start using a natural progesterone cream see results within days, such as increases in energy, feelings of equanimity and even-mindedness, a feeling of warmth throughout the body, rosier skin, youthful vitality, and a renewed sex drive. Progesterone is also a natural diuretic and helps use fat for energy. The addition of this natural progesterone cream also protects against fibrocyctic breasts, endometrial and breast cancer, helps restores proper cell oxygen levels (which help burn more fat), functions as a natural antidepressant, builds bone, and is protective against osteoporosis.

Progesterone, which is a precursor of other sex hormones, including estrogen and testosterone, increases energy production, helping the thyroid hormone work more efficiently, causing a slight rise in body temperature. This is called the 'thermogenic' effect of progesterone.

If, like many of my friends and clients, you feel that you're eating a healthy diet, avoiding junk food, and exercising as much as you can fit it in your schedule, but you still have to battle the bulge or that extra fat that just won't seem to go away no matter what you do or don't do, it could simply be that your progesterone level is low and you would benefit from some natural progesterone cream.

13. Get some sun! The sun has been getting a lot of bad press lately. Actually, sunlight in moderation is very good for the body in a variety of ways. It increases your metabolism, as documented in the excellent book, *Sunlight*, by Zane Kime, M.D. Dr. Kime states, "There is conclusive evidence that exposure to sunlight produces a metabolic effect in the body very similar to that produced by physical training, and is definitely followed by a measurable improvement in physical fitness." He also explains in this book how a plant-based diet (vegan—no dairy or eggs) will greatly decrease the risk of skin cancer.

14. Nourish your spirit. To maintain a healthy body, you must first nourish your spirit. The real epidemic in our culture is spiritual heart disease—the feelings of loneliness, isolation, and alienation that pervade our culture. This is addressed beautifully in the book, *Love and Survival: The Scientific Basis for the Healing Power of Intimacy,* by Dean Ornish, M.D. Many people who suffer from spiritual malaise use food or stimulants such as drugs, caffeine, alcohol, sex, or overwork to numb the pain and get through the day.

Stretching, deep breathing, and meditation will relax your mind and you will experience a greater sense of peace and well-being. Then you'll be able to make eating and exercise decisions—and other lifestyle choices—that are life enhancing rather than self-destructive.

Dieting alone doesn't work. Dieting combined with regular aerobic exercise is better, but it won't replace the muscle tissue that's lost in aging. ***When you combine strength training, aerobic exercise, and sensible eating and nourishment for your spirit, you have an unbeatable combination for reaching and maintaining your ideal weight, improving your metabolism, creating a fit, lean body, and celebrating life.***

SUCCESS

Chapter 6

SUPERFOODS & SUPPLEMENTS THAT HEAL & REJUVENATE THE BODY

Let your food be your medicine and medicine be your food.
—Hippocrates

More and more studies are now being done to substantiate what many have known for years—that a plant-based, whole foods diet offers the highest amount of health-providing substances, including phytonutrients, chlorophyll, vitamins, minerals, and fiber all of which help to heal and rejuvenate the body.

Since I get hundreds of letters each year asking me what supplements I take and recommend, I will also include my favorite ones in this chapter. By adding these superfoods and supplements to your whole foods based diet, you will be getting the very best nature has to offer us to support radiant health.

Fruits & Vegetables

The USDA recommends that we eat at least 5 servings of fruits and vegetables every day, but I say go for 7 to 12 servings a day. (Sorry. French fries, chips, and ketchup don't count.) Why? Most vegetables contain more nutrients per calorie than any other food. In fact, many vegetables contain more protein per calorie than meat and more calcium per calorie than milk. For example, romaine lettuce, which gets 18% of its calories from fat and almost 50% from protein, is a rich treasure-trove of hundreds of cancer-fighting phytonutrients. (Beware, however. Not all lettuces are created equal. Iceberg, for instance, is virtually nutrient free.)

Nutrient Density Comparison

100 calories of each	Broccoli	Sirloin Steak
Protein	11.2 gm	5.3 gm
Calcium	322 mg	2.4 mg
Iron	3.5 mg	.7 mg
Magnesium	74.5 mg	5 mg
Potassium	1084 mg	88 mg
Fiber	4.7 gm	0
Phytochemicals	very high	0
Antioxidants	very high	0
B_2	.71 mg	.04 mg
Niacin	2.8 mg	1.1 mg
Zinc	1.04 mg	1.2 mg
Vitamin C	350 mg	0
Vitamin A	7750 IU	24 IU
Vitamin E	26 IU	0
Weight	10.6 oz	0.84 oz

In a review of more than 200 epidemiological studies, raw vegetable consumption shows the strongest protective effects against cancer compared to all other beneficial foods. However, fewer than 1 in 500 Americans consume enough calories from vegetables to ensure this defense. An easy way to get enough vegetables is to eat two large salads daily. This simple practice will do more for improving your health than just about anything else you can do. Make fruit salads, too, because fruit will help satisfy your sweet tooth.

Fruits and vegetables are the highest water-content foods, are the most nutritious per calorie foods you can eat, especially when you eat them raw. Plus, they are low in fat and saturated fat and contain no cholesterol. *In terms of weight loss, you can eat as many raw fruits and vegetables as you want. In fact, the more raw vegetables you consume, especially leafy greens, such as spinach, romaine, and other greens, the faster you will lose fat.*

Diabetics can significantly lower their blood sugar—and maybe even reduce their need for medication—simply by eating lots of fruits, vegetables, and high-fiber grains. This was shown in a recent study at University of Texas Southwestern Medical Center in Dallas. Diabetics spent six weeks on the diet recommended by the American Diabetes Association (ADA) and another six weeks on an "experimental," high-fiber diet. The ADA diet is designed to keep blood sugar under control. The experimental diet reduced blood sugar levels by about 10%, which is comparable with the results from an oral diabetes drug.

The high-fiber diet also reduced concentrations of cholesterol and triglycerides, which have been strongly linked to heart disease. Heart disease is a major cause of death among diabetics—accounting for about 50% of all deaths. In a study of 652 participants on the Pritikin Program, 39% of adult-onset diabetics on insulin left the program insulin-free, while 70% of the diabetics on oral agents left the program free of these medications. Participants who diligently continued the program were able to stay off the medications.

In numerous studies, people who eat more fruits and vegetables have a lower risk of cancers of the lung, colon, stomach, esophagus, throat, and mouth. Other studies show that a diet rich in fruits and vegetables lowers blood pressure and can lower risk of stroke, heart disease, and diverticulosis.

So increase consumption to 7 to 12 servings each day and you'll feel better within hours. What's a serving? One average piece of fruit or 1/2 cup of cooked vegetables or 1 cup of raw.

Antioxidants and other phytochemicals in fruits and vegetables may help prevent up to 20% of all cancers. The following foods have been found to have the most protective effects against cancer (these findings were based on 83,234 participants in the Harvard Nurse's Study): garlic and onions, carrots, green vegetables, tomatoes, cruciferous vegetables like Brussels sprouts, broccoli, cauliflower, and cabbage, soy, and fruit, including citrus. Just three or more servings of vegetables may cut your risk in half for prostate, breast, and colon cancers.

The potassium in fresh fruits and vegetables may lower blood pressure, help maintain fluid balance in the body, and prevent muscle cramps. Here are a few natural ways to boost your intake.

Food	Serving Size	Potassium
Red beans	1 cup, canned	650 mg
Orange juice	1 cup	475 mg
Banana	1 medium	476 mg
Spinach	½ cup, cooked	420 mg
Baked potato	1 medium, w/ skin	330 mg
Strawberries	1 cup, sliced	275 mg

Lycopene, a cousin of beta carotene that gives the red color to tomatoes and watermelon, is also associated with reduced risk of breast and prostate cancers, and carotenoid-rich foods are associated with better cancer survival. Vitamin C and carotenoids protect eyes against disease.

Fruits and vegetables, for the most part, are alkaline-forming foods. As you'll read in Chapter 7, it's best to shoot for 80% alkaline-forming foods and no more than 20% acid-forming foods. Besides being the best foods for detoxification and rejuvenation, they also increase the flow of electrical energy throughout the body, which when low, causes lethargy and depression.

Perhaps most importantly, fruits and vegetables contain lots of *fiber*. If there is any "nutrient" that people in the U.S. are deficient in, it is *fiber*. The recommended intake for fiber is anywhere from 35 to 50 grams per day. Currently, the average intake among Americans is only about 10 to 12 grams, which is one of the main reasons that 50% of Americans are considered obese.

Choose Fiber for Health

Because dietary fiber—from fruits, vegetables, and grains—remains largely undigested in the gastrointestinal tract, experts believe that it slows the progress of food through the gut, reducing the absorption of food, and keeping insulin secretion at low or moderate levels.

A recent study reported in the *Journal of the American Heart Association* examined the diets of over 2,900 individuals between 18

Food	Fiber per serving	Serving amount
Vegetables	2-3 grams	1/2 cup cooked vegetables
		1 cup raw vegetables
Fruits	2-3 grams	1 medium piece of fruit
		1/2 grapefruit, banana
		1/2 cup diced or cut, frozen
Beans	4-7 grams	1/2 cup cooked beans
Nuts & seeds	1-2 grams	1 ounce (2 tablespoons)
Unrefined complex carbohydrates	3-5 grams	1/2 cup cooked, starchy veggies (peas, corn, potatoes, yams) 1/2 cup cooked whole grain (rice, oatmeal, barley)
Refined carbohydrates	1 gram	1 ounce bread (1 slice whole wheat bread, 1/2 whole wheat pita or bagel)
		1 ounce dry cereal*

*Many dry cereals show misleading amounts of fiber because a lot of it is supplemental fiber that has been added to the "refined" cereal. This is NOT the recommended form of fiber.

and 30 years of age for cardiovascular risk factors. Researchers found that high-fiber diets were associated with "lowered insulin levels, accelerated fat loss, and reduced other risk factors for cardiovascular disease in young adults." High-fiber intake also was associated with lowered blood pressure.

The type and source of fiber is very important. There are two broad categories of fiber that you will see on food labels, called **insoluble** and **soluble**. This simply refers to the ability of these to dissolve in hot water. We need a mix of both types of fiber in our diets: Insoluble fiber assists in maintaining regular bowel movements, while soluble fiber lowers blood cholesterol levels and can help regulate blood sugar concentrations and insulin levels.

The best source of fiber is from whole natural foods rather than processed foods or supplements. The more a food is processed, the lower its fiber content, and the less effective its fiber.

This classic experiment was done more than 20 years ago: You can squeeze 2 apples, drink the juice in 30 seconds, and feel hungry half an hour later. You can cook 2 apples and make applesauce, eat it in a few minutes, and feel hungry an hour or two later. But if you eat 2 whole apples, it will take you 20 to 30 minutes, and you won't be hungry for several hours because you won't have the swings in blood sugar that the juice or applesauce will cause.

The previous guide will help you estimate the fiber in your diet. The recommended minimum is 35 grams.

Sprouts for Life

One of the healthiest foods you can eat is sprouts, especially if you grow them fresh at home. During germination, seeds become alive and undergo a host of internal changes that greatly increase the number of nutrients. Water absorption swells the sprouting seed from 6 to 10 times its normal size, under tremendous dynamic pressures per square inch. Proteins are converted into free amino acids and starches are changed into simple plant sugars. Minerals chelate, or combine in a way that increases their assimilation and the vitamin content increases from 3 to 12 times. Chlorophyll and carotene content increase dramatically when they are exposed to sunlight.

Wheat sprouts, for example, contain 4 times more folic acid and 6 times more vitamin C than unsprouted wheat. In studies at the University of Pennsylvania, vitamin C content in some seeds was found to increase up to 700% in just the first 72 hours of sprouting! For this reason some fresh sprouts contain more vitamin C than citrus juices. This also applies to vitamins A, E, the B complex, and others, depending on the variety of seed sprouted.

Sprouts are complete foods, with proteins known as "complete proteins" because they contain all the essential amino acids. Sprouts also contain all other essential dietary nutrients, along with live enzymes to help assimilate them. Simple plant sugars such as maltose are easily digested and enter the bloodstream quickly; for this reason, sprouts are also classed as "quick energy" foods.

Sprouting Guide

VARIETY OF SEED	SOAKING TIME (HOURS)	FULL TIME RINSE & DRAIN (PER DAY)	AVERAGE TIME TO HARVEST (DAYS)	SPECIAL HANDLING	SUGGESTED USES
Alfalfa	8	3	3–4	None	Juices, Salads, Sandwiches
Beets	8	3	3–5	None	Juices, Salads
Buckwheat	8	3	2–3	Remove remaining husks	Juices, Pancakes, Salads
Chia	8	No	3–5	Mist	Casseroles, Salads, Sandwiches
Corn	8	3	2–4	None	Soups, Tortillas Vegetable Casseroles, etc.
Cress	No	No	3–5	Mist gently with water 3 times a day or mix with other seeds	Breads, Salads, Sandwiches
Dill	8	3	3–5	None	Juices, Salads, Sandwiches
Fenugreek	8	3	3–5	Mist gently with water	Salads, Snacks
Flax	No	No	3–5	Mist gently with water 3 times a day or mix with other seeds	Juices, Salads
Garbanzo	8	3	3–4	None	Soups, Vegetable Casseroles
Lentil	8	3	2–4	None	Juices, Salads, Soups, Vegetable Casseroles, etc.
Millet	8	3	3–5	None	Juices, Salads, Soups, Vegetable Casseroles, etc.
Mung Bean	8	3	3–4	None	Omelets, Oriental Dishes, Salads, Snacks, Soups
Mustard	No	3	3–5	Mist gently with water 3 times a day or mix with other seeds	Juices, Salads
Napa Cabbage	8	3	3–4	None	Juices, Salads
Oats	8	3	2–3	Remove remaining husks	Breads, Granola, Snacks
Peas, Alaskan	8	3	3–4	None	Omelets, Salads, Snacks, Soups

Sprouting Guide (continued)

VARIETY OF SEED	SOAKING TIME (HOURS)	FULL TIME RINSE & DRAIN (PER DAY)	AVERAGE TIME TO HARVEST (DAYS)	SPECIAL HANDLING	SUGGESTED USES
Peas, Special	8	3	3–4	None	Omelets, Salads, Snacks, Soups
Pichi Bean	8	3	3–4	None	Omelets, Oriental Dishes, Salads, Snacks, Soups
Porridge Pea	8	3	3–4	None	Omelets, Oriental Dishes, Salads, Snacks, Soups
Radish	8	3	3–4	None	Juices, Salads, Sandwiches
Red Clover	8	3	3–5	None	Juices, Salads, Sandwiches
Rye	8	3	2–3	None	Breads, Granola, Snacks
Sesame	8	3	2–3	None	Breads, Granola, Snacks
Soybean	24	3	3–5	Change soaking water every 8 hours	Casseroles, Oriental Dishes, Salads
Sunflower (Green	8	3	3–5 5–7)	Remove remaining husks	Salads, Snacks
Triticale	8	3	1–2	None	Breads, Granola, Pancakes, Snacks
Wheat (Wheat Grass	8	3	2 5–7)	None	Breads, Granola, Pancakes, Snacks

If you don't know how to sprout, I recommend the Handy Pantry's Basic Sprouting Starter Kit (see the Resource Directory), which makes sprouting easy and fun and provides a daily supply of all types of sprouts from seeds, nuts, grains, and legumes. I also buy my sprouting seeds from Handy Pantry along with their Sprout Spray, which is also a fruit and vegetable wash.

Alfalfa sprouts are one of the most popular, nutritious, and delicious of all sprouting seeds. They are high in protein, essential amino acids, and eight digestive enzymes; vitamins A, C, B complex (including B_{12} often missing in vegan diets), D, E, and 5 minerals: iron, phosphorous, calcium, magnesium, and potassium. When exposed to light, they are also high in chlorophyll. Alfalfa sprouts have a sweet, nut-like flavor and sprout easily in combination with other seeds, making a lively addition in salads, sandwiches, or as a snack by themselves.

Because sprouts have a very limited shelf life (old sprouts may develop salmonella) and you don't always know how old store-bought sprouts may be, I encourage you to grow your own. It's easy and lots of fun. Children can even do it. The Sprouting Guide chart will help you.

Some of Susan's Favorite Health Foods

Flax Seed: Nature's Medicine

Often referred to as 'nutritional gold,' flax seed is rapidly becoming the wonder grain of health. It has the potential to improve and prevent cardiovascular disease, cancer, diabetes, and many other degenerative conditions, as well as to improve skin and vitality.

Its history is as rich as its medicinal benefits. For more than 7,000 years, flax seed (also known industrially as linseed) has been consumed by humankind. It is one of the oldest known cultivated plants used not only for food, but also for making linen.

Flax fiber was used by Stone Age people for making ropes and fish nets, and the flax seed was used for food. Flax was cultivated in Babylon in 5000 B.C. and by 3000 B.C., the ancient Egyptians used it to make linen mummy wrappings; the oil was used as a cosmetic and applied to wall paintings for the tombs and temples. In the 5th century B.C., Hippocrates wrote about using flax to relieve inflamed mucous membranes, abdominal pains, and diarrhea. Ancient East Indian scriptures state that a yogi must eat flax daily in order to reach the highest state of contentment and joy. More recently, Mahatma Gandhi observed: "Whenever flax seed becomes a regular food item among the people, there will be better health." In Vedic medicine, flax is considered a 'cooling' oil, used to reduce inflammation.

Today edible flax seed and its healing oil are being hailed as the latest cure in the fight against cancer and coronary heart disease by plant biochemists and health researchers. A real powerhouse, this seed packs a quadruple whammy: a high dose of LNA (omega-3) fatty acids, a healthy fat which helps lower cholesterol; a proper ratio of LNA to LA (omega-6) fatty acids; fiber, especially cholesterol-lowering soluble fiber; and lignans, a kind of fiber that is looking more and more like a potent blocker of some kinds of cancer. All this and it tastes good, too!

PROTEIN: Flax seeds contain high-quality, easily digestible protein with *all* the amino acids (the building blocks of protein) essential to health, making it a complete protein. From this, the body can manufacture the other dozen amino acids required to make proteins essential for building muscles, blood, skin, hair, nails, and internal organs, including the heart and the brain.

COMPLEX CARBOHYDRATES: Flax seed provides instant calories for energy and assists in digestion and regulation of protein and fat metabolism.

FIBER: An excellent source of both soluble and insoluble fiber, flax keeps the digestive tract from becoming clogged with mucus by keeping everything moving, maintaining healthy intestinal flora, and keeping the colon clean. It also helps keep cholesterol and bile acids from being re-absorbed into the body through the intestinal walls. When foods progress into the small intestine, the gall bladder secretes bile acids to assist in breaking down fats. Bile is actually produced in the liver and concentrates in the gall bladder as a dietary fat emulsifier. Bile is rich in enzymes that break apart triglycerides. A healthy person's bile excretion will absorb 95% of fat consumed. However, the liver and gallbladder can become taxed and less efficient from a diet of too much fat. Fiber from flax helps in binding excess fats and allowing their excretion into the large intestine and ultimate expulsion from the body.

MUCILAGE: Mucilage is a thick gum found in many plants, especially flax seed (12% to 15% of volume), which makes flax seed one of the best natural laxatives available. Like the pectin found in apples, mucilage in flax is important in maintaining bowel regularity. Due to the presence of essential fatty acids in the mucilage, it tends to soothe and protect the delicate stomach and intestinal linings and keeps the contents moving progressively along.

Many degenerative diseases start in the colon through the toxic effects of constipation and poor peristaltic action of the colon muscle. When flax seed (oil and ground meal) is taken with fluids, the mucilage assists in alleviating constipation, increasing stool bulk and softness, and speeding up transit time out of the body, preventing toxic buildup in our bowel. As a result, stools smell less foul, breath is fresher, and there is less stress on the liver and eliminative organs, including the kidneys and skin. Flax seed can be chewed, but the small seeds can get stuck in your teeth. I prefer the oil and freshly ground meal.

Flax mucilage also has the ability to buffer excess acid in sensitive stomachs, and its absorptive properties help to stabilize blood glucose. When the pancreas isn't being force-cycled through the dramatic highs and lows from excess sugars in the diet, which results in either overages or shortages of blood saturated or starved glucose levels, then insulin production is more stable. Sufficient quality fiber from foods such as flax, retards the cycles of sugar highs and lows frequently associated with such progressive diseases as hypoglycemia and late-onset adult diabetes, both of which have a defective glucose metabolic factor.

MINERALS: Flax seed contains most known major and trace minerals: phosphorous, magnesium, potassium, calcium, sulfur, sodium, chlorine, zinc, and iron and adequate trace amounts of manganese, silicon, copper, fluorine, nickel, cobalt, iodine, molybdenum, and chromium.

VITAMINS: Flax seed contains fat-soluble vitamins E and carotene, and water-soluble vitamins B_1, B_2, and C. The tocopherol compounds found in vitamin E act as antioxidants in the body, protecting other molecules and cell components from damaging reactions with oxygen. Vitamin E is an antioxidant substance that works as a synergistic ally with vitamins A and C and as a regulator of cell respiration. Flax is particularly high in minerals and vitamin co-factors.

LIGNINS and LIGNANS: Unlike many other plant fibers, flax seed is high in both lignin and lignan. Lignin is an insoluble fiber that our bodies convert to several kinds of lignans (cellulose-like materials that form the cell walls of plants). Flax seed is the richest known source of lignans, containing 100 times as much as the next best source, which is wheat bran. While all vegetables provide lignin precursors to some degree, flax provides much more, about 800 micrograms per gram, as compared to only 8 micrograms per gram in common fiber such as bran. Lignans have recently attracted the attention of researchers because they have been found to be useful in treating viral, bacterial, and fungal infections as well as cancer. In fact, high levels of lignans in the bowel are associated with reduced rates of colon and breast cancer.

The lignans formed from flax are pseudo-estrogens that block estrogen receptors in the body. The molecular shape of the lignans is such that they bind with the estrogen receptors, thus 'smoothing out' the hormonal and metabolic effect of estrogen release in the body. Over-production of estrogen is known to stimulate colon and other forms of cancer: 30% to 50% of all malignant colon tumors contain numerous estrogen receptors. Significantly, the rate of colon cancer tends to correlate with those of breast cancer, and both seem to be more prevalent in people with low-fiber diets.

Studies reveal that lignans resemble estrogens and attach to estrogen receptors in the body, but do not have the tumor-stimulating effect of hormonal estrogen. Normally induced syndromes, like hot flashes or elevated body temperature, are slightly mitigated by these lignans and lignins. Further, research shows that lignans derived from flax can also reduce levels of unbound estrogen in the blood, which explains how they can also help prevent breast cancer. Perhaps the presence of lignans, derived from plant fiber, may be one of the main reasons why vegetarians have substantially lower cancer rates than meat eaters.

ESSENTIAL FATTY ACIDS (EFAs): EFAs are part of every cell in our bodies, where they play important roles in maintaining the structure of the cells and in producing energy. Our glands need EFAs to carry out the minute secretion of hormones and other biological regulating substances. EFAs help muscle cells to recover from use and abuse. EFAs are critical to infants' prenatal and postnatal development, especially brain development, and for growth spurts throughout childhood.

Our bodies do a remarkable job of creating most of the nutrients we need from the resident cell materials on hand, but the nutrients our bodies can't synthesize are called the essential nutrients, and these must be adequately supplied in our diets. Of the 45 essential nutrients, 2 are fatty acids: LNA (alpha-linolenic acid or omega-3) and LA (linoleic acid or omega-6). Besides being an excellent source of the essential LNA fatty acids, flax seed also contains important trace nutrients such as phospholipids, phytosterols, and beta-sistosterin. These naturally occurring compounds assist in the digestion of fats and are just beginning to be recognized for their immune-enhancing properties.

The Modern Diet & LNA Deficiency

In the past 100 years, developments in modern food processing have drastically reduced the nutrient value, including the LNA content, of many of the foods we eat. In his book, *The Omega-3 Phenomenon*, Dr. Donald O. Rudin explains that modern food processing and food selection opportunities severely distort the availability of many essential nutrients—especially limiting the LNA essential fatty acids. Whenever high heat and caustic agents are used to sterilize food, the incidence of diseases such as cancer, heart disease, and arthritis sky-rocket. Heart disease and many cancers are linked to distortions of dietary fats. Dr. Rudin calls LNA "the nutritional missing link" and attributes its profound absence in most foods to the cause of many degenerative conditions.

Americans who eat a lot of highly refined and processed foods consume excess amounts of refined LAs and insufficient amounts of unrefined LNA fatty acids. Fast food restaurants usually cook with highly refined, unstable polyunsaturated oils such as corn, sunflower, safflower, and soy oils containing highly concentrated LA fatty acids and deadly trans-fats. The physiology of fast food consumers remains in a perpetual state of fatty acid imbalance, increasing their risk of some 50 degenerative diseases such as heart attacks, cancer, arthritis, stroke, kidney impairment, liver disease, auto-immune disorders, and skin disorders.

These so-called American degenerative diseases have risen over the past 100 years in a near perfect linear fashion with the elimination of omega-3, and the concentration of omega-6 in the food chain. In many regards, saturated fats may have been ruled guilty by association as the genesis of cardiovascular disease appears to be more closely related to a rise in vegetable oil ingestion than it does to saturated fat.

Japanese researchers have been studying the leading cause of westernized degenerative diseases in Japan and the world. Their work has gone far to confirm the landslide of emerging scientific research revealing that the genesis of degenerative diseases can be traced to a drastic reduction in the ingestion of omega-3 in relation to increased ingestion of omega-6. Perhaps most powerful and convincing are the words of the Japanese researchers themselves excerpted from the study summary:

"In this review, we summarize the evidence which indicates that increased dietary linoleic acid (omega-6) and relative omega-3 deficiency are major risk factors for western-type cancers, cardiovascular and cerebrovascular diseases, and also for allergic hyper-reactivity. We also raise the possibility that a relative omega-3 deficiency may be affecting the behavioral patterns of a proportion of the young generations in industrialized countries." It is proposed that dietary intervention with omega-3 supplementation, and the reduction of omega-6 in the diet could successfully reverse the rising trend toward westernized degenerative diseases in Japan, and the world.

Fish oils have been touted for the 'heart saving' LNA fatty acids found in the flesh of deep-sea fish, such as salmon and mackerel, which they obtain from the algae of plankton that comprise the foundation of the ocean's food chain. Unfortunately, research shows that along with a concentration of LNA, fish also concentrate in their bodies traces of pesticides, heavy metals, and other industrial pollutants such as PCBs. According to Ralph Nader and other respected environmental activists, even our deep-sea waters are now polluted, and fish store the pollutants in their livers and fatty tissues. Organic flax seed contains no such toxic residues.

The Proven Benefits of LNA

Research and clinical experience demonstrate that regular consumption of flax seed and oil has been correlated with the successful treatment of:

CANCER: Recent research in breast, lung, and prostate cancer cell lines shows that LNAs kill human cancer cells in tissue cultures without harming the normal cells. Research evidence also suggests that lignans may fight off chemicals responsible for initiating tumors and block estrogen receptors, which may reduce colon cancer risk. According to Dr. James Duke of the U.S. Department of Agriculture, flax seed contains 27 identifiable cancer preventive compounds. Additional studies show that LNAs inhibit tumor formation (smaller tumors, less metastasis, longer survival time). The National Cancer Institute is currently researching flax seed for its potential ability to prevent cancer.

HEART DISEASE: One of the unique features of flax seed oil is that it contains a substance which resembles prostagladins, which may well be part of its potent therapeutic value in preventing heart disease. The prostaglandins regulate blood pressure and arterial function, and have an important role in calcium and energy metabolism. No other vegetable oil examined so far matches this property of flax seed oil.

DIABETES: Late-onset adult diabetes is suspected to originate partially from a deficiency of LNAs and an excess of saturated and trans-fats in the diet. Although this syndrome can take as long as 30 years to emerge as a full blown disease, reversal of symptoms can occur with positive changes in the diet and proper supplementation of LNAs from flax seed oil. A concurrent lack of vitamins and minerals makes the disease worse. LNAs may also lower the insulin requirement of diabetics.

INFLAMMATORY TISSUE CONDITIONS: LNA fatty acids decrease inflammatory conditions of all types. Inflammatory conditions are the diseases that end in 'itis,' including bursitis, tendonitis, tonsillitis, gastritis, ileitis, colitis, meningitis, arthritis, phlebitis, prostatitis, nephritis, splenitis, hepatitis, pancreatitis, and otitis, as well as lupus. Many of these inflammatory conditions may be eased by use of LNAs.

SKIN CONDITIONS: Pedigree show animals are fed linseed oil, made from flax seed, to keep their coats glossy. Along the same lines, recent research has shown that skin conditions in humans, such as psoriasis and eczema, have improved dramatically when flax seed and flax seed oil was added to the diet. These skin conditions are exacerbated by lack of LNAs in the diet. Taking flax seed oil regularly in your diet is helpful for treating dry skin, dandruff, and sun-sensitive skin.

SEXUAL DISORDERS: The most common physical cause of impotency of men and non-orgasmic response in women is blockage of blood flow in the arteries of the pelvis. Decrease of blood flow prevents full expansion (erection) of the penis and/or the clitoris. Thus ejaculation and/or orgasm cannot occur. The solution is to unblock narrowed arteries in general, and the consumption of flax seed oil will help.

STRESS: Many people find increased calmness to be the most profound effect of using fresh flax seed oil. This may be partly due to that fact that, under stress, LNA fatty acids appear to slow down the over-production of stressing biochemicals such as arachidonic acid. The 'fight or flight' stress response is mitigated by the LNAs, which compete against the arachidonic acid cascade that happens when we are chronically stressed. Arachidonic acid in the blood thickens blood platelets in anticipation of wounding and bleeding, which is an ancient natural defense mechanism. The LNA fatty acids keep these in check.

WATER RETENTION: The LNA and LA fatty acids in flax seed oil help the kidneys excrete sodium and water. Water retention (edema) accompanies swollen ankles, some forms of obesity, PMS, and all stages of cancer and cardiovascular disease.

OTHER CONDITONS: LNAs are necessary for visual function (retina), adrenal function (stress), and sperm formation. LNAs can improve symptoms of multiple sclerosis (MS) and research shows that when LNA consumption is high, MS is rare. Flax seed oil can also help symptoms of cystic fibrosis by loosening viscous secretions and relieving breathing difficulties; some cases of sterility and mis-carriage; some glandular malfunctions; some behavioral problems (schizophrenia, depression, bipolar disorder); allergies; addictions (to drugs or alcohol); and weight loss programs.

In addition to disease treatment, one of the most noticeable signs of improved health from the use of flax seed oil is progressive and increased vitality and energy and stamina. Fatigued muscles recover from exercise more quickly. Flax does have a cooling effect on inflammatory conditions, but it also generates a healing 'heat energy' in the body due to the fact that the fatty acids are burned up for energy production, speeding up biochemical processes like metabolism. In simple terms, flax increases metabolic rate and the efficiency of cellular energy production. It stimulates respiratory and cellular oxidation, producing energy that we experience as warmth. For athletes, or anyone wishing to reduce fat and create a fit, lean body, this is great news!

Using & Storing Flax Seed Oil

Producing the oil from flax seed without damaging or destroying the vital LNA is no simple task. It is most healthful when consumed fresh. Ideally, the oil should be expeller cold pressed in the absence of heat, light, and oxygen with no post refinement measures such as filtration or exposure to excess heat and other damaging environmental factors. Choose a flax oil that is delivered manufacture-direct to health food stores. Flax oil should be packaged in a special dark (HDPE) opaque plastic (not glass) container that won't interfere or leech into the oil. Just because it says flax oil on the bottle does not mean that you are getting a fresh, unrefined/unfiltered product. Therefore, look for products that include a "freshness" date stamp.

Make sure you keep flax oil refrigerated after you purchase it from the refrigerator section of the health food store and use it up within the time stamped on the bottle, usually within 4 months. You can also keep it in the freezer as it still remains a liquid and lasts longer—up to 5 months—although if you're using it regularly you will probably go through a couple of bottles each month. I use flax oil in smoothies, on grains and potatoes, in salad dressings, and in juices as well as part of my massage oil, skin moisturizer and hair conditioner.

In addition to flax seed oil, I keep organic flax seeds on hand to freshly grind directly in a smoothie or juice or over a food dish or meal. Flax seed grinders are inexpensive, small, and very easy and convenient to use. (Refer to the Resource Directory for more information on my favorite brand, Barlean's Organic Flax Oil. See the listing under the Grain & Salt Society for a flax seed grinder.) Or, for the convenience of having fresh ground flax seed without the grinder, you may want to consider Barlean's pre-ground flax seed product, "Forti-Flax" (1 to 2 tablespoons of flax oil or 2 to 4 tablespoons of flax meal).

Chlorella: The Daily Detoxifier

In our modern society, there are so many chemical and environmental dangers that we are either not aware of, or don't like to think about. Pesticides in foods, parasites and fungi, chemically-laden paints and solvents, insecticides, aerosols, metals, cosmetics, hair dyes, deodorants, first- and second-hand tobacco smoke, corrosives from air conditioning units; the list is endless.

The toxic contaminants in our drinking water include nitrates, bacteria, pesticides, radon, metals, and lead. Lead in drinking water is linked to 680,000 cases of high blood pressure and over 10,000 bladder and rectal cancer cases each year, and is tied to trihalomethanes (odorless combustible gas) found in tainted water.

The air we breathe, both indoors and outdoors, is laden with dangerous ozone, carbon monoxide, pesticides, and sulfur oxides. Over 75 million Americans are affected by indoor air pollution in both homes and offices from toxins contained in paint, furniture, carpeting, adhesives, solvents, even our clothing.

The FDA lists over 2,800 "intentional" food additives, many of which are sulfur or tar-based. Many commercial food manufacturers use hormones, antibiotics, preservatives, dyes, and pesticides, all with potentially dangerous symptoms and side effects.

Environmental toxins can build up over time, paralyze the immune system, and damage the cells in the body. To a degree, the body has its own defense system to combat and eliminate toxins, but the overwhelming quantities that bombard us on a daily basis are more than the average person can handle. These toxins can be stored in the body for many years until they create a *toxic overload* that taxes the liver and can undermine your body's ability to efficiently burn fat. In other words, as the toxic load builds up, it becomes harder to lose extra fat.

Detoxification, which we'll look at more extensively in the next chapter, refers to the removal of toxic substances from the body. Chlorella is considered to be nature's most powerful detoxifying, natural discovery. Chlorella is a microscopic, green, single-celled freshwater algae. Its many nutrients work in harmony with one another, helping to balance and stabilize the processes of the body on a cellular level.

Chlorella is nutrient rich whole food which contains more than 20 different vitamins and minerals, all of the essential amino acids, fiber, and life-giving chlorophyll. It provides an abundance of naturally occurring beta carotene and is nearly 50% protein. It also contains iron (more than spinach), iodine, zinc, lysine and many other substances that are lacking in many vegetarian diets.

Though the whole chlorella cell is packed with nutritional benefits, perhaps the greatest value of chlorella lies deep inside the cellular core, a nucleic-peptide complex known as the Chlorella Growth Factor, or CGF which is responsible for cell repair and regeneration. Chlorella is 10% ribonucleic acid (RNA) and 3% deoxyribonucleic acid (DNA), the highest nucleic acid content of any known food source. It has 17 times more RNA (the anti-aging powerhouse) than canned sardines and 510 times as much as steak).

Chlorella will not interfere with any prescription or over-the-counter medications and is a perfect complement to any multivitamin or nutritional supplement. I recommend taking chlorella daily.

Each chlorella cell is a complete plant in itself with all of its living enzymes intact, allowing you to consume it wholly and naturally. Cultured in pure, mineral water and uncontaminated by chemical additives or pesticides, chlorella is naturally protected by a tough outer cell wall that, in its natural state, is difficult to process. In order to improve digestibility, chlorella manufacturers use various techniques to break down the cell wall. The brand I prefer is manufactured by the Dyno-Mill process, which is a patented mechanical process that does not involve heat or chemicals. It leaves a live, whole food, with all of its life-giving enzymes. The company that utilizes the Dyno-Mill process is Sun Chlorella. I've been taking their product for 17 years. It comes in tablet, granule, or liquid form in most natural food stores (see the Resource Directory).

Great Garlic!

Numerous studies shows that garlic—especially an aged garlic extract called Kyolic—may help prevent several types of cancer, reduce the risk of heart disease, lower cholesterol, help prevent Alzheimer's disease, improve memory, boost the immune system, and much more.

Over 150 studies on aged garlic extract have been presented at various symposiums and published in various scientific journals with some of the exciting findings.

CANCER RISK: Research has shown that garlic can significantly lower the risk of developing breast and prostate cancers and can slow its progress in subjects already suffering from either disease. Several Chinese studies have found garlic also helps prevent stomach cancer and a researcher in Australia showed greatly reduced skin cancer in mice by applying aged garlic extract on affected rodents. Other studies suggest that garlic slows the activity of carcinogens linked to colon, rectal, intestinal, stomach, and esophagael cancers.

HEART and CIRCULATORY DISEASE: Garlic has been shown to reduce the risk of heart disease and stroke by unclogging blocked arteries, preventing cholesterol and other deposits from sticking to the arteries, and reducing plaque formation.

Researchers at Flinders University of South Australia in Adelaide recently analyzed 7 placebo-controlled studies involving more than 400 people who took garlic. They found that a daily dose of 600 mg to 900 mg of garlic powder pills significantly lowered systolic pressure (the first number in a reading) in 3 studies. Diastolic pressure (the second number) was significantly lowered in 4 studies.

Kyolic Aged Garlic Extract™ was recently patented for its ability to reduce elevated homocysteine. Elevated homocysteine levels have been shown to be a much stronger risk factor for heart disease than even elevated cholesterol levels, smoking, or elevated blood pressure.

The aorta is the large artery that delivers oxygen-rich blood from the heart to the rest of the body. It becomes less elastic with age, a factor contributing to high blood pressure. A two-year study at Ohio State University tracked the progression of aortic stiffness in 100 people 50 to 80 years of age. They found daily doses of 300 mg of garlic powder pills markedly reduced the progression.

ALZHEIMER'S DISEASE and AGING: Garlic enhances blood circulation to the brain, which helps prevent senility, Alzheimer's, and even Parkinson's disease. A Japanese study showed that garlic can combat age-related memory loss and brain cell deterioration, and a French study found that garlic improves memory and relieves symptoms of depression and fatigue.

IMMUNE SYSTEM: Garlic contains compounds that boost the activity of white blood cells, which are the cells that help ward off disease. More than 20 studies have shown that garlic inhibits the growth of bacteria, viruses, and fungi.

I could go on and on. Suffice it to say that aged garlic extract, or Kyolic, is a supplement worth taking daily to help heal and rejuvenate the body. I have been taking Kyolic aged garlic extract for more than 30 years, longer than any other supplement. While I recommend cooking with fresh garlic and include it in many of the recipes in this book, too much raw garlic is irritating to the digestive system, not to mention its effect on the breath. Kyolic is not a commercial food additive or a flavoring, it is a nutritional supplement. Kyolic is organically grown and aged naturally without heat so it's a 'living' food and retains all its life-giving enzymes. During aging, the concentrated active compounds are mellowed and the harsh, irritating, odorous compounds found in raw garlic are converted to dozens of valuable, stable, safe, and odorless compounds, including S-allyl cysteine, that make Kyolic so beneficial. It is the only truly odorless garlic product available.

Kyolic comes in a variety of excellent formulas, including both capsules and liquid, that are available in natural food stores (see the Resource Directory).

Ascorbate Power

Vitamin C is fundamental for health and disease prevention. In fact, many researchers believe that the role of vitamin C in the body goes far beyond that of a nutrient. The evidence comes from studies of animals and the health benefits people derive from taking high doses of vitamin C. Most animals produce their own vitamin C, literally hundreds of times the amount people routinely obtain from food. Scientific studies on people show that a high intake of vitamin C extends life span, fights infections, lowers blood pressure and cholesterol, as well as reducing the likelihood of dying from heart disease and cancer. According to Linus Pauling, "Vitamin C is different because, at one time, all animals made their own vitamin C in their livers. All of this extra vitamin C must be important—otherwise, the majority of animals wouldn't be producing so much of it." So, why don't people make their own vitamin C? One theory holds that a genetic accident millions of years ago left the ancestors of human beings and a handful of animals—including the guinea pig—unable to produce this vitamin in their bodies.

In animals—and in people—vitamin C maintains homeostasis, the term biologists use to describe staying on an 'even keel' when faced with stress, infections, heart disease, cancer, and other conditions. Vitamin C is essential for a smooth-running immune system, is an antioxidant, and may even help prevent Alzheimer's disease. A study of 633 persons, ages 65 years and older, at Rush University for Healthy Aging and Harvard Medical School, found that 91 of the sample participants, after the follow-up period of 4.3 years, were diagnosed with Alzheimer's disease. Yet, none of the 27 vitamin C supplement users had the disease.

Mineral Ascorbates

There is a big difference between vitamin C ascorbic acid and vitamin C mineral ascorbates. In high levels, ascorbic acid is irritating to the kidneys, bladder, and urethra. If intake is suddenly increased, the cells can't process it, and it heads for the kidneys and spills over in the urine.

Mineral ascorbates are more readily accepted by the cells because the minerals often serve as ascorbate transporters to aid in assimilation of the ascorbate by the cell. Studies show the countless advantages of vitamin C, in the form of mineral ascorbates, over pure ascorbic acid. Mineral ascorbates are neutral (nonacidic) and have no adverse side effects, unlike high levels of ascorbic acid, which may cause heartburn, nausea, flatulence, diarrhea, and excess urination, inducing loss of minerals. Many health enthusiasts are unaware that ascorbic acid is only an intermediate form of vitamin C.

In animals, the ascorbic acid produced in the liver promptly reacts with minerals before circulation in the bloodstream to form mineral ascorbates. Jay Patrick, chemist, president, and founder of Alacer Corporation has developed a full line of vitamin C products that deliver fully reacted mineral ascorbates. I've been taking one of his products, Emer'gen-C™, which is a tangy, nonacidic, effervescent drink mix, for *22 years*. It offers these ascorbates: Calcium ascorbate, molybdenum ascorbate, chromium ascorbate, magnesium ascorbate, copper ascorbate, manganese ascorbate, potassium ascorbate, and zinc ascorbate.

Unlike ascorbic acid, which lowers the pH of the urine, mineral ascorbates are essentially pH neutral and far more effective to the 70 trillion cells of the body. Emer'gen-C replenishes valuable electrolytes. A 6-ounce drink of Emer'gen-C furnishes 200 mg of potassium—8 times more than 8 ounces of the popular sports drink, without unnecessary sugars or salts. I take it with me to drink before, during, and after my workouts. Another product, Triple Power, incorporates 1,000 mg vitamin C as mineral ascorbates with 500 mg glucosamine and 400 mg chondroitin. This is an excellent formula for improving or maintaining healthy joint structures and cartilage tissues. I like to keep some on hand in my home, office, purse, briefcase, and automobile. For more information, please refer to the Resource Directory.

The following are a few more products I have been taking for years.

ALL ONE: is a 100% pure multivitamin/mineral dietary supplement in powdered form that I've been taking for over 25 years. Every molecule is nutritive: a complete whole food with high-potency antioxidants, B-complex, chelated minerals, and a broad spectrum of vitamins and essential trace elements—all in optimal balance—including a complete profile of amino acids to ensure the proper assimilation of nutrients. Simply shake one tablespoon into your morning juice or water and you're done for the day. It assimilates and digests just like food. ALL ONE formulas contain no fillers or binders, and no sugars, sweeteners, or flavorings. When I need an extra dose of calcium or fiber, I use ALL ONE's formulation booster powders and mix them with the ALL ONE in juice or smoothies.

LIVING FOOD: created by SineQuaNon, Living Food is a superlative blend of powdered whole, fresh "living" organic foods, including flax seed, sunflower seeds, millet, quinoa, dulse, alfalfa leaf, nori, parsley, aloe vera, and barley grass. It contains enzymes, amino acids, chlorophyll, antioxidants, phytonutrients, and fiber, and is designed to be blended into a variety of convenient, nourishing, high energy recipes. It contains no additives, preservatives, colorings, dairy, yeast, gluten, sugar, salt, corn, wheat, or hydrogenated oils (trans fatty acids). I add this daily to my juices or smoothies, as you'll see in many of the recipes. I also use Living Cleanse and Living Enzymes. Living Cleanse helps purify the blood and cleanse the colon. The herbs in this formula, including organic milk thistle, organic Indian pennywort, and organic aloe vera, are nonabrasive and nonhabit-forming and provide a body purification without extensive lifestyle modifications. Living Enzymes helps to enhance enzyme reserves and intestinal fortitude. Like an inherited bank account, if we spend and never replace our resource metabolic enzymes, they will become depleted and eventually run out. The way we manage our enzymes has a direct effect on our energy, health, and longevity. For more information or free samples, refer to the Resource Directory.

An All-Natural Herbal Tonic

Bio-Strath is an easily absorbable whole food herbal yeast tonic that provides the body with 11 vitamins, 19 minerals, and 20 amino acids (including all the essential and branched chain amino acids), along with a variety of other immune enhancing co-factors. The beauty of Bio-Strath lies in one simple fact: It is completely natural. No chemicals, heat, or preservatives are used in making Bio-Strath.

Due to the structural similarity of the *Saccharomyces cerevisiae* yeast cell to that of the human cell, the nutrients present are in similar proportions to how they occur in our cells and are already in a bioavailable and metabolically active form. This readily allows our cells to absorb the nutrients they may be lacking and reach their natural state of balance known as homeostasis. When the body is in this balanced state, it is less susceptible to fatigue, illness, and lethargy.

Bio-Strath herbal yeast has NO relation to the parasitic strain of yeast known as *Candida albicans*, which is linked to a number of health problems. On the contrary, Bio-Strath is recommended to help boost vitality and immunity for people with candida overgrowth, and has been proven (via invitro studies) to neither provoke nor sustain a yeast infection: In fact, Bio-Strath herbal yeast inhibits candida growth (as well as many other microbes).

While many products claim to support the immune system, improve concentration and memory, fight fatigue, and boost physical efficiency, Bio-Strath has confirmed these benefits in over 35 clinical studies. It's also excellent for children, particularly those needing additional seasonal support or improvement of concentration levels. Furthermore, it has been proven to have a strengthening and revitalizing effect on senior citizens and pregnant women.

I've taken this superlative product for more than two decades and highly recommend it to everyone. It's available from natural foods stores or refer the Resource Directory.

SUCCESS

Chapter 7

SIMPLE WAYS TO DETOXIFY & REJUVENATE YOUR BODY & YOUR LIFE

Each patient carries his own doctor inside.
—Albert Schweitzer

I have learned never to underestimate the capacity of the human mind and body to regenerate—even when prospects seem most wretched. The life force may be the least understood force on earth.
—Norman Cousins

Steve hadn't seen a physician for several years. When his family, friends, or associates got the flu or a cold, he always stayed healthy. This was the story he related during one of my weekend seminars. But all of a sudden Steve's luck changed. A year earlier he caught a bad cold that stayed with him for a couple of weeks. Then a month later, he developed a sore throat that turned into a deep, wracking cough that lasted close to 3 months. Was it coincidence that his illnesses blossomed only a few months after a brief separation from his wife, along with dissatisfaction on the job?

Benjamin Franklin said, "Anything that hurts, instructs," so when you feel sick, it can be nature's way of getting your attention and letting you know when you need to make better choices. As I described in detail in Chapter 1, quite often illness, in one way or another, is related to stress. I know that I used to catch colds when I was under extra stress. I can also recall times when I have felt sure I would not get sick even though a virus was running rampant and almost everyone I knew had it. And I didn't. Perhaps you felt that you simply could not afford to get sick because of some commitment you wanted to keep. It was as if you asserted your will to keep going and your immune system cooperated.

The fact that you have control over your wellness and can choose to be healthy and functioning fully is the foundation of a new science that's rapidly gaining in popularity. Around the world immunologists, psychiatrists, endocrinologists, neuroscientists, microbiologists, and psychologists are bringing together their expertise in this new field called psychoneuroimmunology (PNI). PNI deals with all aspects of how the mind can affect the immune system's complex network of organs, vessels, and white blood cells. Research in this fascinating area indicates that the immune system, brain, and other vital body systems communicate with and influence one another.

Uncontrolled stress can have a detrimental impact on the immune system, suppressing its ability to fight disease. In other words, if you are chronically distressed or anxious or tense, these emotions may manifest themselves as arthritis, heart disease, a kidney ailment, asthma, even cancer. On the other hand, well-managed stress can help keep your immune system healthy. That is to say, if you are happy and well-adjusted, your body can maintain its disease-fighting forces at peak capacity.

The bottom line is this: Consciously choosing how you live your life and how you take care of mental or physical challenges is essential. I have an unshakable belief in the power of will, faith, and hope but at the same time, I recognize that one of the first steps to achieving and maintaining radiant health in body, mind, and spirit is by opening the channels for detoxification and rejuvenation.

For more than two decades, I've practiced holistic health and lifestyle counseling individually, with families, and in groups; some of my clients have major illnesses. My approach includes seeing the positive side of all circumstances, choosing to be in charge and to not feel hopeless, and of course, lots of laughter. These all help to rejuvenate and cleanse the body. Rather than sitting indoors, many of my sessions are conducted outside in nature, walking by the beach, hiking in the mountains, or sitting by a stream. Being in a peaceful, beautiful environment helps my clients feel peaceful inside, to let go of negative emotions, and to open themselves up to the spirit of life and the steps needed to bring about a healing and balance in their lives. During these sessions, I always talk about the importance of detoxification. Since the body reflects the spirit and the spirit reflects the mind, we must first start by cleansing and purifying the body. But no treatment will be successful without the patient's faith, hope, will, and positive attitude. As Albert Schweitzer once said, "We doctors do nothing. We only help and encourage the doctor within."

Our cells produce toxins naturally as the waste product of metabolism. In addition, bacteria, parasites, and yeasts in the body create more waste that we must eliminate. The Environmental Protection Agency estimates that in 1999, in the United States, 1.3 billion pounds of emissions were pumped into the air and 218 million pounds of industrial byproducts were emptied into surface waters. From there, pollutants get into our food.

Normally, the body does an efficient job of eliminating harmful substances. The channels of toxic elimination include the urine, stool, and mucus; in the breath we exhale (one of many reasons it's important to frequently breathe slowly and deeply); in the sweat that passes through our skin (yes, the skin is an organ, in fact it is the biggest organ of elimination). All of these exit routes for toxins depend on the liver, which usually does an excellent job. However, when it's overloaded—when you're stressed out, lack sleep, eat junk food, consume alcohol, caffeine, and sugar, live in a smoggy environment, etc.—these situations impair the liver's ability to function, slowing it down, which, in turn, leads to toxic build-up. This is acutely evident when the liver breaks down as a result of years of alcohol abuse.

There are several symptoms associated with toxic overload. These include fatigue, depression, irritability, muscle and joint pain, cardiovascular irregularities, sinus irritation, mental confusion, gastrointestinal tract irregularities, insomnia, headache, flu-like symptoms, sneezing, coughing, runny nose, allergic reactions, and a general negative attitude about life. I know what you're thinking: We've all had one of these symptoms at one time or another. So how do you know if you need to detox? Well, unless you live in a stress-free environment out in the country where the air is clean, eat all organic food with most or all of it raw, sauna daily, are at your perfect weight, and drink pure alkaline water along with organic fresh fruits and vegetable juices daily, chances are you need to find ways to detox.

Detox programs are very beneficial and you'll find a combination Detox/Rejuvenation retreat described in detail in Chapter 20. But in addition to making time for the occasional retreats, where you accelerate the process, it makes good sense to live day-to-day in a way that doesn't encourage a toxic build-up. Here are some of the best ways I know to detoxify and rejuvenate your body and your life.

Drink Your Way to Harmonious Health & Youthful Vitality

We've already discussed the salutary effects of water. Its importance to healing, health, and vitality can not be overestimated, and alkaline water has particular benefits for detoxifying and rejuvenating.

Without water, life does not exist. Before scientists look for any form of life on other planets, they first look for any sign of water. Over 70% of our body weight is water; which is about 10 gallons of water for a 120 pound person. We are bundles of water wrapped in skin standing on two feet.

Water is a strong solvent that carries many invisible ingredients: minerals, oxygen, nutrients, waste products, pollutants, etc. Inside the human body, blood (90% of which is water) circulates throughout the body distributing nutrients and oxygen, and collecting wastes and carbon dioxide. Every substance deep in our body was brought there by blood and can be carried out by blood. When a person loses 20 lbs. of weight through a diet program, that 20 lbs. of substance comes out of the body through urine, which is why any diet program requires drinking a lot of water. Many of you already know this. Unfortunately, doctors and other health professionals do not specify what kind of water to drink. You may think it's all the same, but some water is actually more effective than others in the function of carrying out waste products from the body.

Acid Water & Alkaline Water: A Brief Lesson in pH

Everybody knows that water is 2 hydrogen atoms to 1 oxygen atom, H_2O. (In real life, water molecules resemble more like $H_{12}O_6$, most of them forming a hexagonal structure and a small amount forming a pentagon shape, $H_{10}O_5$. A water molecule is heavy, that is why it stays in liquid form at room temperature.) At room temperature, 1 out of 10 million H_2O molecules is electrically split (ionized) into a hydrogen ion (H^+) and a hydroxyl ion (OH^-). This water is called neutral water and its pH value is said to be 7. The 7 denotes that there is one H^+ ion per 10^7 H_2O molecules. When substances are dissolved in the water, depending upon the substances, the water can have more H^+ ions than OH^- ions, and vice versa. Water with more H^+ ions is called acid water; water with more OH^- ions is called alkaline water. (The law of nature dictates that when H^+ ion density is 1 in 10^x power, the OH^- ion density is 1 in 10^{14-x}. The index of density for H^+ ion and that for OH^- ion always adds up to 14. For that reason, we only measure the hydrogen ion density and call it pH. When the pH is 7, the water is neutral; higher than 7 is alkaline, and lower than 7, acid.)

In a 10-oz glass of water, there are 10^{25} number of H_2O molecules: that is, 1 followed by 25 zeros. If that 10-oz glass of water has a pH value of 10, there are 10^{21} number of OH^- ions in that water, and the number of H^+ ions is 10^{15}, which is negligible compared to the number of OH^- ions. The following table compares the pH values and the number of H^+ ions and OH^- ions per 10-oz of these liquids:

	pH	H^+	OH^-
Popular brand cola	2.5	3.162×10^{22}	3.162×10^{13}
Diet soft drink	3.2	6.310×10^{21}	1.585×10^{14}
Popular brand beer	4.7	1.995×10^{21}	5.012×10^{15}
Distilled water	7.0	1.000×10^{18}	1.000×10^{18}
Bottled mineral water	7.8	1.585×10^{17}	6.310×10^{18}
High pH tap water	8.0	1.000×10^{17}	1.000×10^{19}
Alkaline water	10.0	1.000×10^{15}	1.000×10^{21}

Note that water with a pH value of 10 has 100 times more OH^- ions than water with a pH value of 8. This means that water with a pH value of 10 is 100 times more effective than water with a pH value of 8 in neutralizing acid radical H^+. (From the above chart, **we can see that it will take 32 glasses of pH 10 alkaline water to neutralize a glass of cola with a pH value of 2.5.**)

How We Age

When foods are eaten they are broken down into small nutrients and delivered to each and every cell in the body. These nutrients are burnt with oxygen in a slow, controlled manner to supply the necessary energy for us to function. After oxidation, these nutrients become waste products. Gourmet or junk food, *all* foods make waste products. The difference between healthy food and unhealthy food is the amount and kind of wastes produced: acid or alkaline. Human cells die in about four weeks: some regenerate and some are destroyed. Dead cells are waste products. All waste products must be discarded from the body, mostly through urine and perspiration. Most of these wastes are acidic, therefore when we excrete them our urine is acidic and our skin is acidic.

Most of us overwork, stay up late, and get up early, and stress ourselves to the limit without giving ourselves time to rest. We also like to eat meat and grain, and enjoy colas and other soft drinks, which are all highly acidic foods and drinks. Furthermore, the polluted environment kills our healthy cells, thus producing more acidic wastes. This means that we cannot get rid of 100% of the acidic wastes that we make daily; these leftover wastes are stored somewhere within our bodies.

Since our blood and cellular fluids must be slightly alkaline (pH value of 7.3 to 7.5) to sustain life, the body converts liquid acidic wastes into solid wastes. As long as these wastes are not dissolved in liquid, they do not influence the pH value of the liquid. Solidification of liquid acid wastes is the body's defense mechanism to survive. Some of these are: cholesterol, fatty acid, uric acid, kidney stones, phosphates, sulfates, urates, gallstones, etc., and they accumulate in many places throughout our body.

One of the biggest problems caused by the build up acidic wastes is the fact that *acid coagulates blood*; blood becomes thicker and clogs up the capillaries, which is why so many adult diseases require blood thinners as part of treatments. It is commonly known that degenerative diseases are caused by poor blood circulation. Where there is an accumulation of acidic wastes, and the local capillaries are clogged, any organ(s) in that area will not be getting an adequate blood supply, eventually leading to dysfunction of that organ(s).

The Connection Between Degenerative Diseases & Acidic Wastes

As we age, we accumulate more acidic wastes. Depending upon the individual, the storage places are different and we display different kinds of disease symptoms. Some of the diseases caused by excess acidic wastes, or the lack of alkalinity are:

Allergies	Arthritis	Asthma
Atherosclerosis	Cancer	Chronic diarrhea
Constipation	Diabetes	Fibromyalgia
Gallstones	Gout	Hangovers
Hay fever	Headaches	Heart disease
Hemorrhoids	High altitude sickness	High blood pressure
Hives	Hyperacidity	Indigestion
Kidney diseases	Kidney stones	Leg cramps
Morning sickness	Nausea	Neuralgia
Obesity	Osteoporosis	

Neutralizing Acid: The Importance of Alkaline Water

The fact that alkaline neutralizes acid is a basic natural phenomenon that requires no double blind test. Alkaline water has no nutritional or medicinal value; all it does is neutralize the acidic wastes in the human body and liquefy them for elimination by the kidneys. If you touch chicken or meat, your hands become sticky with fat. Washing the fat off your hands with regular tap water does not work unless you use soap. Soap liquefies the fat and makes it easier to clean. Fat is acid, soap is alkaline; same idea.

How to Make Alkaline Water

A water ionizer electrically splits regular tap water into alkaline and acid water. Connected to the faucet and plugged into the electrical outlet, it makes alkaline water instantly. One drawback is the fact that if the original tap water contains only small amounts of alkaline minerals, the alkalinity of the water would be very weak. Another drawback is the cost; prices range from about $900 to $1,300. (See Ionizer Plus® in the Resource Directory for the water purifier/ionizer I use and recommend.)

An alternative solution that I use and recommend is an inexpensive alkaline concentrate known as AlkaLife® that is added to ordinary drinking water. It contains a patented combination of minerals and will not upset the mineral balance in our body when consumed on a long-term basis. For more information, please refer to the Resource Directory.

The Connection Between Acidic Wastes & Pain

When we over-exert ourselves or are under severe stress, we create concentrations of acidic wastes in particular areas of the body too fast for the normal processes to disperse them. Because acid coagulates blood, the capillaries around the concentration get clogged, so blood cannot get into that area to carry out the wastes, causing pain that can last for a long time. We may take painkillers but they aren't removing the cause of the pain, only fooling the brain into thinking we don't feel it. When the effect of the medicine wears off, the pain returns and some of these medications can create negative side effects.

The only way to eliminate the cause of the pain is to disperse these concentrated wastes. An efficacious method for dispersing concentrated wastes is to use a localized far-infrared (FIR) heating pad near or on the area of pain. Far-infrared rays penetrate deep into the body; the heat expands the clogged up capillaries to allow warm blood to penetrate into the area and pull out the concentrated acids (such as lactic acid) and disperse them to a cooler area by blood circulation and heat transfer.

We commonly misunderstand that an inflamed area is hotter than the rest of the body, so we use an ice pack to bring the swelling down. Actually, the inflamed area is cooler than the rest of the body because blood is not circulating there. The only reason why the ice pack seems to work is by providing extreme cold to the affected area, the body tries to even out the temperature by forcing blood flow. However, since an ice pack does not help expand clogged up capillaries, it takes longer for the pain to subside than by using a FIR pad.

Hot baths and far-infrared sauna also help relieve pain, but because they heat the whole body, the process of heat transfer is slow. Massage, vibrators, and magnets can also help but since they do not contribute to the expansion of clogged up capillaries, their effectiveness is also slow. Alkaline water neutralizes acids but it cannot penetrate into the trapped areas. Once FIR heat pulls the acids out, alkaline water can then neutralize them and dispose of them safely through the kidneys. The Thermotex company manufactures FIR heating pads in various sizes. They are FDA-approved medical devices for pain relief. For a more detailed explanation of the relationship of acid/alkaline and diseases and the scientific explanation of the far-infrared technology, refer to the insightful book *Reverse Aging* by Sang Whang or to AlkaLife in the Resource Directory.

To sum up: Aging, degenerative diseases, and pain are all caused by poor blood circulation caused by the accumulation of acidic wastes, which coagulate blood, resulting in clogged up capillaries and even blocked arteries. Medicine cannot reduce the acid level to eliminate the fundamental cause of pain and diseases; it can only treat symptoms. Drinking alkaline water is the fastest and cleanest way to neutralize acidic wastes and help the body eliminate them safely. When the concentration of wastes in an area builds to the point of pain, we need the help of a far-infrared heating pad to disperse the concentration. If the wastes are not eliminated, they will accumulate somewhere else and accelerate the aging process. The double-prong attack of far-infrared heating pad and alkaline water is very effective for eliminating these problems.

Sleep Your Way to Harmonious Health & Youthful Vitality

There is nothing more restorative for your body than a good night's sleep, night after night after night. Consistent lack of sleep can lead to a variety of health problems including toxic build-up, weight gain and aging, depression, irritability and impatience, low sex drive, memory loss, lethargy, relationship problems, accidents, and at least 1,500 reported "drowsy driving" fatalities each year. Studies reveal that **driving on only 6 hours sleep is like driving drunk**. Cars are so cozy and comfortable these days and cruise control doesn't help. The instant you feel drowsy at the wheel of an automobile—when your eyelids get heavy—get off the road!

People are sleeping less now than they did a century ago, thanks to electric lighting, the shift to an urban, industrialized economy, not to mention late-night television. The result is a disruption of basic body metabolism. With workloads and daily stress increasing for many Americans, sleep issues loom larger than ever for both individuals and society.

The first doctor to observe REM (rapid eye movement) sleep back in the 1970s, Dr. William C. Dement, says that sleepy people are dangerous to themselves and others. The National Highway Traffic Safety Administration estimates that sleep deprivation plays a role in nearly 100,000 traffic accidents each year; it has also been cited as a leading cause of workplace mishaps and has contributed to such disasters as the Chernobyl nuclear reactor meltdown and the Exxon Valdez oil spill.

Let's take a brief look at sleep and how lack of it affects us as individuals and as a society.

Karine Spiegel and colleagues at the University of Chicago asked research participants to stay in bed just 4 hours per night for 6 nights, then 12 hours per night for the next 7 nights. When sleep deprived, blood sugars, cortisol, and sympathetic nervous system activity rose, and thyrotropin, which regulates thyroid function, fell. In other words, the results of this study show that chronic sleep deprivation forces the body into a fight-or-flight response, pushing blood sugars and other hormone-related functions out of kilter.

Higher cortisol levels, among other things, lead to memory loss, an increase in fat storage, and a decrease in muscle: the perfect combination if you want to lower metabolism and gain weight easily. But if you want to increase muscle mass, which is necessary to create a fit, lean body, you need at least 8 hours of sound sleep nightly to encourage muscle maintenance and growth and the release of the human growth hormone, which helps keep us youthful and strong. Put another way, sleeping more can make you slimmer.

Sleep deprivation may also accelerate the aging process. In the same Spiegel study, participants who only slept 4 hours per night for 1 week metabolized glucose 40% more slowly than usual, which is similar to the rate seen in elderly people. Glucose metabolism quickly returned to normal after getting a full night's sleep every night for a week.

So how do you know if you are sleep deprived? Dr. Dement says that if you become sluggish, drowsy, or fatigued, particularly after lunch or in the middle of the afternoon, you are sleep deprived. If you have difficulty getting up in the morning—one of my clients often sleeps through two alarms—you're sleep deprived.

Ninety-five percent of Americans suffer from a sleep disorder at some time in their lives and 60% suffer from some persistent sleep disorder, according to Dement's research. When it comes to sleep, he says, **most people require a minimum of 8 hours nightly**. Every hour you lose adds to your sleep indebtedness, and you cannot expect to catch up by sleeping late 1 day a week. The lost sleep accumulates progressively and contributes to long-term health problems. And this doesn't just pertain to adults. Children and teens actually need even more sleep than adults. Sleep loss affects how they learn, increases the chance of accidents, or depression, and violent or aggressive behavior.

Recognizing that many of us simply can't get to bed any earlier or get up any later, Dement recommends napping. A few enlightened businesses are adopting the pioneering view that napping actually can promote productivity. Some companies even provide special nap rooms for employees. Naps should be recognized as a powerful tool in battling fatigue.

However, if you have insomnia, naps can actually aggravate your night's sleep. By taking the edge off your sleepiness, an afternoon nap may make it even harder for you to get to sleep at night. In other words, if you are sleepy because of insomnia, napping should be *avoided*.

Naps are also *not* recommended after meals. It's natural to want to nap after eating because distention of the stomach from the meal increases the deep-sleep drive. The problem is that if you overeat, the digestive process may interfere with the *quality* of your sleep, and conversely, sleep may interfere with the digestive process. You are better off to allow digestion to occur *before* sleeping as both digestion and sleep tend to work better when performed separately.

5 Tips for Better Sleep

1. Morning exercise helps sleep at night: Exercise helps you sleep better but you don't want to engage in strenuous exercise too late at night because it accelerates the body's metabolic rate, which remains "revved up" for a few hours, making it tough to sleep. Morning exercise routines or, if you've got insomnia, exercising 4 hours before bedtime, will help you sleep much better.

2. *Increase evening body heat for deeper sleep:* Normally, your body temperature hits a peak 2 hours before bedtime. As your body temperature drops, melatonin is released and your body gets physiologically ready for sleep. The bigger the drop in temperature, the deeper the drop into deep sleep. People with insomnia do not have the normal drop in temperature so they aren't as ready for deep sleep. Heating the body up with exercise 4 hours before bedtime (to give it enough time for the adrenaline release caused by exercise to wear off) can assist the physiological drive into deep sleep. A hot bath 2 hours before bedtime or a sauna early in the evening can be helpful alternatives. This overall increased body temperature, with its accompanying big drop back to normal, helps promote sound, deep sleep.

3. *Make sure the bed is for sleep and sex only:* Avoid working, eating, or watching TV in bed. Reading until you fall asleep is okay but try to read inspirational, uplifting, or calming books. Here are some good nighttime reading suggestions: My book, *Choose to Live Peacefully,* has 40 short chapters that will uplift and inspire you, and put you in a positive, peaceful frame of mind as you drift off to sleep. You may also enjoy *The Promise of Sleep* by William C. Dement, M.D., *Power Sleep* by James B. Maas, Ph.D., and *Steve Martin: The Magic Years* by Morris Walker. Finally, I also highly recommend *Casandra's Angel* by Gina Otto.

4. *Create a conducive environment:* Sleep in natural fiber pajamas in a dark and quiet room, with fresh air and green plants. (I believe that all that extra oxygen from green plants promotes sound sleep.) A cool room and pillow are also helpful. You can place a zip-top bag filled with ice on top and remove it when you go to bed. Two or three drops of pure essential lavender oil on your pillow case promotes relaxation and calm. And of course, a good mattress and a few pillows are essential. When side sleeping, place a spare pillow between your legs, and under your knees when you're on your back. Avoid sleeping on your front side (stomach) as this can lead to severe lower back pain and wrinkles on your face.

5. *Don't eat too close to bedtime:* A big, spicy meal may cause sleep-inhibiting indigestion and excessive hunger will make you restless. Choose your evening meals wisely. Carbo-rich foods help send the amino acid tryptophan to the brain, which may induce sleep. Proteins inhibit tryptophan's journey to the brain, making you more alert. So if you are really hungry in the evening, after your dinner meal, choose a healthy carbohydrate snack instead of protein. Alcohol is a stimulant and blocks the restful sleep experienced during the REM cycle. Get a balance of minerals throughout the day, especially calcium, magnesium, and iron, because these have a sedative effect; deficiencies may keep you awake.

SWEET DREAMS!

Sunbathing Your Way to Radiant Health

The sun is the source of light and warmth and sustains our existence. It provides the energy for plants to photosynthesize the products necessary for growth. This energy is then stored in plants in the form of carbohydrates, proteins, and fats and is transferred to us upon consumption. In a sense, the cycle of life can also be called the cycle of light. Raw plant foods are so beneficial for us because we're taking life-giving sunlight into our bodies.

But the sun has also been getting a lot of bad press lately, and while baking in the sun is clearly not good for us, the latest research shows that short bouts of exposure without sun block may yield significant health benefits, from helping to prevent some cancers, to warding off depression, and increasing fitness and libido, lowering cholesterol, blood sugar, and blood pressure, to name only a few.

There seems to be conclusive evidence that sunlight produces a metabolic effect in the body that is very similar to physical training. Just 10 to 15 minutes in the sun, without sunscreen, 2 to 3 times per week, supplies 90% of the recommended dose of disease-preventing vitamin D, which is also needed for calcium absorption, and thus plays an important role in protecting against osteoporosis, bone fractures, and PMS. Preliminary findings further indicate that because vitamin D may affect mood, lack of sun may play a role in all types of depression—not just in the most serious seasonal-affective disorder, which tends to strike during winter months.

The sun/cancer link stems from research that found that women who live in the Northeast are 40% to 60% more likely to die from breast cancer than those who live in "sunnier" West Coast or southern areas. A new study by epidemiologist Esther John, Ph.D., at the Northern California Cancer Center, suggests that the incidence of cancer has as much to do with geography as with behavior: She found that women who either lived in the South or said that they were frequently outdoors were 30% to 40% less likely to develop breast cancer than women who didn't fit that profile. Other research indicates that sunlight may help prevent prostate and colon cancers as well.

Experts attribute the lower risk to high levels of vitamin D, which the body produces when UVB rays penetrate the skin. Most of us don't get enough of this nutrient through diet alone. "If you live in the north, or are indoors a lot, you're at a greater risk for being vitamin D-deficient," says Susan Thys-Jacobs, M.D., director of the Osteoporosis Center at St. Luke's Roosevelt Hospital, in New York.

Recent evidence reveals that sunlight also stimulates the thyroid gland to increase hormone production, which increases metabolism, which means you'll burn up more energy or calories.

When sunlight strikes the skin, it also increases the tone of the muscles under the exposed skin which, in turn, burns more calories to increase weight loss.

I have practiced safe sunning for 30 years. You'll see in Chapter 20 that it's also part of the 7-Day Rejuvenation program. Of course, *baking* in the sun is still not advisable, and morning and afternoon are better times to bask in the sun, especially during the summer. If you're in the sun longer than 20 to 30 minutes, apply a sunscreen with an SPF of 15 or above. But for those 10 to 20 minute sessions a few times a week, expose as much of your body to the sun as possible. If you can sunbathe "au naturel," do it, as you'll reap more benefits of increased vitamin D and sex hormones when more skin is exposed.

Sweating Your Way to Radiant Health

For thousands of years, people have enjoyed the therapeutic benefits of saunas, from the elaborate bath/sauna/exercise complexes of the ancient Romans, to the simple but effective sweat lodge structures of the Scandinavians and Native Americans.

Sweating is not only an important part of our physical well-being, but in this world full of water and airborne pollution, toxic chemicals, heavy metals, and poor dietary and exercise habits, the therapeutic internal cleansing of regular sweating is critical to maintain a healthy body and mind.

The hot, dry air of the sauna is therapeutically different from the steam room: The dry sauna causes profuse sweating, with the air itself absorbing the sweat, but the water-saturated air of the steam room doesn't readily accept the sweat released by the body. The steam room makes you feel hotter because your sweat doesn't evaporate and carry away the heat, which raises a question: Is it better to be warm on the inside or sweaty on the outside?

That depends on what you want from either system. When exposed to heat of any kind, blood vessels in the skin dilate and allow more blood to flow to the surface activating the millions of sweat glands that cover the body. The fluid in the blood hydrates the sweat glands, which pour the water that we know as sweat out into the skin's surface. As the water evaporates from the skin, it draws heat from the body. It's nature's cooling system.

Either the sauna or the steam room can be used to relax and unwind, but the dry sauna clearly has more therapeutic benefits. By causing the sweat to evaporate and get carried away, the dry sauna helps the kidneys rid the body of more toxic metals picked up from the environment.

If you want to lose weight, the sauna is more beneficial than the steam room because it places a greater demand on the body in terms of using up calories. Because the heart has to work harder to send more blood to the capillaries under the skin, the energy required for that process is derived from the conversion of fat and carbohydrates to calories. The sweat glands must also work to produce sweat, which requires energy and more calories. A person can burn up to 300 calories during a sauna session, the equivalent of a 2- to 3-mile jog or an hour of moderate weight training.

Don't forget that sweating can be very dehydrating. You can lose up to a quart of water during a 20-minute sauna. Without replacement, such a high water loss can lead to disruption of normal heart rhythms, and cause fatigue and nausea. I recommend drinking fresh juice or water before, during, and after the sauna. Any attempt to lose weight by depriving your body of replacement fluid is extremely risky and can land you in the hospital on i.v. fluids. I also suggest eating plenty of leafy greens and a variety of other vegetables to replace essential minerals such as iron, zinc, copper, and magnesium that are lost in sweat.

Sweating by overheating the body in a dry sauna has a number of beneficial effects: It speeds up metabolic processes of vital organs and inhibits the growth of pathogenic bacteria or virus. The vital organs and glands, including endocrine and sex glands, are stimulated to increased activity.

The immune system is strengthened by creating a "fever" reaction that kills potentially dangerous viruses and increases the number of leukocytes in the blood, which is important for fighting colds, flu, and even cancer, and for bolstering resistance to infections and allergies. Sweating increases and accelerates the body's own healing and restorative capacity. It also produces a drop in diastolic blood pressure by making the heart pump harder. Dry heat also stimulates vasodilation of peripheral vessels, which relieves pain and speeds healing of sprains, strains, bursitis, peripheral vascular diseases, arthritis, and muscle pain. And finally, a daily sauna promotes relaxation, thereby lending a feeling of well-being.

We now know that to maintain a healthy body and mind, everyone needs to regularly eliminate and flush out the toxins that accumulate in their bodies. Athletes experience this through sweating. Those of us who are unable to exercise heavily for whatever reason need to create a regular sweat and daily (or at least a few weekly) saunas is the best method of doing this.

The Best Sauna for Home or Office

Many health clubs and hotels have saunas, and if they're all you've got, use them. But I don't want to sit in a public sauna where countless other people have been sweating out their toxins. This may sound crazy, but a personal sauna could be the most important investment you can make in your own health. I attribute the fact that I haven't been sick in years to the fact that I have been taking several saunas a week.

After years of research into portable saunas, the ones I use—and the best ones on the market—are made by Heavenly Heat and Finnleo, the world's leaders in saunas. Please refer to the Resource Directory for more information

Massage: The Healing Touch

Skin is the human body's largest organ, accounting for 19% of our body weight and covering approximately 20 square feet depending on our size. From the ancient Greek gymnasium and Roman baths to modern day spas and health clubs, massage has been recognized for its health enhancing effects. This age-old healing practice has enjoyed a renaissance in the last quarter century. Today, massage is a flourishing art form.

From infancy to old age, massage enhances general health and well-being. I've been getting massages for the past 25 years, and for me it's the equivalent of a long nap, in terms of refreshment. Not only does it calm my nerves, release stress, and make me glow from the inside out, it energizes my body in a way that makes me feel youthful.

Therapeutic massage has many applications, variations, and techniques. Many of the therapeutic effects of massage recognized by personal and clinical experience over the years have been supported by scientific research. In addition to the commonly known benefits of relaxation and stress relief, new applications for therapeutic massage are surfacing in areas related to mental and emotional well-being, infant care, aging, athletics, and other special situations. Exciting new discoveries link touch, and therapeutic massage, to over-all body rejuvenation/detoxification and improved immune system function.

Therapeutic massage reduces stress and tension, improves circulation, relieves muscle spasms, helps to rid the body of toxins and retained fluids, and improves the skin. In terms of weight loss, the person massaging you is burning more calories than you are, but as your stress is massaged away your hormones will be more balanced, which aids in fat reduction. Some people claim it aids in cellulite reduction. While I've never seen any good studies to prove that, I have seen impressive results in clients. Best of all, I know that massage feels terrific.

Science is now confirming that massage is good medicine. Dr. Diana J. Wilkie, associate professor at the University of Washington School of Nursing, is a nationally recognized pain researcher. Together with her colleagues, Wilkie has documented the intensity of pain (as well as the pulse and respiratory rates) of hospice residents with cancer, before and after they received massage therapy. Wilkie's group found that massage therapy provided immediate relaxation as well as pain relief. Their study results will be used to help plan a larger study of massage therapy as a means of relieving cancer pain and stress.

The University of Miami's School of Medicine opened what they call "the first institution in the world for basic and applied research on the sense of touch"—The Touch Research Institute (TRI). More than 50 TRI studies have shown massage to have positive effects on conditions from colic to hyperactivity to diabetes to migraines—in fact, on every malady TRI has studied thus far. Their projects have included researching the impact of massage on immune functioning in AIDS and cancer patients, the effects of touch on patients with addictions, and the effects of touch on physical and emotional development. TRI staff collaborates with researchers at several universities, including Miami, Duke, and Harvard and reports some impressive results: Premature "crack babies," each given 3 fifteen-minute massages a day for 10 days, suffered fewer complications, displayed markedly more mature motor behavior, and gained an astounding 28% in weight by the end of the 10 days. Abused children living in a shelter become more sociable and active with regular massage. Preschoolers were more focused when given massages, and adult office workers were more alert when given regular massages. HIV-positive males who received 5 massages a week for a month showed improved immune function and significantly reduced anxiety and stress.

Based on all their empirical research, TRI worries that Americans aren't getting enough touch, especially with growing concerns about sexual harassment and abuse in school and workplaces. Even in preschools, touch has become taboo. (The National Education Association, which represents 2 million teachers, sums the matter up in a slogan: teach, don't touch.) "The implications for children involve significant effects on their growth, development and emotional well-being," observes psychologist Tiffany Field, staff director at TRI. She says America is suffering from an epidemic of "skin hunger" and talks about a "dose of touch" as if it were a vitamin. I would agree.

Variations

There are many types of massage. The best way to discover your favorite massage styles is to try a variety of techniques and decide for yourself.

SWEDISH is a classic, relaxing and soothing, yet stimulating massage. It's the one I recommend if you are new to massage.

ACUPRESSURE is a traditional healing treatment developed in China, consisting of pressing on certain points related to all parts of the body and to different health problems. For example, the Chinese claim that a toothache can be relieved by pressing certain points underneath the eyes.

Shiatsu is a more modern version of acupressure, developed in Japan. In this form, the ball of the thumb is usually used. Refer to the Shiatsu-Aid Massage Board in the Resource Directory.

POLARITY THERAPY is said to be derived from yogic and spiritual practices in India. Often, the therapist's hands are held far apart while applying pressure and rocking motions to specific 'poles of energy' in the body.

TRAGER massage usually involves vibratory and shaking motions, and, like Polarity, may be performed while the recipient is clothed.

ZONE THERAPY or FOOT/HAND REFLEXOLOGY is not really a complete massage because only the feet or hands are treated. Its practitioners believe that every part of the body is mapped into a specific area of the feet and hands, and that by massaging the hands or feet only, effective benefits are obtainable. For example, the technique claims to affect remote parts, such as the eyes, by massaging the junction between the second and third toes.

REICHIAN massage is intended to break down 'body armor,' which is said to be formed as a defense against releasing emotions and built-up tensions. Much attention is paid to breathing and verbal analysis.

PROSKAUER massage also works with breathing, and is usually

light and subtle. The more advanced techniques such as deep tissue and lymph massage and Rolfing should not be attempted by people not specially trained in these methods. It is important for the masseuse not to work beyond his or her understanding.

AROMATHERAPY massage utilizes different essential oils extracted from plants, many of which are effective for everything from bacteria fighters to mind and body relaxers. Aromatherapy massage is my favorite way to relieve stress. Some of my favorite pure essential oils include rose, lavender, chamomile, sandalwood, lemon, sage, rosemary, and eucalyptus (also great used in the sauna).

- Lavender, one of the most versatile essential oils, has relaxing and anti-inflammatory properties. It eases tension and headaches, and promotes restful sleep. I put a couple drops on my pillow most nights before bedtime.

- Lemon is an uplifting antimicrobial oil that revitalizes the skin and adds a freshness to any oil blend.

- Rose, sometimes called the queen of essential oils, is a calming oil. This gentle antiseptic is also beneficial for dry and aging skin.

- Rosemary oil has astringent properties and increases circulation and relieves muscle pain.

- Peppermint oil relieves nausea and indigestion and offers an invigorating wake-up when you're feeling foggy and less than energetic.

For best results, choose high-quality essential oils extracted with pure steam or a nontoxic oil; avoid essential oils extracted with industrial solvents like hexene. (You may need to call the manufacturer to find this out.) Most essential oils must be diluted before you apply them to your skin. Pregnant women should avoid most essential oils (rose, lavender, and peppermint are fine).

To make a simple, skin-softening, essential oil aromatherapy rose facial mask, add 2 drops rose oil to 1/4 cup of thick, plain yogurt. Apply to a clean face, massage in for a couple of minutes, then wait 15 minutes, and rinse with tepid water, ending with cold. You can also do this with lavender oil or a combination of lavender, rose, chamomile, and yogurt.

More Closeness & Intimacy

Massage is also an excellent way to become comfortable being touched by another person. This may sound elementary, but for many, being touched in a nonsexual, caring fashion is not a part of our daily lives.

Massage is an ideal way to express one's love and caring for another person through the hands. To be touched lovingly, without feeling like someone is trying to excite you, can create a great deal of trust and intimacy. One of the most frequent complaints I hear from women is that they don't get enough nonsexual touching and caressing. Massage is not only a wonderful way to receive that healing, rejuvenating touch, but also a way to teach your partner how you like to be touched.

14 Tips for Getting the Most from Your Massage

1. **Get a good, adjustable massage table** to eliminate some of the bending and stooping as you work so if you are giving a massage, your own back is less likely to get tired. My favorite table and the one I use and recommend is by Golden Ratio (see the Resource Directory). It will make it easy to change positions around the person being massaged without a break in the flow of your massage.

2. **Try to make the room as quiet and comfortable as possible.** Any outside noise and bustle can be extremely disconcerting, so dim the lights, and play some tranquil, soothing music or have it quiet.

3. **Make sure the massage room is warm enough,** ideally about 70°F or even slightly higher, and free of drafts.

4. **It is insignificant whether you start at the top or bottom of the body.** As long as you have some methodical way of covering every part of the body that is to be massaged, the massage will be complete with no obvious omissions.

5. **Allow the person being massaged to choose whether to first lie face down or face up.** It's helpful to have a clock or watch within view so that various areas of coverage can be timed. If you are giving a 30-minute massage, ask the receiver to turn

over after 15 minutes. During all phases of the massage, check your posture and make adjustments for any difficulties you are experiencing.

6. **Make sure that you feel good before you work on another person.** If you are rundown physically or emotionally, you should be receiving, not giving.

7. **Make sure the person being massaged is relaxed and comfortable before you begin.** Massage therapist Jackie Day in Bandon, Oregon, says, "I think draping is necessary most of the time, except if you know someone very well. Never assume that because you are 'dressed' friends you are also 'undressed' friends. Issues of abuse, boundaries, sexuality, being able to say what your needs are, and self-image can all arise." Day suggests telling a person to take off as much as they are comfortable taking off. Not everyone feels relaxed or safe when nude, which are primary considerations in therapeutic massage.

8. **Fingernails should be trimmed as short as possible and filed smooth,** otherwise acupressure becomes acupuncture! Remove all jewelry. Avoid loose clothing or long hair that will trail over the body. The recipient should also remove contact lenses and jewelry.

9. **Ask about cuts, bruises, recent scars, or other injuries to avoid touching these spots.** Find out which areas are the most tense so you can concentrate on them. If in doubt, wait until after a physician has been consulted before massaging. If there are any serious medical problems such as cancer or heart disease, check with a physician before proceeding.

10. **Deep tissue work is contraindicated in the elderly;** however, gentle massage can be most beneficial. Be very careful with senior citizens who bruise more easily, with bruises that can last for weeks. Atherosclerosis is a common condition among senior citizens so care must be taken to stay away from the carotid arteries located on each side of the neck.

11. **Be sure to establish a communication code for pain.** You'll want to apply pressure to the edge of pain, not past it. Ask the person to say 'good' when the pressure is best and don't press any harder.

12. **Make sure your center of gravity (two inches below the navel) is directly over the area you are massaging,** whenever possible. Position yourself right next to the body part you are massaging and move your entire body, not just your hands. Let your legs—not your lower back—support and move you.

13. **If your have never given or received a massage, see what feels good to you:** fast or slow, soft or hard? Try massaging your own body parts that you can reach comfortably without straining. A good area for practicing on yourself, as well as your first attempts with another person, is the foot.

14. **There are many excellent books and video tapes available on massage,** which you might wish to consult before you begin practicing on yourself or someone else. (See Golden Ratio in the Resource Directory.)

Getting Started

If you are new to massage, before you give someone else a partial or full massage, experience a few yourself. I also recommend reading a book or two on the subject and perhaps watching some videos on massage and how to do it.

For couples or for others sharing the same life and home, the 10-minute massage can open the door to something extraordinary: doing massage together every day. Even 10 minutes a day sounds hard if your life is a busy one until you get in the habit of it. Consider making it one of your 21-day agreements (see Chapter 2). **Nothing else in the world requiring so little effort will as effectively change (over the course of time) the mood and tempo of your entire life.** And what could be a nicer gift for someone you love, a gift that keeps on giving. With loving intentions, your therapeutic touch can truly be a rejuvenative, magical one.

Naturally Beautiful Skin

The skin is the largest single organ of the body and comes in many colors, textures, and patterns. Imagine a material that is waterproof, yet can let out water and oil, that can protect like a suit of armor, and yet is infinitely sensitive to touch, that remains strong yet penetrably flexible. It is also a beautiful material—whether pink and white, brown, yellow, or black.

It's amazing to think that all we ever see of one another—and the basis of so many of our judgments about each other—is skin surfaces and hair. The skin is continually growing from within, creating new cells that push their way outward. The skin on the palm of your hand renews every 24 hours, your face every 7 days, and on the rest of your body every 30 days. Yet the skin, perhaps more than any other part of the body, tells the world how we feel mentally and physically as well as how we care for and respect our bodies. American Indians used to diagnose body ailments by the lines in the face.

The skin of an adult covers a surface area of about 18 to 21 square feet. Weighing in at approximately 6 pounds, the skin is about $1/8$ of an inch thick, varying at different areas of the body. It is well supplied with a variety of glands, blood vessels, and nerves, and consists of three distinct layers: the epidermis (which is composed of four sublayers), the dermis, and the subcutaneous fat. The dermis layer relies on the protein collagen to keep it in mint condition by acting as a supporter and major building block of the skin. Elastin, another protein, gives the skin its supple elastic quality.

In an average square inch of skin, there are approximately 200 blood and lymph vessels, more than 100 oil glands, over 650 sweat glands, 28 motor nerves, 13 sense receptors for cold, 78 for heat, 1,300 tactile receptors, and 65 hairs, plus millions of independent cell forms. Isn't that amazing?

Functions of the Skin

Two million pores cover the body's surface and function together as an efficient cooling system. Exercise can raise internal temperature up to 7 degrees above normal. The body dissipates that excess heat through perspiration, which evaporates on the skin.

Besides cooling and protecting the body, the skin also serves as a sense organ. The fetus probably receives most sensations through the skin. From the moment of birth, humans require touching and physical affection as much as food.

Yet, what is so remarkable to me is that no two people on earth have identical skin formation—not even twins—as demonstrated in the science of finger printing. The skin is an organ of amazing complexity, which we are only beginning to understand. Believe it or not, we know more about the brain than the skin.

In a previous section, I wrote about how small amounts of sun are beneficial for your skin. The sun is the body's most effective, efficient, and least expensive source of vitamin D, appropriately termed the "sunshine" vitamin because the action of the sun's ultraviolet rays activates a form of cholesterol, which is present in the skin, converting it to vitamin D. Most of the body's needs for vitamin D can be met by sufficient exposure to sunlight and from eating small amounts of certain foods, such as sprouted seeds, mushrooms, and sunflower seeds.

On the other hand, many people still feel that a deep, golden tan is the mark of the leisure class, portraying health and beauty. The sun does have some beneficial effects, such as clearing up acne, relaxing tired muscles, and creating a positive psychological effect, but too much of this good thing can be the skin's worst enemy.

According to Lisa Ray, of the Sylvia Skin Care Salon in Brentwood (Los Angeles), "Overexposure to the sun can break down the collagen and elastin components of the skin, causing loss of moisture, flexibility and tautness. The best proof of this is to observe the skin after a few years of constantly maintaining a suntan, as I see with some of my clients. Now they come to me to ask what can be done to improve the quality of their skin as a result of sun damage." Ray teaches her renowned clientele how to restore and maintain youthful, healthy skin at any age.

Beautifying Your Skin

Besides using common sense when it comes to sun exposure, here are a few more proven tips you can use to rejuvenate and revitalize your skin.

DRY SKIN BRUSHING is one of the best ways to create beautiful skin all over your body. It's been popular in Europe for decades and is finally beginning to catch on here. Not only does it improve the appearance of your skin, giving you a healthy glow, but it also helps your body eliminate toxins. As your biggest eliminative organ, when the skin is dry-brushed, it assists in sloughing off the dead skin cells that lie on the skin's surface. This enables toxins to be released more efficiently.

Look for a dry brush at your local natural food store or bath and beauty supply store. Make sure it has natural bristles (as opposed to nylon or other synthetics) and a long handle so you can reach all those hard-to-get places on your body. You want to start off very gently for the first couple of weeks until your skin gets used to it.

Brush in circular motions, always moving toward the heart. If you have patches of eczema, skin eruptions, or any other skin condition, avoid brushing the affected areas. Also, avoid brushing the face. Try this process of dry brushing daily (do it before you shower or bathe) and you'll see and feel a difference before the first week is up.

Try combining dry skin brushing with regular saunas. You'll be amazed at how invigorated you feel.

EXERCISE improves circulation throughout the body and creates an increase in body heat. Heat draws blood into the skin surface increasing dermal capillary circulation. And with a greater blood flow to the capillaries of the skin comes more nourishment and better complexion. Your skin benefits from most types of heat: saunas, exercise, aromatherapeutic baths, and massage.

SLEEP is not only good for overall health, as discussed above, it is imperative for healthy skin. Like so many other organs, the skin regenerates and heals most effectively while we sleep, so getting adequate sleep will help keep your skin healthy and beautiful.

DIET is also essential for healthy skin. Nutrients in plant-based foods nourish the skin and provide all the elements necessary to keep skin looking youthful. Not only do these fiber-rich foods help keep the digestion system moving smoothly, but they are also rich in antioxidants—like vitamins C and E, various carotenoids, and flavonoids—all beneficial to the skin. Eating an antioxidant-rich diet also bolsters our protection against disease.

WATER is as important as diet to keep your skin healthy. In fact, you'll see a difference in the appearance of your skin in less than 3 days if you drink at least a half gallon (64 ounces) of purified water daily (use 2 drops of AlkaLife in five of the glasses of water). I usually drink at least 80 ounces of water daily, and even more if I work out for more than 2 hours that day. Increased water consumption will make your skin softer, smoother, and even more toned. When you fly, take a small bottle of Evian mist and spray your skin every 15 minutes. The spray mist will refresh your skin and increase the spirit-lifting negative ions around you. You'll arrive at your destination with a healthy glow and more positive attitude, especially if your bring your own fruits and vegetables to eat while flying.

VITAMIN C is one of your skin's best friends. Collagen and elastin, which are two of the building blocks of the skin, are only made by the fibroblast cells with the use of vitamin C. Sags, bags, droops and puckers, blotches and spider veins are signs of vitamin C deficiency in the skin. You can apply vitamin C directly to your skin (it comes in lotions, creams, serums, and oils) and should also ingest it.

Living a stress-filled life increases your need for vitamin C. Excellent sources include oranges, strawberries, tomatoes, grapefruit, and dark green leafy veggies. I also keep Emer'gen-C packets (see Resource Directory) with me all the time to add to my water or juice so I get an ample amount of the best form of vitamin C: as mineral ascorbates.

POSITIVE ATTITUDE and MEDITATION bring more vitality to our lives by reducing stress, anxiety, depression, and pain. Scientists are finding that meditation also helps keep us wrinkle-free and healthy. One study showed that people who had been meditating for more than 5 years were biologically 12 to 15 years younger than non-meditators. It reduces tension in the body and helps foster a positive attitude. (For more information on how to meditate, refer to my book-on-tape, *Wired to Meditate: Making the Connection with Your Divine Source* and my book *Choose to Live Peacefully*.)

Surround Yourself with Beauty

An essential part of rejuvenating your body and life is to surround yourself with beauty to feed your soul. Spending as much time as possible out in nature, breathing in the negative ions from the natural environment (such as by an ocean, lake, or stream, or in the mountains), will lift your spirit and bring you a sense of peace.

Make your home a sanctuary. Whether you live in a mansion or a studio apartment, a country house or a trailer, there are countless things you can do to enrich the quality of your environment. Don't feel compelled to fill up all the spaces. Space is a luxury and having pure space will give some of you a serene feeling, like a refreshing walk in the country.

Fill your spaces with things that give you joy and peace—fresh flowers and plants, natural baskets, light, beautiful colors on your walls, and great fragrances. You don't have to have lots of money to create a sanctuary. Maybe all you need to do is paint a room, bring in some fresh plants, wash your windows, or clean out some closets! When you decorate your home, don't settle for someone else's taste. Your home should be your sanctuary and express your feelings, emotions, and imagination. Think about the location, furnishings, and decorations so they satisfy you emotionally and express your soul's individuality.

And don't forget to have a room, or a corner of a room that's just for you—a meditation area, a sacred place, where you visit daily to turn within to find the peace of your own company.

Yes, it's wonderful to be out in nature and to delight in her beauty. But you don't have to be in nature to see beauty all around you. If you keep your thoughts high and your heart pure, you will see beauty all around you everyday. You can see beauty in your work, while driving, when visiting or talking with others, and in even the most common things. When your heart is filled with love, or God, beauty is your constant companion.

Love, Honor & Respect Yourself

The final aspect of rejuvenating your body and life, which really ought to be at the top of the list, is to celebrate your magnificence. Love, honor, and respect yourself and your life. You are one special being born from the joining of one sperm out of approximately 500 million, and one egg. You are already a winner, a divine being comprised of a body, mind, and spirit. You already have everything you need to live your highest potential, to live fully.

It starts with taking loving care of yourself. Cherish, love, and respect your body temple unconditionally no matter what its current shape. If you'd like to make some change, make that commitment today. The information in this book is designed to help you begin and maintain a healthy lifestyle.

Never put yourself down or tolerate any kind of abuse. Never think or say anything negative about yourself. Trust yourself and tune into the inner voice that really knows what's best for you—that loving guidance that's always there to support and guide you. Let go of your dependence on external things. Turn to the inner knowledge of your own Higher Self, the light within. Meditation is the best way I know to feel the inner connection with the Divine. Take a few minutes every day and practice loving yourself, tuning into the loving light within, and honoring your divinity. Breathe deeply. Practice and live with great reverence. That's how you honor yourself and God. Remember: **When you are loving yourself, by taking care of yourself and living a balanced life, you are loving God.**

And from this day forward, think of your body in a new light. Realize that it's a magnificent temple and deserves the best life has to offer. When you live with this awareness, it is much easier to choose to live a wellness lifestyle, and when you do, you will find that your body responds favorably and every aspect of your life is enriched.

Part II:

SAVORY RECIPES

Chapter 8

JUICES & SMOOTHIES

Juicing is one of the easiest, most efficient, and delicious ways to ensure you're meeting your daily produce quota (remember, I recommend 7 to 12 servings per day). Fresh juices or a smoothie can serve as a meal or a snack or something you can eat quickly when you don't have much time. While I don't advise eating on the run—it's terrible for the digestion—I know we all have to do it sometimes, but we don't need to eat poorly just because we're eating quickly! I've been drinking fresh juices for nearly 30 years. In fact I make a habit of doing a weekly "juice fast" to give my digestive system a rest, and I always wake up the next day feeling more energetic, lighter, and more positive.

When shopping for produce, go for organic whenever possible and choose the freshest fruits and vegetables possible. If you can't buy organic, make sure to wash your produce well. Even if you buy organic, you'll want to be sure to rinse your vegetables to get rid of stray dirt. While there are a variety of produce washes available in natural food stores and supermarkets, you can also make your own. Here's my recipe:

Produce Wash

Fill your sink with cold water, add 4 tablespoons of salt and the juice of a lemon. Soak the fruits and vegetables for 10 minutes, then rinse under cold water. You can also substitute 1/4 cup of white vinegar for the lemon.

After your produce is washed, all you need to do is cut it into pieces to fit the size of your juicer or blender and you're ready to roll. I am a big fan of the Green Life® Juicer, which is manufactured by the Tribest Corporation. (For more information, see the Resource Directory.)

Before I prepare fresh juices, whether fruit or vegetable based, if I know I will drink a glass right away, I usually drink a glass of water first. Doing this gives me the diluting benefits of a chaser (dilutes the concentrated fruit sugars) but allows me to drink my juices full strength, which means I get the full flavor and all the nutritional benefits.

Make sure you sip slowly and don't gulp down your juice. Try using beautiful goblets and glasses that you've kept frozen in the freezer. The chilled glass helps keep the juice cool and adds a touch of simple elegance.

Weight Loss Express

Serves 1 to 2

This easy-to-prepare, delicious juice supercharges metabolism, helps normalize body chemistry, and rejuvenates skin because it supplies an abundance of synergistically balanced nutrients that the cells can use immediately to energize the body. If you like carrot juice, you'll love this weight loss special.

1 medium apple, peeled and quartered
2 large or 3 medium carrots, cut to juicer size
2 stalks celery
3 inches cucumber, peeled and halved
1/2 cup parsley, stems and tops
1/2 small lemon with peeling, if organic
1 to 2 inches fresh ginger
1 to 2 tablespoons Living Food powder (see Resource Directory)

Juice all produce ingredients, blend in the powder, and serve.

Strawberry Citrus Deluxe

Serves 1 to 2

This fruit juice blend is as beautiful to look at as it is delicious to drink. Enjoy it any time of day.

1 ruby red grapefruit, outer skin peeled (leaving pithy part on) quartered

2 tangerines, cut in half

1 orange, quartered

6 large strawberries, green tops included

1/4 inch fresh ginger (optional)

Juice all ingredients and serve.

• **F Y I**

Strawberries

Strawberries are a good source of vitamins A and C, beta carotene, folic acid, and potassium. They are also anti-cancer, antiviral, and antibacterial.

Top of the Morning

Serves 1 to 2

If you don't have much time for breakfast but want a healthy start to the day, this vegetable and fruit combination fits the bill. I've enjoyed this drink several times each week for three decades.

3 medium carrots

1 apple

1 large stalk celery

1 stalk broccoli, with florets

1/3 cup parsley

1/4 sweet bell pepper (orange, red, or yellow)

1/2 small beet (scrubbed)

1/4 lemon wedge with peeling, if organic

1/4-inch piece of ginger

Juice all the ingredients, and serve.

Calcium Cooler

Serves 1 to 2

This juice is bright green and has a super-fresh taste. It's not only a great source of calcium, but it is loaded with the antioxidant power of the leafy greens.

3 organic green apples

2 medium leaves kale

1 stalk broccoli with florets

4 large leaves spinach, washed well (dirt loves to cling to spinach)

3 sprigs fresh mint

1/4 wedge lemon with peeling, if organic

Juice all the ingredients, and serve.

• F Y I

Apples

Apples are a super health food. They help to relieve constipation, reactivate beneficial gut bacteria, reduce total cholesterol, and help detoxify the body.

Carotene Cocktail

Serves 2

3 medium carrots

1 large red apple

1 large ripe tomato, quartered

1/2 yellow, red, or orange sweet bell pepper

1/2 cup baby spinach

1/4 cup parsley

1/4 wedge lemon with peeling, if organic

1/4-inch piece fresh ginger

Juice all the ingredients together, and serve.

• F Y I

Ginger

Ginger has a long and honored tradition in folk medicine. Some of its benefits include preventing motion sickness, quelling nausea and morning sickness, and relieving menstrual cramps. It's also great for improving circulation, which is one of the reasons I add it to many of my juices. To help relieve the chills and congestion of a cold, you can make ginger tea by simmering one or two slices of fresh ginger root in a few cups of water for 10 minutes. I like to add a pinch of cinnamon and a few drops of fresh lemon juice for piquancy.

Tropical Fruit Cocktail

Serves 1 to 2

This colorful juice helps reduce inflammation in addition to providing vitamin C, calcium, magnesium, and potassium.

2 cups pineapple (peeled, if not using the Green Life or Green Power Juicers or if not using an organic pineapple)

1 ruby red grapefruit (peel the outer skin but leave pithy part on)

2 firm kiwi, peeled

4 strawberries with green tops

Juice all the ingredients together, and serve.

• F Y I

Pineapple

Pineapple contains bromelain, a potent digestive enzyme that scavenges bacteria and parasites. Rudy red grapefruit has more beta carotene than pink or white grapefruit.

Berry–Cherry Zing

Serves 1 to 2

Believe me, it's worth the time it takes to pit the cherries for this recipe.

30 cherries, pitted
3 red apples
1 cup fresh blueberries
1 cup strawberries, tops removed

Juice all the ingredients together, and serve.

• **F Y I**

Cherries

Cherries are excellent sources of calcium, phosphorus, and vitamin C. Blueberries also provide vitamin C and are an excellent laxative, improve circulation, benefit eyesight, and have antioxidant and anti-bacterial properties.

Energizing Tonic

Serves 2

This spicy drink stimulates circulation and helps rev up metabolism by creating heat and energy. I usually double or triple this batch and keep it on hand. Pour some into ice trays and freeze, using the frozen cubes in water or tea. If you're familiar with Yogi tea or chai, this is like a minty version of these popular Indian teas.

3 cups purified water
4 slices (1/4-inch) fresh ginger root
4 cinnamon sticks, cut in half
1 tablespoon dried peppermint, either loose or in a tea bag
1/2 teaspoon cardamom seeds
1/8 teaspoon whole cloves

In a medium saucepan, combine all the ingredients and simmer for about 10 minutes. Strain and drink hot or cold.

Peppermint

Peppermint reduces gas, nausea, and the spastic symptoms of irritable bowel syndrome. Caution: Peppermint leaf is strictly off-limits for those who are pregnant or have gallstones or hiatal hernia.

Rejuvenation Tonic

Serves 2

First thing in the morning, as an afternoon pick-me-up, or to use throughout the day as a one-day rejuvenating cleanse, this simple-to-make tonic will make your cells sizzle with enthusiasm and vitality.

2 cups purified water, cold

1 tablespoon Living Food (see the Resource Directory)

1 tablespoon fresh lemon juice

1 to 2 teaspoons 100% pure organic maple syrup

1/8 teaspoon organic cayenne pepper

In a blender or food processor, blend on slow speed and serve.

VARIATION: You can substitute 1 cup fresh pineapple or apple juice for 1 cup of the water.

• T I P

One–Day Cleanse

One day a month or more, on a day when you don't have to work and can take it easy, drink this rejuvenation tonic 3 times during the day combined with juices made from a blend of 2 to 3 vegetables and fruits (as opposed to all fruit). This is a great way to cleanse, detoxify, and rejuvenate the body, mind, and spirit. Also, create opportunities during this day to get extra sleep, breathe deeply, take a long bubble bath, spend time in nature, and meditate.

Antioxidant Express

Serves 2 to 3

This free-radical scavenger cocktail will do wonders for boosting immunity and restoring youthful vitality.

1 cup organic green tea, freshly brewed and chilled

4 medium carrots, washed but not peeled

1 red or green apple

1/2 cup broccoli sprouts

1 stalk broccoli, including florets

1/2 cup cauliflower

3 leaves romaine lettuce

1/4 red bell pepper

1/4 yellow or orange bell pepper

1/4 wedge lemon with peeling, if organic

1/4-inch piece fresh ginger root

1 heaping tablespoon Barlean's Organic Greens powder
  (see the Resource Directory)

Juice everything but the Barlean's Greens powder. Once all the fruits and vegetables have been combined, blend in the Greens powder. Serve with lemon wedge.

• F Y I

Green Tea

While all the vegetables in the Antioxidant Express are rich in antioxidants, green tea takes the prize. The antioxidants found in green tea are among the highest found in any food or beverage. These body-friendly companions aid in the prevention of disease by battling free radicals, which are believed to be a major cause of cancer, heart disease, and aging. All black and green teas comes from the same bush. The differences between teas exist in the different times of harvesting and different methods of processing.

Natural Beauty Cocktail

Serves 2

Drink this daily for a week. Your skin will glow, your eyes will sparkle, and your energy will soar.

1 medium red or green apple

1 red, yellow, or orange bell pepper

3 medium carrots

3 leaves romaine lettuce

2 stalks celery

1/2 medium cucumber

1/4 wedge lemon with peeling, if organic

1/4- to 1/2-inch piece fresh ginger root (optional)

Juice all the ingredients together, and serve.

Easy Sleepytime Cocktail

Serves 1

Taken an hour before bedtime, this delicious combination is guaranteed to help you fall asleep without having to count sheep.

1 cup freshly brewed chamomile tea

2 apples

2 stalks celery

1/4 cup parsley

Juice the apples, celery, and parsley, then mix with the tea. Sip slowly.

• **F Y I**

Chamomile Tea

Teas made from the mildly sedating herb, chamomile, are useful in treating insomnia and soothing gastritis, an inflammation of the stomach lining. Caution: Chamomile belongs to the same plant family as daisies and dandelion. If you are allergic to those plants, you should avoid chamomile.

Peaceful Cocktail

Serves 2

If you're feeling irritable or anxious, this colorful drink will lift your spirits and lower your stress levels.

1 ruby red grapefruit, outer skin peeled (leave pithy part on)
1 pear
8 large strawberries, with green tops
1 cup freshly brewed lemon balm tea
1/4-inch piece fresh ginger root (optional)

Juice all the fruits (and ginger, if using) and mix with the tea.
As you drink this cocktail, make sure to breathe slowly and deeply.

• F Y I

Lemon Balm

This herb is a member of the mint family. Lemon balm is reported to help combat mild forms of anxiety and irritability. The tea can also be daubed onto herpes sores on the mouth or genitals. Use it three to six times a day at the first sign of an outbreak to reduce or even prevent symptoms. Some people use it as an adjunct to antiviral medications. Caution: Pregnant women and people with hypothyroidism should not use lemon balm.

Anti–Cancer V–12

Serves 2 to 3

After tasting this delicious vegetable juice, you'll never want to drink the canned varieties again.

4 large ripe tomatoes
3 large carrots
3 stalks of celery
1 bell pepper, yellow, red, or orange

4 green onions

4 leaves of the greenest romaine lettuce

4 large leaves of spinach

2 leaves of kale

1/2 cup of broccoli sprouts

1/2 small beet

1/3 cup parsley

1-3 cloves garlic

1 small lemon with peeling, if organic

1/4 teaspoon living Celtic Sea Salt (see the Grain & Salt Society
   in the Resource Directory)

Juice all the ingredients. Add extra tomatoes at the end if you need
more juice.

• F Y I

Lutein

*Lutein is a carotenoid pigment found in plants. Lutein protects the
colon cells from damage caused by highly reactive compounds called
free radicals. A free radical is a type of oxygen molecule that freely
moves inside cells, reacting with proteins, fats, and DNA, changing
their structure and disrupting their function. Free radicals are generated by the metabolism of oxygen and other chemicals such as cigarette smoke, unsaturated fats, food additives, and environmetal
chemicals such as herbicides, pestcides, and preservatives. In several
recent studies eating a lutein-rich diet was reported to reduce the
risk of colon cancer by as much as 17%. Good sources of lutein
include tomatoes, carrots, oranges, broccoli, kale, romaine lettuce,
and spinach.*

Vitality Shake

Serves 1 to 2

I make this smoothie, or a variation (see below), several mornings a week right after my workout. It really hits the spot and provides a balance of high protein, carbohydrates, and omega-3 fatty acids. This smoothie is also a great meal replacement.

For a Vitality Dessert, pour this or another favorite smoothie into ice cube trays and freeze. Take the frozen Vitality cubes and press through the Green Power or Green Life juicer (see Resource Directory) and you have a very healthy ice cream/sorbet-type dessert or meal.

1 cup purified water (mixed with 1 packet of Raspberry or Tangerine Emer'gen-C)

1 ripe banana, peeled

1/2 cup frozen fruit such as blueberries, strawberries, cherries, peaches, banana plus other frozen fruit, raspberries, papaya, etc.

1 to 2 tablespoons Living Food (see Resource Directory)

1 tablespoon ALL ONE (see Resource Directory)

1 tablespoon Barlean's Flax Oil (see Resource Directory)

Blend, adding extra water, if necessary, to achieve the consistency you desire. Serve immediately.

VARIATIONS: Vary the fruits and instead of water, use a juice as the base, such as apple or pineapple, or soy or rice milk, or nut milk (see recipe below). To increase protein, B vitamins and vitamin E, I add freshly-milled raw wheat germ and nutritional yeast. When I want to add an extra boost of protein, I'll also include a scoop of soy protein powder or blend in 6 almonds or a few pumpkin or sunflower seeds.

• TIP

Freezing Bananas

At any given time, I have about 20 frozen ripe bananas (I store them in zip top freezer bags) that I use in smoothies, to create banana ice cream, or simply to eat frozen as a snack. Frozen banana added to a smoothie makes it colder and thicker.

Easy Nut Milk

Serves 2-4

1/2 cup almonds or cashews

2 1/2 cups purified water (for soaking the nuts)

Soak the nuts in the water overnight to release and increase the nutrients and make the protein more digestible. Drain and reserve the water. In a nut or coffee grinder or Vita Mix (see the Resource Directory), grind the nuts to a meal. Place the liquid and meal in a blender and blend at high speed for about 2 minutes. Strain the resulting liquid through a fine mesh strainer. Chill and serve.

VARIATIONS: Sweeten with a touch of maple, barley malt, or brown rice syrup, or add a teaspoon of pure vanilla extract.

For a warm drink on a chilly evening, add a dash of cinnamon, cardamom, and/or nutmeg. For a chocolate flavor, add 1 teaspoon carob powder or organic cocoa powder.

Make seed milk by substituting sunflower seeds for the nuts.

• F Y I

Cashews & Almonds

Cashews provide calcium, magnesium, iron, zinc, and folic acid. Almonds are a great source of protein and are very alkaline. They are the king of nuts, providing calcium, magnesium, phosphorus, potassium, zinc, folic acid, vitamin B_{12}, and vitamin E.

Nut Milk Smoothie

Serves 1

1 cup almond nut milk (see recipe on page 211)
1 ripe frozen banana, cut into chunks
Dash of cinnamon

Blend all the ingredients together, and serve.

VARIATIONS: For a chocolate flavor, add 1 teaspoon carob powder or organic cocoa powder. For more of a complete, nutritious meal, blend in 1 to 2 tablespoons Living Food (see the Resource Directory). For a sweeter taste, blend in 3 medjool dates and a few drops of pure vanilla extract, and for an exotic taste, guaranteed to impress anyone, blend in 2 apricots with a dash of nutmeg and cardamom.

Dried Plum & Apple Smoothie

Serves 1 to 2

Dried plums is really another way of saying prunes, which sometimes get a bad rap. This is a refreshing afternoon pick-me-up guaranteed to keep you in the flow.

1 cup vanilla soy yogurt
8 prunes, pitted
1/2 cup frozen apple juice concentrate
1/4 lemon, peeled (outer layer only, keep pithy part on)
1/8 teaspoon ground cinnamon
3 leaves of fresh mint
5 to 6 ice cubes

In a blender or food processor, blend until smooth and serve.

• F Y I

Prunes

A natural laxative, prunes are a good source of calcium, phosphorus, potassium, beta carotene, and iron. They help to lower cholesterol and are beneficial for blood, brain, and nerves.

Cranberry–Apple Cooler

Serves 1 to 2

12 ounces cranberry-apple juice, freshly juiced
    or from health food store

1 to 2 tablespoons Living Food (see the Resource Directory)

1 large ripe banana

Water and ice to taste (optional)

In a blender or food processor, blend until smooth and serve.

VARIATIONS: Instead of cranberry-apple, try papaya, apple, or orange juice.

• F Y I

Cranberries

Cranberries have abundant antioxidant and antibacterial properties, which is why they are recommended for urinary tract infections. They are also a good source of calcium, magnesium, potassium, manganese, and phosphorus.

Creamy Cinnamon Banana
Serves 1 to 2

8 ounces vanilla almond milk (see page 211)

1 to 2 tablespoons Living Food (see Resource Directory)

1 frozen or fresh ripe banana, peeled

1/4 teaspoon cinnamon

Pinch of nutmeg

Pinch of cloves

In a blender or food processor, blend until creamy smooth, and serve.

• F Y I
Cinnamon

Researchers at Kansas State University have added cinnamon to the growing list of natural bacteria fighters. In lab tests of apple juice samples inoculated with 1 million of the dreaded E. coli bacteria (about 10,000 times the level needed to make you sick), the addition of a single teaspoon of cinnamon knocked out 99.5% of the bacteria in 3 days. When the cinnamon was combined with a small amount of a common preservative, the germs were reduced to undetectable levels—lower than with the preservative alone. So spicing up your next glass of juice or cider or smoothie with cinnamon may be a good idea for reasons beyond great taste.

Tropical Fruit Smoothie
Serves 2 to 3

2 ripe bananas, peeled

1 mango, peeled, seeded, and cubed

1 papaya, peeled, seeded, and cubed

1 cup fresh pineapple chunks

Ice cubes to taste

In a blender or food processor, blend until smooth. Serve.

• **F Y I**

Bananas

Bananas are a terrific health food, complete with their own colorful and protective wrapping. They provide potassium, tryptophan, vitamin C, beta carotene, vitamin K, and vitamin B_6. Not only do they promote sleep and remove toxic metals from the body, they act as a mild laxative, are antifungal, and are a natural antibiotic. The pectin in bananas helps heal ulcers and lowers cholesterol. The best way to eat them is ripe, i.e., when there are spots on the skin.

Mixed Melon Ambrosia

Serves 2 to 3

Melons provide a treasure trove of vitamins A, B, and C, along with trace minerals and enzymes. On a hot summer day, everyone loves this beautiful, delectable smoothie.

2 cups watermelon chunks
2 cups honeydew melon chunks
1/2 cup cantaloupe chunks, frozen
1/2 cup strawberries, frozen
1 tablespoon maple syrup (optional)

Juice the watermelon and honeydew together. Pour the melon liquid into the blender and blend with the frozen fruit. Sweeten to taste. (I like it best without any sweetener.)

VARIATION: Substitute frozen pitted cherries or blueberries for the strawberries.

• **F Y I**

Melons

Because of their high water content, melons are excellent rehydrators and cleansers. For maximum benefit, eat melons alone when you're not creating a smoothie. Cantaloupe is one of the best sources of beta carotene and vitamin C.

Mango Coconut Cream Smoothie
Serves 2 to 3

2 medium mangos (about 1 cup), cut into chunks

1 cup orange, lemon, vanilla, or peach soy yogurt

3/4 cup lite coconut milk

3/4 cup vanilla soy milk or nut milk

2 tablespoons frozen orange juice concentrate, thawed

Juice of 1/2 lime

In a blender or food processor, blend until creamy smooth, and serve immediately.

VARIATION: To increase protein to almost 20 grams per serving, increase soy milk to 2 cups and add 2 tablespoons of soy protein powder.

• F Y I
Coconut

Coconut contains iron, fiber, and lauric acid, an antimicrobial and antibacterial fatty acid also found in human milk. An 8-ounce serving of fresh milk has only 60 calories, mostly from sugars. Try it, instead of water or vegetable stock, to cook grains and cereals.

• F Y I
Fruits, Vegetables & Blood Pressure

Eating more fruits and vegetables helps to lower high blood pressure and reduce bone loss that leads to osteoporosis. In a recent study of more than 3,500 elderly women, it was found that those with the highest systolic pressure (the upper number in the blood pressure reading) lost almost twice as much bone mass each year as did those with the lowest systolic pressure. In other words, high blood pressure hastens bone loss promoting calcium excretion.

Kiwi–Melon Smoothie

Serves 2 to 3

3 kiwi, peeled and cut into chunks

1 cup crenshaw, honeydew, or cantaloupe cubes, frozen

1 cup lemon, kiwi-lemon, or similar soy yogurt

1 cup nut milk or soy milk

1 tablespoon frozen orange juice concentrate, thawed

In a blender or food processor, blend and serve immediately.

VARIATION: In many smoothies that have a juice or soy or nut milk base, you always have the option of using water. That's what I usually do unless I want the extra calories or nutrients in the liquid base. For example, if I want more protein, I'll use the soy milk and even add two scoops of soy protein.

Very Strawberry–Banana Smoothie

Serves 2 to 3

The combination of high vitamin C strawberries and high potassium banana is a nutritional winner and the beautiful rose color of this smoothie also nourishes the soul.

8 frozen strawberries

1 ripe frozen banana, cut into chunks

2/3 cup fresh strawberry juice

1/2 cup vanilla soy yogurt

2 tablespoons frozen apple juice concentrate, thawed

In a blender or food processor, blend and serve. Add 1 to 2 scoops of Living Food or soy protein powder to increase protein.

Peach Smoothie

Serves 3 to 4

What could be finer than the taste of fresh summer peaches?

4 fresh ripe peaches, peeled, pitted, and cut in to chunks

1 ripe frozen banana, peeled and cut in to chunks

1 cup vanilla or peach soy yogurt

1$\frac{1}{3}$ cups almond nut milk or vanilla soy milk

2 large ice cubes

$\frac{1}{2}$ teaspoon pure vanilla extract

In a blender or food processor, blend and serve immediately.

VARIATION: Substitute nectarines, apricots, or pears for the peaches.

• F Y I

Peaches

A favorite summertime treat, peaches are a good source of calcium, magnesium, phosphorus, vitamin C, potassium, beta carotene, and folic acid. They are a mild diuretic and laxative, are very alkalinizing, and are cleansing for the kidneys and bladder.

• F Y I

Pears

Pears are not only delicious but are a good source of pectin, which aids peristalsis and the removal of toxins. They are also a good source of calcium, magnesium, phosphorus, potassium, beta carotene, folic acid, and are high in iodine, which makes them an excellent food for weight loss. Pears are also a natural diuretic.

Positively Pear Smoothie

Serves 1 to 2

1 cup pears, peeled, cut in to chunks and frozen

1 ripe frozen banana, cut in to chunks

3/4 cup vanilla nut milk or rice milk

In a blender or food processor, blend until smooth.
Serve immediately.

Cantaloupe–Berry Smoothie

Serves 2 to 3

1/2 ripe cantaloupe, cut into chunks

1 cup frozen berries (blueberries, strawberries,
blackberries, or raspberries)

1 cup berry soy yogurt

1 cup vanilla nut milk or soy milk

In a blender or food processor, blend and serve immediately.

VARIATION: To increase protein, add 1 to 2 scoops of soy protein
powder or Living Food (see Resource Directory).

Veggie Smoothie

Serves 3 to 4

Here's a great way to "eat" your vegetables! The combination of miso and mint may sound odd but they add a wonderful balance of flavors to this veggie drink.

2 cups carrot juice (about 8 to 10 carrots)

1 cucumber, peeled if not organic

1 bell pepper, red, yellow, or orange

6 leaves romaine lettuce

3 leaves cabbage, green or purple

3 ounces silken tofu

1/2 small lemon, with peel if organic

1 to 3 cloves garlic (optional)

2 tablespoons Living Food (see the Resource Directory)

2 tablespoons Barlean's Flax Oil (see the Resource Directory)

1 teaspoon organic miso

Fresh mint sprigs, for garnish

Juice enough carrots to make 2 cups. Continue to juice the other vegetables and the lemon. Pour this mixture into a blender and add silken tofu, Living Food, flax oil, and organic miso. In a blender or food processor, blend until creamy smooth. Pour into chilled glasses and garnish with a sprig of mint.

VARIATION: Instead of this juice, you can use any other vegetable juice you've made. Simply blend it with silken tofu, Living Food, and miso for a delicious and nutritious high protein salad in a glass.

• F Y I

Miso

Miso is a fermented soybean paste made by combining soybeans, a fermenting agent, salt, and various grains, then fermenting for 6 months or longer. Because miso is partially digested by fermentation, the body easily assimilates its nutrients. Miso also contains live enzymes that benefit the microbial balance of the digestive tract.

Creamy Cherry Smoothie

Serves 2 to 3

This beautiful smoothie really hits the spot. It will fill you up and leave you energized for hours.

1 cup frozen pitted cherries

4 to 5 large ice cubes

1 1/2 cups vanilla soy or almond nut milk

2 ounces silken tofu

1 tablespoon Barlean's Flax Oil, optional (see the Resource Directory)

1/2 teaspoon pure vanilla extract

1/8 teaspoon pure organic peppermint, orange,
    or lemon extract

In a blender or food processor, blend until smooth and serve immediately.

Watermelon–Ginger Refresher

Serves 3 to 4

5 cups watermelon, seeded and cut into chunks

1 1/2 tablespoons fresh ginger root juice (put through your juicer)

1 1/3 cups purified water

Fresh mint sprigs

In a blender or food processor, blend and serve.

VARIATION: To create a slushy version, freeze 3 cups of watermelon chunks and blend with the remaining 2 cups of unfrozen watermelon. Pour into glasses that have been chilled in the freezer and garnish with fresh mint.

• T I P

Toasted Watermelon Seeds

Remove the seeds from the watermelon, rinse, season, and toast them for a delicious snack.

Fruit Power Shake

Serves 2 to 3

1¹/3 cups fresh orange juice or apple juice

¹/2 orange, cut into chunks (peel removed)

1 ripe banana, cut into chunks

6 frozen strawberries, green tops removed

10 frozen pitted cherries

¹/3 cup apple, peeled

¹/2 cup vanilla soy milk

1 to 2 tablespoons Living Food (see the Resource Directory) or vanilla soy protein powder

1 to 2 tablespoons Barlean's Flax Oil

In a blender or food processor, blend until smooth and serve right away.

Fresh Fruit Slushes, Sorbets & Ice Cream

I use my Green Power or Green Life Juicer (see the Resource Directory) to make fresh fruit ice cream and sorbet. Nothing could be easier to make than these tasty and healthful frozen desserts. When you've got the time, just make lots of fruit juice and freeze it in ice cube trays. My favorites are orange, tangerine, cantaloupe, watermelon, honeydew, apple, and grape. Just take 7 or 8 of the cubes and put them in a blender with a glass of fresh juice and blend. This makes an incredible drink that can double as a rich dessert by adding more juice cubes. I sometimes make this my meal.

You can also peel and seed a cantaloupe or honeydew and put the entire fruit into a blender and blend a few seconds, until smooth. Then pour the liquid into ice cube trays and freeze. You'll always have a low-calorie, nutritious snack on hand. These melon cubes are closer in consistency to hard ice cream than ice cubes made from just juice.

Chapter 9

BREAKFASTS & BRUNCHES

I know that many of you are chronically pressed for time and feel lucky if you find the time to wolf down a muffin and coffee on your way to the office. Unfortunately, skipping breakfast or eating empty calories serves to lower metabolism and energy and sets up a body chemistry that tends to turn food to fat more easily and to store that fat throughout your body. **There's no more important meal than breakfast.** A good breakfast stokes the fire; it gets the metabolic machinery out of inertia from your night's rest. When one of your goals is to accelerate fat loss, make sure you eat breakfast.

The word breakfast literally means 'breaking a fast,' so you want to start the day off with the healthiest foods possible to feed your 70 trillion cells. Simple, light, and nutritious are the keys to remember for your first meal of the day. Fresh fruit in season is one of the most nutritious breakfasts you can have since we digest fruit quickly and can readily reap its high energy benefits in a matter of minutes. Fruit is the highest water content food so it rehydrates your body and fills you up without adding lots of calories. As you adopt this habit of eating fresh fruit for your morning meal, you will see how it helps give you an energetic start to the day without feeling stuffed.

In addition to fresh fruit, fruit smoothies are quick and easy and the perfect breakfast when you want to lose weight. And remember, it's best to eat several smaller meals throughout the day instead of 2 or 3 larger meals if you want to lose fat and restore youthful vitality. This is called grazing.

In this chapter, I've included some of my favorite breakfasts that are not too heavy and will give you a balance of carbohydrates, protein, and essential fatty acids. (I didn't bother with too many fruit recipes since these are so simple to make.) Some of you might prefer a bigger meal in the morning. Most of the recipes that follow would also work well for those weekend brunches when more food might be appropriate.

Pinwheel Citrus Delight

Serves 2 to 4

This is one of my favorite breakfasts because it's very nutritious and it's as beautiful to look at as it is delicious to eat.

2 ruby red grapefruit

1 large, juicy navel orange

4 large ripe kiwi

Berries in season, such as blueberries or raspberries

1/3 cup raw almonds, raw walnuts, and/or raw cashews (alone or combined)

Fresh mint sprigs, for garnish

Peel the fruit with a knife. Be sure to remove all the white pith that's just under the skin of the citrus. Slice the fruit into circles, as opposed to sections. Arrange the circles of fruit on a plate in a way that looks great and shows off all the colors. Sprinkle the berries around the other fruit. In a nut grinder, coarsely grind the nuts then mix them together in a bowl. Sprinkle 1 tablespoon of the nut mixture over each plate and garnish each with a sprig of mint.

VARIATION: Try the same thing with other fruits you love such as melons, pineapple and tangerines, papaya and mango, pears and apples, or peaches, apricots, and nectarines.

• F Y I

Grapefruit

Ruby red grapefruit contains more nutrients than the white or pink varieties. A good source of vitamin C, potassium, magnesium, and calcium, grapefruit also contains salicylic acid, which helps arthritis. Grapefruits are also good for allergies and infections of the throat and mouths.

Berry Salad with Fruit Sauce

Serves 3 to 4

3 cups berries in season—strawberries, blueberries, raspberries, blackberries or any combination, rinsed well

3 ripe bananas, sliced

1 tablespoon vanilla soy milk

2 to 3 drops pure peppermint extract

Fresh mint sprigs, for garnish

In a bowl, mix 2 of the bananas with 2 cups of the berries. Blend together remaining bananas, berries, soy milk, and peppermint extract. Arrange fruit in the bowls (slice strawberries, if large) and top with the sauce. Be creative: Drizzle the sauce in a pattern that pleases your eye and suits your own personal style.

• **F Y I**

Berries

Berries provide us with calcium, magnesium, phosphorus, potassium, vitamin B_3, and vitamin C, and also help expel mucus, phlegm, and toxins. They are excellent for female reproductive health and help relieve menstrual cramps. Raspberry-leaf tea reduces nausea in pregnancy. Berries, in general, are low in calories, and are very nutritious, so keep your refrigerator and freezer stocked with lots of scrumptious berries.

Muesli

Serves 2 to 3

This unroasted granola treat is very nourishing and versatile.

5 medium apples

1/2 lemon

1 1/3 cups rolled oats

1/4 cup rye flakes

1/4 cup prunes, pitted

2 medjool dates, pitted, or 3 to 4 regular soft dates, pitted

2 tablespoons raw sunflower seeds

1/4 cup walnuts or almonds

1/4 cup small raisins, sprinkle on top

Dash of cinnamon

Core and quarter the apples. Juice the wedges and save 1 1/2 cups of the juice and all the pulp. Juice the lemon, set aside the juice. In a food processor, process oats, rye flakes, prunes, dates, and the seeds/nuts and cinnamon until coarsely ground. Put this mixture in a large bowl. Add the apple pulp, after discarding any large pieces of skin. Add the apple and lemon juices to the ground mixture and mix well. Let it sit for about 15 minutes. Serve with fresh fruit on top, such as sliced strawberries. Also, try it with vanilla soy milk or a large dollop of soy yogurt or apple sauce.

• TIP

Freezing Muesli

I often make a large batch of muesli without the apple juice or pulp and freeze it until needed. Then I add the liquid and apples when I'm ready to eat. Sometimes I combine the ground mixture with some soy milk or grated apple. Right before eating, I might also add some freshly milled, raw wheat germ and freshly ground flax seed.

Sensational Spicy Granola

Serves 12 to 16

3 apples

1 small lemon

1 small orange

8 cups rolled oats

2 cups unsalted, raw nutmeats, such as almonds, walnuts, pecans, cashews, pine nuts, or pistachios, or a combination of any or all

1 cup wheat bran

1 cup raw wheat germ

1/2 cup raw, unsalted sunflower seeds

1/2 cup unsweetened shredded coconut

¹/₄ cup sesame seeds

¹/₄ cup unrefined sesame or canola oil

¹/₄ cup brown rice syrup

3 tablespoons maple syrup

1 tablespoon pure vanilla extract

1 tablespoon apple concentrate

1 teaspoon pure almond extract

2 teaspoons cinnamon

1 teaspoon cardamom

1 teaspoon ground ginger

¹/₂ teaspoon coriander

¹/₂ teaspoon nutmeg

¹/₂ teaspoon Celtic Sea Salt (see the Grain & Salt Society
   in the Resource Directory)

1 cup chopped, dried fruit such as prunes, raisins, dates,
   cherries, peaches, or apples, or a combination

Preheat oven to 300°F. Juice the apples, lemon, and orange, reserving the combined juice. In a large bowl, combine the rolled oats, nutmeats, wheat germ and bran, coconut, seeds and all the spices.

In a small saucepan, stir together the combined juice, oil, maple and brown rice syrups, apple concentrate, and vanilla and almond extracts over low heat until well blended and heated through. Pour the hot liquid over the dry mixture and combine until very well mixed. Spread the mixture on 2, 11 x 17-inch jelly-roll pans and bake for 25 to 30 minutes, stirring to re-layer it every 5 to 7 minutes, or until the oats are crisp and brown, but not burned. When done, remove from the oven and pour into a large cool bowl to stop the cooking. Add the dried fruit and combine thoroughly. Set aside to cool completely. Store in an airtight container.

• T I P

Storing Granola

I keep my granola in zipper lock bags to snack on. It also freezes well so consider doubling or tripling the recipe so you always have some on hand.

Banana Applesauce Muffins

Makes 12

These make a great snack or on-the-go-meal.

1¹/4 cups oat flour (you can grind your own
    by putting oatmeal through a Vita Mix)

1 cup rice flour

1 teaspoon baking soda

1/2 teaspoon baking powder

2 teaspoons cinnamon

1/4 teaspoon nutmeg

1 very ripe medium banana (lots of spots please)

2/3 cup applesauce

1/2 cup apple juice

1/3 cup orange juice

1 large apple, peeled, cored, diced

1/2 cup raisins

Preheat the oven to 350°F. In a large bowl, combine the flours, baking soda, baking powder, and spices. In a food processor, combine the banana, applesauce, and juice. A little at a time, add in the dry ingredients. Transfer to the large bowl and fold in the diced apple and raisins. Using a nonstick muffin tin, fill the cups about 2/3 full and bake for 12 to 13 minutes. Serve with Apricot, Prune, or Apple Butter Spreads (see recipes, pages 234-235).

Creamy Coconut Millet Cereal

Serves 4

1 cup millet

1 cup purified water

1/2 cup lite coconut milk

1/2 cup vanilla soy milk

1 tablespoon maple syrup

2 tablespoons brown rice syrup

1/3 cup unsweetened shredded coconut

1/8 teaspoon cinnamon

1/3 cup raisins, chopped pitted dates, diced apples,
or dried cherries, or a combination (optional)

In a blender, process the millet until it is very fine. In a saucepan,
bring water and soy and coconut milk to a boil. Add the millet and
stir. Lower heat to a simmer and add syrups, cinnamon, and fruit.
Cook until smooth and soft, about 3 to 5 minutes. Top with the
shredded coconut and serve with vanilla soy milk. Add raisins,
dates, dried apples, or dried cherries, as desired

• **F Y I**

Millet

This gluten-free grain is highly alkaline and easily digestible.
Rich in fiber and a low allergenic food, millet is rich in magnesium,
potassium, phosphorus, and vitamin B$_3$.

Oatmeal Deluxe

Serves 5 to 8

Here's one of the tastiest oatmeal recipes you'll ever make.

5 cups purified water

3/4 teaspoon cinnamon

1/8 teaspoon powdered ginger

1/8 teaspoon nutmeg

1 teaspoon coriander

3 1/4 cups rolled oats

1/2 cup raw sunflower seeds

2 cups vanilla soy milk

2 cups apples, peeled, cored and grated

1 tablespoon maple syrup

1/2 cup raisins, dried cherries, chopped dates, or combination

In a large saucepan, combine the water, cinnamon, nutmeg, ginger, and coriander and bring to a boil. Add the remaining ingredients and reduce heat to low. Cook until thickened, stirring occasionally. Serve with vanilla soy milk

VARIATION: Top with rice syrup, maple syrup, or applesauce.

• F Y I

Oats

Oats, an outstanding antioxidant grain, are packed with a high fiber content, which ensures a mild laxative and cholesterol-lowering effect. Oats are excellent for bones and connective tissue because they are a good source of calcium, magnesium, and phosphorus. Add to the mix manganese, iron, vitamin B_5, folic acid, and silicon.

Top of the Morning Quinoa Cereal

Serves 4 to 5

Pronounced "KEEN-wah," this versatile food is a "newly discovered" ancient grain that originated with the Aztec Indians. It has an impressive nutritional profile and a nutty, distinctive flavor. Some folks call it the "super grain." Its easy-to-digest protein, calcium, iron, potassium, magnesium, lysine, and B_3 make it a winner on any health enthusiast's menu.

1 1/3 cups quinoa

2 cups fresh apple juice

1 teaspoon unrefined sesame oil

1 teaspoon brown rice syrup

1/8 teaspoon Celtic Sea Salt (see the Grain & Salt Society in the Resource Directory)

2 tablespoons pecans, cashews, walnuts, or pistachios, roasted and finely chopped

Put the quinoa in a large bowl and cover with cold water to wash. Gently rub it between your palms for about 10 seconds to wash off the saponin, a bitter, naturally occurring substance that acts as a pesticide.

Drain it in a fine-mesh strainer. Repeat the washing process 3 times. Run cold water through quinoa until the water runs almost clear.

In a medium saucepan, combine the juice, oil, syrup, and salt and bring to a boil. Make sure it doesn't boil over. Add the washed quinoa, cover and lower the heat. Simmer for 12 to 15 minutes, or until all the liquid has been absorbed. Remove from the heat and let stand for 5 minutes. Add the nuts and fluff with a fork. Serve warm or chilled. Top with vanilla soy milk, applesauce, or a dash of cinnamon.

VARIATION: Instead of apple juice, you can substitute orange juice, vanilla soy milk, coconut milk, rice milk, nut milk, water, or any combination.

Scrambled Tofu

Serves 4

I love breakfast food anytime of the day and this great protein dish has no cholesterol. Most scramble recipes call for sautéing. In this recipe you cook everything in a light vegetable broth or water.

1/4 cup vegetable broth (or water)

1 small red pepper, diced

1 zucchini (optional)

3/4 cup mushrooms, diced

1/2 red onion, diced

1/2 cup finely chopped green onions

1 clove garlic, finely minced

1 pound firm to extra-firm silken tofu, drained,
    pressed dry, and crumbled

1 1/2 teaspoons curry powder or 1 teaspoon turmeric
    for color if the curry is too spicy for you

1 tablespoon Bragg liquid aminos or tamari

Set the sauté pan over high and add vegetable broth to scald. Add the vegetables and Bragg or tamari, garlic, and sauté until tender. Add the tofu and spices, mixing everything well—for about 5 minutes.

VARIATION: Most vegetables work well, such as carrots, broccoli, or cauliflower. Serve with salsa and warm whole grain pita bread to make a Tex-Mex delight. Add some roasted or hash brown potatoes and you'll never miss eggs again.

• F Y I

Tofu

Made from soybeans, tofu is a perfect vegetarian source of protein and has anti-cancer and cholesterol-lowering properties. Besides amino acids, it is also packed with iron, potassium, calcium, magnesium, vitamin A, and vitamin K. Caution: If you have a history of breast cancer in your family, check with your doctor about consuming tofu and other soy products, or feeding soy formulas to your infant.

Orange–Blueberry Buckwheat Pancakes

Serves 2 to 4

3/4 cup vanilla soy milk (or rice milk or nut milk)

1 tablespoon fresh orange juice

1 teaspoon orange zest (use an organic orange)

2 tablespoons maple syrup

1 cup buckwheat flour

1/8 teaspoon Celtic Sea Salt

1 teaspoon baking powder

Dash cinnamon

1/2 cup blueberries

Maple syrup, applesauce, or all-fruit preserves, for topping

In a small bowl, mix together milk, syrup, orange juice, and zest. In another large bowl, mix together flour, baking powder, salt, and a dash of cinnamon. Pour liquid into the dry mixture and fold in the blueberries. Lightly coat a nonstick skillet or griddle with vegetable spray and set over high heat. Pour batter and cook 1 to 2 minutes over medium heat or until the tops bubble. Turn the pancake and cook briefly on second side. Serve with a topping of your choice.

• **F Y I**

Buckwheat

Buckwheat contains all 8 essential amino acids, making it an excellent plant-based protein. It strengthens capillaries and helps detoxify the body. It's rich in phosphorus, beta carotene, vitamin C, calcium, magnesium, phosphorus, potassium, zinc, manganese, and folic acid. Caution: If you have skin allergies or cancer, check with your doctor before eating buckwheat.

Tofu Pancakes

Serves 3 to 4

This recipe is so tasty, you'll never believe that it's both oil- and egg-free! Make them for a healthy, festive brunch.

1 12-ounce package soft lite silken tofu

2/3 cup vanilla soy milk

1/2 medium ripe banana

1/2 cup whole wheat pastry flour

1/4 cup flax seed meal

1 tablespoon brown rice syrup

Dash cinnamon

In a blender, combine all ingredients and blend until smooth. Heat a nonstick griddle over medium heat and lightly mist with vegetable spray. Pour batter onto the hot griddle. When bubbles appear, turn the pancake over. Don't be concerned if the first couple of pancakes don't look great. They're priming the griddle for the best to come. Serve with soy yogurt, maple syrup, or applesauce.

Chapter 10

Spreads, Sauces, Dips & Marinades

When you emphasize more plant-based foods in your diet, it's helpful to have a variety of different sauces, dips, spreads, and marinades that you can use to create a wide variety of flavors, textures, and colors. The recipes in this chapter are easy, healthy, and delicious and will allow you to create a whole new array of healthy dishes and expand your menu repertoire.

Don't be afraid to experiment by adding or subtracting a little bit of this or that to come up with your own mouth-watering creation. Like making smoothies and fresh juices, it's hard to mess up these recipes. Use each within 3 to 5 days.

Apricot & Prune Butter Spreads

These butters are great on whole grain bread or toast, pancakes, waffles, or as a topping for fruit. Use the prune, apple, and apricot butter spreads as a replacement for butter and oil in baking recipes.

1½ cups dried apricots and/or prunes (unsulfured)
3 cups purified water

Soak the dried fruit in a bowl of the purified water overnight. In the morning, transfer the water and fruit mixture to a saucepan, adding enough additional water to cover the fruit. Simmer for 10 minutes. Strain and save the cooking water. In a food processor or blender, purée the fruit and, if necessary, blend in some of the cooking water to smooth out the texture.

VARIATIONS: To add sweetness, blend in a couple of chopped medjool dates. For some extra zing, add a dash of cinnamon or nutmeg when puréeing, or add a cinnamon stick to the simmering process.

• **F Y I**

Apricots are rich in copper, calcium, magnesium, potassium, folic acid, vitamin C, beta carotene, boron, and iron. They are a good laxative, potent antioxidant, and a natural sweetener.

Also a laxative, prunes help to lower cholesterol and provide calcium, phosphorus, potassium, beta carotene, and iron to your diet.

Apple Butter Spread

Try this healthy topping on whole grain toast, pancakes, waffles, muffins, or fruit. Or use this delicious spread in place of oil and eggs in your baked goods to lower fat.

6 medium apples, organic, if possible
Purified water
Dash sea salt

Peel, quarter, and core the apples. Grate them into a heavy stockpot and add a pinch of salt and enough water to barely cover the grated apples. Simmer over low heat for 2 hours, or until the mixture is thick and deep brown in color, stirring occasionally to prevent burning.

VARIATION: Try adding some ground cinnamon, cloves, nutmeg, or allspice.

Date–Apple–Berry Butter Spread

This sweeter fruit butter spread is quicker to make than the one above and especially favored by those who prefer to eat more raw, living foods, like I do. I triple the recipe so I have lots on hand to use as a topping, spread, or simply as a snack.

2 apples

1/3 cup blueberries, strawberries, raspberries,
   or a combination

2/3 cup purified water (you may need a little extra)

1 cup pitted dates (I use medjool)

Dash of cinnamon

In a blender, combine all the ingredients and pulse to desired consistency. Chill before serving.

VARIATIONS: Adjust the amount of water to reach the best consistency for the dish you're serving. For example, if you're using it to top whole grain pancakes or to drizzle over fresh fruit, you might want to add a little extra water. If you're using it as a spread on toast or crackers or to spread on pear, apple, or banana slices, keep it a bit thicker.

• **F Y I**
Pectin, a phytochemical found in abundance in apples and other fruits, is a type of fiber that has been shown to be effective in lowering cholesterol levels.

Carrot–Tahini Spread

This easy-to-prepare, colorful spread is delicious on sandwiches, on top of whole grain toast, or used as a dip for raw vegetables. Instead of carrots, substitute butternut squash, acorn squash, or combinations of carrots, parsnips, onions, garlic, and cabbage.

4 cups carrots, cut into 1-inch pieces

3/4 cup purified water

11/4 teaspoons kuzu (available at natural food
   or Asian specialty stores)

1 to 4 tablespoons tahini

In a steamer, steam carrots for 15 to 20 minutes or until tender. Reserve the liquid. In a food processor or blender, purée the carrots until smooth, adding 1/2 cup of the cooking liquid. In a small bowl, mix kuzu in 1/4 cup cold water. Add it to the carrot purée and reheat it until it thickens and the mixture bubbles. Stir in the tahini. Set aside to cool.

• **F Y I**

Tahini

High in calcium, omega-3's, iron, zinc, magnesium, vitamin E, and folic acid, tahini (sesame seed butter) is the perfect creamy ingredient for salad dressings, soups, and sauces. The possibilities of tahini are endless. Traditionally used in hummus, the rich nutty flavor and creamy texture of tahini (which tastes terrific combined with lemon juice) is an essential kitchen ingredient. Rejuvenative Foods (see the Resource Directory) make the best raw tahini I know. Also look for their raw almond, cashew, sunflower seed, hempini, and pumpkin seed butters in addition to their four scrumptious Pure 100% Organic Chocolate Spreads using raw nut and seed butters along with Rapunzel 100% Pure Organic Cocoa Powder.

Veggie Millet Spread

Looking for a different spread to serve with tabbouleh or hummus or to stuff in celery, bell peppers, or Belgian endive? This highly alkalinizing, health-promoting spread is perfect.

1/2 cup cooked millet

1/2 cup silken extra firm tofu

1/2 cup grated carrot

2 tablespoons grated zucchini

2 teaspoons Barlean's Flax Oil (see Resource Directory)

2 tablespoons fresh parsley, minced

1 1/2 tablespoons light yellow miso

1 tablespoon almond or cashew butter

2 1/2 tablespoons nutritional yeast

In a bowl, combine all ingredients and serve with warmed whole grain pita triangles.

• F Y I

Nutritional, or brewer's, yeast is a very rich source of B vitamins, chromium, selenium, all the essential amino acids, RNA, DNA, manganese, choline, inositol, potassium, and PABA. It can be added to sauces, dips, spreads, smoothies, soups, breads, or sprinkled on grains and salads to nutrify your meal and body.

Quick High Protein Bean–Tofu Spread

This versatile spread can be flavored any number of ways. Try it on raw vegetables or whole grain crackers or breads.

2 cups beans, cooked and mashed (black, navy,
    lentils, garbanzo, pinto, and/or split peas)
1 (12.3 ounce) package of lite silken firm tofu

Season to taste (some of my favorites include Bragg liquid aminos, roasted garlic, chopped parsley, cayenne, dill, thyme, sea salt, tamari, shoyu, celery seed, or miso)

In a food processor, combine all ingredients and mix until smooth.

VARIATIONS: The possibilities are endless, so be creative!

Blend in 2 tablespoons tahini, sunflower seed, almond, or cashew butters, sautéed garlic and onions, roasted bell peppers*, or garlic. Or blend in ground, unsalted pistachio nuts, steamed carrots, celery, parsnips, squash, or cured olives.

*Roasted peppers are easy to make. Simply place peppers directly on a gas stove-top burner or under a preheated broiler. Cook peppers on all sides, turning with tongs, until the skin blackens and blisters. Transfer to a heavy-duty plastic or paper bag (closed) and steam for about 5 minutes. When cool enough to handle, peel away the charred skin with your fingers. Don't rinse them under water as that will wash away some of the flavor. Cut away any black spots with a small sharp knife.

• T I P

Artichoke Dip

In the mood for artichoke hearts? Would you like a simple, gourmet mouth-watering spread/dip that will be a guaranteed hit at any party or family gathering? Blend thawed artichoke hearts with tofu, tahini, and a dash of shoyu or tamari to taste.

Lemonaise Spread

This is a wonderful, light spread to use in place of mayonnaise in dips, spreads, dressings, or on whole grain sandwiches. Make it thick and use it as a spread, or thin and use it as a dressing, drizzled over steamed asparagus or broccoli florets.

Juice of one medium lemon

1/4 cup cold-pressed walnut oil

1/4 cup agar flakes

2 tablespoons purified water

1/8 teaspoon sea salt

Dash of cayenne and/or garlic powder (optional)

In a blender or food processor, combine all ingredients and blend to desired thickness. You can add more water or oil to create the consistency you want. Refrigerate.

VARIATIONS: To make an herbed lemonaise spread, add any of your favorite herbs such as rosemary, thyme, parsley, dill, tarragon, cumin, chili powder, turmeric, curry, or Herbes de Provence. Or to make garlic lemonaise, add pressed garlic to taste.

Quick & Easy Onion Dip

This dip goes especially well with raw vegetables—cauliflower, carrots, bell peppers, broccoli florets.

1 1/3 cups plain soy yogurt

1/4 cup minced sweet onion

1 teaspoon onion powder

1 tablespoon minced green onion

2 teaspoons minced fresh parsley

1 teaspoon fresh lemon juice and 1 teaspoon lemon zest—
use an organic lemon

2 teaspoons Barlean's Flax Oil (see Resource Directory)

Sea salt to taste

In a blender or food processor, blend all the ingredients together until smooth. Chill before serving and keep refrigerated.

• F Y I

Long regarded as a super health food, onions are antiseptic, anti-spasmodic, and antibiotic. They help detoxify and remove heavy metals and parasites from the body. Whether sweet or not, onions provide us with calcium, magnesium, phosphorus, potassium, beta carotene, folic acid, and quercetin. Quercetin, found in red and yellow onions and broccoli, fights cancer, viruses, bacteria, and fungi. This antioxidant bioflavonoid also lowers cholesterol and reduces the risk of blood clots. If you don't digest onions very well, try small amounts and chew well. Sweet onion is usually better tolerated.

Tofu–Cilantro "Cream" Sauce

If you want to jazz up baked potatoes, steamed vegetables, whole grains, or organic leafy greens, drizzle this sauce as you lovingly toss.

1 pound soft tofu (organic silken works best)

1/4 cup fresh minced cilantro

1/4 to 1/2 cup plain soy milk (depending on desired consistency)

2 garlic cloves, minced

1 green onion, minced

1 teaspoon fresh lime juice

1/4 teaspoon nutritional yeast

Dash sea salt

In a blender or food processor, blend all ingredients, beginning with ¹/4 cup soy milk and adding a little at a time, as needed, to get the consistency you desire.

VARIATIONS: Instead of cilantro, substitute fresh dill, basil, parsley, or even some mint.

• F Y I

A phytochemical called genistein, which is an isoflavone present in soybeans, soy flour, tofu, and textured soy protein, helps reduce blood cholesterol and fights cancer. It may also ease menopausal problems, including hot flashes, and may help in building bone density.

Emerald Green Sauce

Are you looking for a healthy, colorful sauce that even kids love? Try this flavorful one on mashed potatoes, steamed vegetables, grains, or noodles, or thicken it up with blended tofu or soy yogurt and use it as a dip for raw or lightly steamed cold vegetables.

4 large stalks celery

¹/4 pound baby leaf spinach (when steamed, baby leaf spinach is more tender and more flavorful)

¹/3 cup soy milk

¹/3 cup raw, unsalted cashews

1 tablespoon sunflower seeds

1 tablespoon yellow or white miso

1 teaspoon nutritional yeast

Juice the celery and spinach. Reserve ²/3 cup of the combined juice. If you're short, add extra celery to make ²/3 cup of juice. In a blender or food processor, purée all ingredients until smooth and creamy. Transfer to a saucepan and bring to a boil, stirring constantly. Lower the heat and simmer, stirring occasionally for about 2 to 3 minutes. If you'd like this sauce thinner, add extra soy milk. If you'd like it thicker, blend in soft organic silken tofu.

• F Y I

Spinach helps regulate blood pressure, boosts the immune system, and supports bone health. It's rich in beta carotene, folic acid, potassium, iron, vitamin B_6, vitamin C, calcium, magnesium, and the phytochemical lutein. Lutein, also found in abundance in kale and collard greens, is an antioxidant carotenoid with more power than its better known cousin beta carotene. It fights free radical damage and has been shown to reduce the risk of macular degeneration, a common cause of blindness in older people.

Homemade Sunny Ketchup

Unlike most store bought ketchup, this easy-to-prepare and satisfying ketchup is low in sodium and sugar, and it's fat free. You may want to double or triple the recipe. It also makes a lovely gift when you put it in a beautiful glass jar with a ribbon around the top.

12 ounces organic tomato paste

1/2 cup purified water

1/2 cup fresh organic tomato juice

2 tablespoons fresh apple juice

1 to 2 cloves garlic, minced

1 teaspoon nutritional yeast

2 teaspoons apple cider vinegar

1/2 teaspoon onion powder

1/8 teaspoon dried oregano

Combine all ingredients thoroughly. Store in a covered container in the refrigerator.

VARIATION: Add fresh chopped herbs such as cilantro, parsley, basil, or tarragon to give it a different flavor.

• F Y I

Tomatoes are an excellent source of the phytonutrient, lycopene, which has antioxidant properties, protects against cancer (notably prostate and pancreatic cancers), and stimulates the brain. All tomato products such as ketchup, tomato sauce and paste, and tomatoes are rich in lycopene.

Sensational Salsa

Besides using salsa as a dip for tortilla chips and raw vegetables or a variety of Mexican dishes, I use salsa on everything from brown rice, millet, or quinoa, as a topping on baked potatoes or steamed vegetables, or wrapped in lettuce leaves with some avocado slices, grated carrots, and other vegetables.

1^1/2 cup diced tomatoes, organic if possible, diced

2 tablespoons finely diced white onion

1 tablespoon finely diced red bell pepper

1 tablespoon finely diced yellow bell pepper

1 tablespoon fresh cilantro, chopped

2 teaspoons fresh lime juice

1 jalapeño chile, seeds and white rib removed, minced

1 teaspoon minced or pressed garlic

1/8 teaspoon minced ginger

Sea salt to taste (I usually use about 1/2 teaspoon)
(Add the salt just before eating since it draws out the tomato juices.)

Combine all the ingredients thoroughly in a bowl. Refrigerate until ready to serve.

VARIATIONS: For Corn Salsa, add 1/2 cup corn kernels cut right off the cob. For Mango Salsa, add 1/2 cup diced mango. For Avocado Salsa, add 1/2 to 3/4 cup diced avocado.

• T I P

What Makes Chiles Hot?

Most of the chile's heat is in the white tissue (the ribs), not the seeds as most people think. If you want a hotter salsa, leave in the white tissue and seeds and mince the whole thing. I recommend wearing gloves when you do this and keep your fingers out of your eyes.

Shiitake Mushroom Sauce

You'll find numerous ways to use this fat-free, delicious sauce, such as drizzled on whole grain pasta or noodles, over tofu steaks, or on top of vegetables or grain burgers.

1/4 cup fresh juice from a potato (I use a medium
    Yukon Gold or Finnish potato but any kind will do—
    just press it through your juicer)

1 cup fresh carrot juice (4 to 6 carrots)

1/3 cup fresh spinach juice

2 1/4 cups shiitake mushrooms, cleaned and thinly sliced

1 tablespoon low sodium tamari

2 teaspoons nutritional yeast

In a saucepan, combine the mushrooms with the three juices. Stir constantly as you bring it to a boil, then lower heat to simmer, stirring occasionally, just until the juice has thickened and the mushrooms are tender. At the last moment, add the tamari and yeast and stir. Yields about 2 cups.

VARIATION: Substitute other mushrooms for shiitake mushrooms and add your favorite herbs such as basil, rosemary, sage, or thyme.

• **F Y I**
Mushrooms help thin the blood, boost immunity, and lower choles-terol. Shiitake mushrooms contain a potent anti-cancer element. Mushrooms are also rich in calcium, iron, magnesium, vitamin B_3, vitamin B_5, folic acid, and zinc.

Great Guacamole

This is one of my favorite toppings on baked potatoes, sweet pota-toes, yams, salads, and grains, and as a dip for raw and steamed vegetables. Leave the avocado pit in the guacamole to keep it green even when serving. Also, store the guacamole in the refrigerator in an opaque, airtight container with the pit in the center.

3 ripe avocados, peeled and mashed

1 small red onion, minced and lightly sautéed

3 cloves garlic, minced and lightly sautéed

1/4 cup chopped green onions

1/3 cup chopped fresh cilantro

1 jalapeño pepper, finely minced (If you like it mild, discard the seeds and white ribs; if you like it hot, mince the whole thing. Be sure to wear gloves.)

1/3 cup tomato, chopped

3 tablespoons fresh lime juice

1/2 teaspoon sea salt to taste

In a small bowl, mix all the ingredients together thoroughly and serve immediately.

VARIATION: While you certainly don't have to sauté the onion and garlic, if you have the time, it gives it a wonderful flavor. I sauté in a few drops of olive oil.

• **F Y I**

Technically a fruit, the magnificent avocado has gotten a bum rap as a fatty food that should be avoided by those desiring to lose weight. Even though 88% of an avocado's calories come from fat, it's primarily monosaturated fat, which accounts for its buttery texture. It has an abundance of nutrients including iron, copper, phosphorus, potassium, beta carotene, folic acid, vitamins B_3, B_5, E, K, and protein. Avocados are easily digested, are good for the blood, and help prevent anemia. If rapid or high weight loss is your goal, limit your avocados to only a quarter at a time and to no more than one each week.

Festive Black Bean Dip

2 cups cooked black beans (if using canned beans, be sure to drain and rinse)

1 cup grated soy jalapeño cheese (you can find it in the cheese section of your natural foods store)

3 cloves garlic, pressed

3 green onions, minced

2 teaspoons chopped fresh cilantro

2 teaspoons ground cumin

1 teaspoon Bragg liquid aminos

In a bowl, combine all the ingredients and serve warm with tortilla chips and salsa.

• **F Y I**

Black Beans

Also called the black turtle bean, black beans are an excellent source of protein and insoluble fiber, which helps to lower cholesterol and normalize blood sugar levels. Add them cold to your salads to increase protein and turn your salad into a main course.

Spicy & Quick Nonfat Bean Dip

Salsa adds a bright flavor note and lovely color to this bean dip.

2 cups (16-ounce can) nonfat black beans, pinto beans,
     or a combination of both, drained and mashed

2/3 cup salsa

Place beans and salsa in a food processor and pulse until desired consistency.

• **T I P**

Bean Dips

It's too bad that commercial bean dips ruin a low fat, high fiber nutritious food into a lard-filled, artery clogging junk food with 60% (or higher) fat-calories. You can buy fat-free mashed beans at your health food store, but it's so easy to make your own. Try stuffing celery or Belgian endive or use as a dip for vegetables or baked tortillas, or topped on grains and salads.

Hummus Delight

Most hummus recipes call for tahini. Tahini tastes great, but it does contain fat, but I don't think you'll miss it in this recipe.

2 cups garbanzo beans (chickpeas), fresh cooked
   or canned (reserve the liquid)

2 tablespoons plus 1 teaspoon fresh lemon juice

1 to 2 cloves garlic, pressed or finely minced

1/4 teaspoon ground cumin

1 tablespoon minced red onion

2 tablespoons minced fresh parsley

1/4 teaspoon sea salt

Cayenne pepper to taste

Cracked pepper to taste

In a food processor, blend the chickpeas, lemon juice, garlic, and cumin with some of the reserved liquid. Add parsley, red onion, and season with salt and pepper. Pulse briefly to mix. Keep refrigerated until ready to serve.

• T I P

Cooking Beans

Beans are not a spur of the moment item. You have to remember to soak them, and it can take an hour or more for them to cook all the way through. Once a month, I cook a large batch of garbanzo beans and store them in the freezer in freezer bags, so I won't run out. Then they're ready whenever I want to make hummus. I love hummus as a spread on toasted whole grain bread with a slice of tomato, onion, and lettuce or sprouts, or wrapped in romaine lettuce leaves with grated carrots and sprouts. I also like to sprinkle whole cooked garbanzo beans on top of my salad or mix them with my grains.

VARIATIONS: Black Bean Hummus: Add 1/2 cup black beans to the recipe when blending. Roasted Red Pepper Hummus: Add 1/2 cup roasted red pepper to the recipe. Roasted Very Garlic Hummus: Add 3 tablespoons roasted garlic (see pages 288-289 for tips on roasting garlic). Roasted Onion Hummus: Add 1/3 cup roasted onion to recipes and 1 tablespoon fresh chives, minced. Dill Roasted Yellow Pepper Hummus: Add 3 tablespoons fresh minced dill and 1/2 cup roasted yellow pepper. Spicy Hummus: Add 1 jalapeño pepper, minced, and 1/8 teaspoon cayenne.

To any of the above recipes, add $^1/4$ to $^1/3$ cup tahini if you want a richer taste and don't mind the extra fat or calories.

• F Y I

Garbanzo beans are a very good source of calcium, magnesium, phos-phorus, potassium, zinc, manganese, beta carotene, and folic acid as well as an excellent source of protein. They help support kidney func-tion and cleanse the digestive system.

Soybean Spread

This is a healthy, versatile, high-protein spread that can be used for raw and steamed veggies, whole grain crackers and bread, or rolled up in Boston or romaine lettuce leaves with grated or julienned vegeta-bles. It's higher in fat than the other spreads, so enjoy it on special occasions until you reach your weight loss goal.

1 pound soybeans (about $2^1/2$ cups dry), cooked (reserve $^1/3$ cup liquid)
$^1/4$ cup Barlean's Flax Oil
$^1/2$ cup mashed ripe avocado
$^1/3$ cup fresh lemon juice
$^1/4$ cup tahini (sesame seed paste)
2 cloves garlic, pressed
2 tablespoons Bragg liquid aminos or low-sodium tamari or shoyu
2 tablespoons minced fresh parsley
$^1/4$ teaspoon ground cumin
$^1/2$ teaspoon onion powder

Mash beans in a blender or food processor, and blend with remaining ingredients. Chill before serving.

VARIATION: For a lighter, sweeter, and higher protein spread, add $^1/2$ cup cooked, mashed sweet potato and 4 ounces firm silken tofu.

• F Y I

Soybeans contain all the essential amino acids, making them a terrific vegetarian food. Soy is a potent phytoestrogen ('phyto' means plant), which may help prevent breast and ovarian cancers. A primary source *of lecithin, which controls cholesterol, soybeans are very rich in calcium, iron, and phosphorus, in addition to vitamins B$_3$ and C, and omega-3 essential fatty acids. Some recent research suggests that soy products are not safe for infants in formulas or for women who have had breast cancer or have a family history of breast cancer. Check with your physician if you're concerned.*

Quick & Easy Fat–Free Garlic Roasted Marinara Sauce

This freezes well in Ziploc freezer bags (1^1/2 cup size works well) so make tons of it to keep on hand for whenever the occasion arises. I use it in a variety of dishes and also as a salad dressing.

^{1}/2 cup vegetable broth, store-bought
    or homemade (see pages 298-299)

2 onions, chopped

3 cloves garlic, minced

2 (28-ounce) cans diced organic tomatoes
    or crushed tomatoes in purée

^{1}/2 cup tomato paste

^{1}/2 teaspoon dried oregano

^{1}/8 teaspoon cayenne

^{1}/2 cup roasted garlic (see page 288 for tips on roasting garlic)

Sea salt and freshly ground pepper to taste

In a large skillet or stock pot, bring the vegetable broth to a boil over medium-high heat. Add the onion and minced garlic and sauté just until the onion is tender, about 5 minutes. Add tomatoes, tomato paste, oregano, and cayenne. Stir and bring to a boil. Reduce heat to a gentle simmer, stirring occasionally as it thickens, about 10 to 12 minutes. Midway through, add the diced roasted garlic. Season to taste.

VARIATION: While this is the basic recipe, I often add frozen artichoke hearts, sliced mushrooms, diced bell peppers, lightly sautéed broccoli and/or cauliflower florets, or diced squash, zucchini, and carrots. Sometimes I add cubed extra firm lite organic silken tofu to increase the protein.

• T I P

Frozen Artichoke Hearts

Look for artichoke hearts in the freezer section of the supermarket. These are fat free and much healthier than artichoke hearts packed in oil. Keep a few packages on hand to throw in salads and to use in sauces, grains, soups, and dips.

Apricot–Ginger Chutney

Chutneys are traditionally sweet and spicy and used in India with meats and grains. I enjoy this mixture of flavors to accompany grains, salads, and even as a dip for vegetables.

1 pound dried apricots (unsulfured Turkish are my favorites), chopped into uniform pieces

$4^1/2$ cups purified hot water

$1^1/2$ cups apple cider vinegar

$1/2$ cup chopped sweet onion

$1/4$ cup chopped garlic

3 tablespoons chopped crystallized ginger

1 tablespoon curry

$1/4$ teaspoon lemon zest from an organic lemon

$1/8$ teaspoon sea salt

1 cup organic raisins

In a large bowl, soak the apricots in hot water overnight or for at least 2 hours. Then transfer them to a medium saucepan. Bring the water and apricots to a boil and add remaining ingredients except the raisins. Reduce heat to low and simmer until the mixture is thick, about 15 to 20 minutes. Add the raisins and simmer for another 15-20 minutes, stirring occasionally, making sure the chutney does not stick. Cool. Store in refrigerator.

Miso–Ginger–Tahini Sauce

For an exotic and winning taste, spoon this sauce over Japanese udon or soba (buckwheat) noodles or drizzled over steamed vegetables, grain dishes, or potatoes.

4 tablespoons white miso

3 tablespoons tahini

1/3 cup vegetable broth or water

2 tablespoons brown rice vinegar

1 1/2 tablespoons fresh ginger juice

1 tablespoon mirin (rice wine)

1 to 2 cloves garlic, pressed

1/2 teaspoon fresh lemon juice

In a medium saucepan, combine miso and tahini. Add the vegetable broth or water, a little at a time, stirring constantly to make a smooth sauce. Add the rest of the ingredients and bring to a simmer, making sure it doesn't boil. Add extra water or broth if too thick or to achieve desired consistency. Serve hot or warm.

• TIP

Mirin

Quality mirin is an ambrosial cooking wine, brewed and fermented from sweet rice, koji, and water. I use it in vinaigrettes, marinades, in vegetable dishes, and in sauces and dips.

AN EXTRA TIME-SAVING TIP: In addition to all the marinade ideas sprinkled throughout this chapter, other great sources for marinades are nonfat or low-fat natural, bottled salad dressings. Look for sweet onion, creamy garlic, toasted sesame, zesty Italian, and Dijon dressings, as these make excellent marinades. (My favorites are made by Spectrum Naturals.) I also use these dressings as dips for artichokes, drizzled over baked potatoes, grains, and steamed vegetables, and in a variety of oven-roasted vegetable and potato recipes.

Chapter 11

Salads

Gone are the days when salad meant a wedge of iceberg lettuce and a few pale pink excuses for tomatoes. Hallelujah! An almost infinite variety of textures, flavors, and colors can be combined to make salads these days. And the more creative you are, the more packed with nutritional benefits your salad can be. They're also easy to make and, unless we drown them in high-fat dressings, salads are generally low in calories. They provide lots of fiber, enzymes, chlorophyll, vitamins, minerals, especially calcium, and antioxidants. I encourage you to eat at least one or two salads every day. They help to fill you up without filling you out. While greens do provide some protein, you can increase the protein content of any salad by adding beans, grains, tofu and other soy foods, seeds, and nuts. I also like to add fresh ground flax seed meal to increase fiber and omega-3's.

Instead of having a small salad as part of your meal, **get in the habit of making the salad your entire meal.** Use a large attractive bowl or let your imagination go and create a masterpiece.

It's well known that most plant-based foods not only help you to maintain a healthy weight, they also may help prevent cancer and heart disease. Here are a few of the best foods that may help prevent both diseases that are easy to bring into your salad meals several times a week: spinach, broccoli, garlic, onions, beans, carrots, flax seed oil and freshly ground meal, beans such as garbanzo, black, kidney, and fresh soybeans (edamame), grains such as quinoa, millet, and brown rice, tomatoes, and most greens, such as romaine lettuce.

Here are some tips to help make the most of your salad greens:

1. *Always purchase greens as fresh as possible, without blemishes, bruises, or discoloring.* They are their best the same day you buy them so don't store them for more than 2 or 3 days. If you have more than you know you'll eat, juice them. Discard any signs of yellowing or discoloring. Whenever you can buy organic, do so.

2. *Choose a variety of greens in different colors.* Romaine lettuce packs 8 times the vitamin A of iceberg lettuce. Arugula has more than twice the calcium of milk, cup for cup. A half-cup of spiky dandelion leaves provides 78% of your daily value of vitamin A. One cup of spicy baby mustard greens provides 10% of your daily value of calcium. The crunchy, tangy leaves of purslane are a good source of omega-3 fatty acids, vitamin C, and iron. Tight heads, such as romaine, radicchio, and Belgian endive, can be cut with a knife; all other greens should be torn. So include a variety of organic greens in your salads and you'll never get tired of eating them.

3. *Always wash your greens.* If they are beginning to wilt from sitting out too long, soak them in a large bowl or sink of cold water. With greens like spinach—where bits of dirt positively cling to the leaves—rinse them 2 to 3 times to make sure all of the dirt is washed away. If you don't use a produce wash, fill the sink with cold water to which you've added 4 tablespoons of salt and some lemon juice. Soak greens for about 10 minutes and then rinse them well. (If you have any doubts about why it's important to wash your vegetables, check back in Chapter 3 on the negative health effects of pesticides and herbicides.)

   When you get your greens and produce home from the market, wash them all at once and dry them thoroughly, then store everything in freezer zipper top bags to which you've added one or two white paper towels. This helps keep your produce fresh and makes it easy and fast to whip up your salads each day.

4. *Make your own dressing,* preferably just before serving the salad, but if you'd prefer to make up a small batch, keep it refrigerated and use it up within a few days. Your dressing will only be as good as your ingredients. Purchase only cold-pressed oils and keep them refrigerated. (The heat used to make commercial oils destroys many of the nutrients and causes the oil to break down more quickly, becoming rancid.) If you purchase bottled dressings, see if there's an expiration date, keep them refrigerated, too, ˙ and don't use bottled dressing you've kept opened in your refrigerator for months.

5. *Don't overdress.* Less is more when it comes to salad dressing. If you're using a dressing that's higher in calories and want to cut

back, keep it on the side and dip. After dressing the salad, toss well. The best instrument you can use is an impeccably clean pair of hands. I like to squeeze a bit of fresh lemon juice onto my salad, even over other dressings. It tastes great and makes the dressing go further. And don't forget, fresh lemon juice makes a simple, light, fat-free dressing for salads, too.

6. *Create some finger salads.* In a bowl, put a few crisp romaine leaves, a carrot, a couple stalks of celery, a half sweet bell pepper, and whatever vegetables appeal to you as close to the way nature made them as possible. Then simply use your hands instead of utensils and chew, chew, chew.

7. *Use edible flowers.* (Note: not all flowers are edible. Please don't pick your own salad flowers unless you have a good guide and know exactly what you're doing. You can find edible flowers in many good produce markets.) Experiment with different flowers and their flavors. Creatively placed around or on what you've made gives an added touch of beauty.

8. *Vary the amounts of the different ingredients* according to your taste. Think of salad recipes as guidelines or a place to start.

Vitality Salad

Serves 3 to 6

You can't get much tastier than this simple, crispy salad.
A great rejuvenator and mild cleanser, this salad lends itself
to any favorite occasion.

2 cups romaine lettuce, torn into small pieces
1 cup baby leaf spinach, torn or left whole, stemmed

THEN ADD:
1/2 cup chopped celery
1/2 cup shredded carrot
1/2 cup shredded beet
1/2 cup diced jicama
1/2 cup diced ripe tomato

¹⁄₂ cup diced cucumber

¹⁄₄ cup diced bell pepper, red, yellow, or orange

¹⁄₄ cup sunflower sprouts

Edible organic colorful flowers (see Mountain Valley Growers in the Resource Directory), for garnish

In a bowl, combine all ingredients and toss with your favorite dressing (see Chapter 12 for suggestions).

• **T I P**

Adding Protein to Your Salad Bowl

Add some beans such as garbanzo beans or black beans, edamame (out of the pods), sunflower or pumpkin seeds, grilled tofu slices, or perhaps a scoop of quinoa or millet, to make this salad a perfect, complete meal in a bowl.

Shredded Rainbow Salad

Serves 4, but you can double and triple these amounts for a larger crowd.

For your next large family gathering or party, make this salad in a large glass bowl in colorful layers, or serve in individual Boston or butter leaf lettuce cups. I guarantee it will be the hit of the party.

¹⁄₂ purple and ¹⁄₂ green cabbage, shredded

1 medium parsnip, grated

2 medium carrots, grated

1 small jicama, grated

¹⁄₂ cup grated daikon radish

¹⁄₄ cup green onion, finely chopped

If serving in a glass bowl, layer the shredded vegetables and drizzle your favorite dressing over the top. If using lettuce cups, toss the shredded vegetables in a large bowl, drizzle with dressing, and spoon into the cups.

• **F Y I**

Parsnips

The parsnip, a pale carrot look-alike, is a splendid superfood as it helps detoxify and cleanse the body, improves bowel action, supports the kidneys and spleen, and is a diuretic. It is rich in potassium, phosphorus, folic acid, calcium, and magnesium. Keep a few in your refrigerator and grate them into salads, soups, casseroles, veggie burgers, or grain dishes.

• **F Y I**

Cultured Vegetables

Cultured refers to the fermentation process. These organic vegetables have been either cut, ground, or shredded and left in a sanitary container for about 7 days at a temperature maintained in the range of 59 to 71 degrees. This process allows for the proliferation of healthful micro-flora (lactobacilli), which help break down the sugars and starches found in vegetables, and in turn aid the pancreas and intestines in proper digestion. The difference between Rejuvenative Foods Raw Cultured Vegetables and commercially available heated sauerkraut is that in the heated sauerkraut, the lactobacilli and healthful enzymes have been destroyed. It's very beneficial to include these cultured vegetables in your diet a few times each week.

Raw Organic Cultured Vegetable Salad

What could be easier? A few scoops of raw cultured vegetables (see note below) on a bed of crisp, organic salad greens. Delectable.

Arrange your favorite greens on individual serving plates. Pick two or three different cultured vegetables (see Rejuvenative Foods in the Resource Directory) and scoop on top of the greens. Be sure to get a bit of the juice as your dressing. A few of my favorites include Raw Sauerkraut, Vegi Delite, and Kim Chi.

Belgian Endive Hummus–Salsa Salad

Another easy and delightfully delicious finger salad that is always a winner whether eating solo or serving at a dinner party.

PER PERSON:

6 to 8 large endive leaves, washed and dried

1/3 cup hummus (see recipe pages 246-247)

1/3 cup salsa (see recipe pages 243)

1 tablespoon fresh flax seed meal

Nest two large endive leaves, one inside the other, to give your finger food more strength. Spread the hummus on the leaves, top that with salsa, then sprinkle flax meal on the top. These endive treats look great on a bed of greens designed in a pinwheel around tomato slices.

Living Nori Salad

Serves 2 to 3

Sea vegetables, like nori, also called seaweed, are the highest source of minerals and are excellent for the cardiovascular and nervous systems. A perfect food for vegetarians, nori helps cleanse the body of toxins and aids digestion. Sea vegetables are rich in calcium, iron, iodine, and potassium.

1 small jicama, grated (about 1/3 to 1/2 cup)

1 medium carrot, grated (about 1/3 to 1/2 cup)

1 medium avocado, diced or mashed

1 green onion, finely chopped

1/3 cup diced red, orange, or yellow bell pepper

1 clove garlic, pressed

1/2 tablespoon Bragg liquid aminos

Romaine lettuce

Nori sheets

Wasabi (optional)*

Pickled ginger (optional)*

Combine the jicama, carrot, avocado, onion, liquid aminos, pepper, and garlic in a bowl. Cover and refrigerate for about 30 minutes. Place a nori sheet on a cutting board and put a large romaine leaf on top of the nori. Spoon the chilled vegetable mixture on the lettuce and roll it up. Seal the nori seam with some dabs of water. Cut into 1 1/2- to 2-inch pieces and serve on a bed of lettuce with a little wasabi and pickled ginger.

*Wasabi, or Japanese horseradish, and pickled ginger, another Japanese specialty, are available in Asian markets and many super-markets with a good Asian foods section. Wasabi is available in powdered form, which can be reconstituted with a few drops of water, or as a paste (in a small tube).

Pear & Arugula Salad with Toasted Walnuts

This hearty salad will serve 2 as a main meal or 4 to 6 as a side salad.

2 small ripe Bartlett or Comice pears, cored and thinly sliced

7 ounces arugula

3 tablespoons cold-pressed extra virgin olive oil

2 tablespoons raspberry vinegar

1/8 teaspoon sea salt

1 tablespoon fresh chives, finely chopped

1/2 cup coarsely broken and toasted walnuts

Place the pears and arugula in a salad bowl. In a separate bowl, whisk together oil, vinegar, chives, and salt. Add the dressing to the pears and arugula and toss to combine.

Arrange salad on individual salad plates and sprinkle with the toasted walnuts. Toast the walnuts in a dry skillet over medium heat for 3 to 4 minutes, stirring constantly.

Crunchy Cabbage, Apple & Turnip Salad with Toasted Cashews

Serves 4 to 6

1/2 medium red cabbage, shredded

1/2 medium green cabbage, shredded

1 large apple, cored and chopped

1 small red onion, finely chopped

1 small turnip, grated

1 cup chopped fresh parsley

1/2 cup ground and toasted cashews

In a large bowl, combine all the ingredients. Toss with a light vinaigrette to which you've added 1 to 2 tablespoons fresh apple juice.

• F Y I

Turnips

A very alkaline vegetable, when eaten raw, turnips aid digestion, are rich in calcium, magnesium, phosphorus, potassium, folic acid, and vitamin C, and they also help clear the blood of toxins.

Hearts of Romaine, Artichokes & Palm Salad

Serves 4 to 6

This elegant simple salad always gets rave reviews.

2 (9-ounce) packages frozen artichoke hearts, thawed, cut in half (approx. 24 hearts)

1 can hearts of palm, drained and sliced 1/2-inch thick on an angle

3/4 cup homemade vinaigrette (see Chapter 12) or bottled nonfat Italian dressing

3 tablespoons chopped fresh parsley

1 clove garlic, minced

2 teaspoons fresh lemon juice

3 heads romaine lettuce hearts,
　　thoroughly washed and dried

1 red bell pepper

1 yellow bell pepper

In a bowl, combine artichoke hearts, hearts of palm, parsley, lemon juice, and dressing. Gently toss and chill. Roast yellow and red peppers*, peel, and slice into thin strips. Now for the fun part. On individual salad plates, arrange first the romaine hearts from the center out in a pinwheel design. With a slotted spoon, scoop the marinated hearts of palm and artichokes in the hub of the wheel. Then place the red and yellow roasted pepper strips in a crisscross pattern over the leaves and hearts. Drizzle some extra marinade dressing over the leaves and serve.

*ROASTING PEPPERS IS SIMPLE: Place peppers directly on a gas stove-top burner or under a preheated broiler. Cook on all sides until the skin blackens and blisters. Transfer to a heavy duty plastic (zip top) or paper bag, close it up, and steam for about 5 minutes. When cool enough to handle, peel away the charred skin with your fingers. Don't rinse them under water as that will wash away some of the flavor. Cut away any black spots with a small knife.

Couscous Garden Salad

Serves 3 to 5

3/4 cup vegetable broth

1/2 cup uncooked whole grain couscous

1/4 cup chopped green onion

1/4 cup chopped yellow bell pepper

1/4 cup chopped mushrooms

1/2 cup chopped Italian plum tomatoes

1 tablespoon chopped fresh basil

1 teaspoon chopped fresh tarragon

2 teaspoons Barlean's Flax Oil
　　or cold pressed extra virgin olive oil

1 teaspoon fresh lemon juice

1 teaspoon organic balsamic vinegar

2 cups baby spinach leaves or head of Bibb
or butter lettuce

1/3 cup ground and toasted cashews, for garnish

3 to 5 lemon slices, for garnish

In a saucepan, bring broth to a boil. Remove from heat and stir in couscous. Cover and let stand until cool, then fluff with a fork. In a separate mixing bowl, combine vegetables, tomatoes, and herbs, oil, lemon juice, and vinegar. Mix well. Add the couscous and combine thoroughly. Cover and refrigerate for about 1 hour or until chilled. Serve on a bed of baby leaf spinach or large leaves of Bibb lettuce. Garnish with lemon slices and sprinkle with toasted ground cashews.

VARIATION: Before steaming the couscous, dry sauté 1/4 cup of the couscous in a skillet for about 2 to 3 minutes. It will turn a darker shade and become imbued with a more nutty flavor. (I usually toast only half so the nutty flavor doesn't overwhelm the salad.) Steam both the toasted and remaining dry couscous together and proceed with the recipe.

• F Y I

Couscous

A delectable, easy-to-digest grain, couscous is feather-light and fluffy and cooks up in minutes. Traditional to North Africa, couscous is made from the endosperm of durum wheat (and therefore must be avoided by anyone with a gluten allergy). Delicious as pilaf, or enjoy it as a dessert by baking with apple juice and your favorite fruits and nuts.

Apricot–Spinach Salad

Serves 2 to 6

This will serve 6 as a side salad, and 2 as a marvelous main course.

4 cups baby leaf spinach, washed and dried

1/2 cup dried unsulphured apricots, chopped (Turkish are the best)

¹/₃ cup chopped green onions

¹/₃ cup diced yellow bell pepper

3 tablespoons toasted sunflower seeds

1 tablespoon toasted sesame seeds

4 tablespoons plain soy yogurt

2 tablespoons organic balsamic vinegar

2 tablespoons fresh orange juice

1 tablespoon fresh lemon juice

1 teaspoon grated orange peel (zest), from an organic orange

1 garlic clove, minced

In a large bowl, toss the spinach, apricots, green onions, bell pepper, sunflower and sesame seeds. In a separate bowl, combine the remaining ingredients. Pour over the salad and toss to combine. Serve right away or chill for about one hour.

VARIATION: Substitute currants, raisins, or dried cherries for the apricots.

• F Y I

Spinach

Spinach is rich in beta carotene, potassium, iron, vitamin B_6, vitamin C, calcium, and magnesium. It helps fight cancer, heart disease, and mental disorders due to its high folic acid content, and also supports bone density and boosts the immune system. Either raw or steamed, this antioxidant superfood is worth making a mainstay of your healthy diet.

Soba Noodle Salad with Garden Vegetables

Serves 4 to 6

Soba, a thin, delicious, high-protein Japanese-style pasta, is often served in a broth or chilled and served with a dipping sauce. Look for either organic whole wheat or buckwheat (my favorite) soba at your natural food store or Asian market.

12 ounces soba noodles

1 cup broccoli florets

1 cup cauliflower pieces

2 carrots, peeled and sliced on an angle 1/4 inch

3/4 cup sliced water chestnuts (you can buy them sliced in a can)

3 green onions, chopped

3/4 cup sliced bamboo shoots, drained

1 cup vinaigrette (see Chapter 12)

2 tablespoons toasted sesame seeds

Cook soba noodles according to the package directions, drain, and chill. Lightly steam the broccoli, cauliflower, and carrots. Chill. In a large bowl, combine the chilled noodles, the chilled vegetables, chestnuts, green onions, bamboo shoots, and dressing of your choice. Refrigerate for at least one hour before serving, mixing occasionally so the flavors blend.

Parsley Lentil Salad

Serves 4 to 6

For color, taste, and an abundance of nutrients, this salad is hard to beat. It's also delicious scooped into warm, whole grain pita triangles.

1 1/2 cups dry lentils (about 10 ounces)

2 cups vegetable broth

1 bay leaf

2 red peppers, roasted and cut into 1/2-inch pieces

1 small red onion, thinly sliced

2 medium organic lemons, see below

1 1/2 cups loosely packed fresh parsley leaves, finely chopped

1/4 cup cold pressed, extra virgin olive oil

1 teaspoon Bragg liquid aminos

1/4 teaspoon fresh coarsely ground black pepper

1/8 teaspoon garlic powder

Rinse lentils well with cold running water; discard any stones or blemished lentils. In a large saucepan, place lentils, bay leaf, and enough water or vegetable broth to cover lentils by 2 inches. Bring to a boil; reduce to simmer and cover for 20 minutes or until lentils are tender. Discard bay leaf. While the lentils are cooking, roast the peppers (see page 290) and cut into bite-sized pieces. Place the sliced onion in a colander and drain lentils over the onion to soften them just a bit and take away their strong bite. Grate 2 teaspoons lemon peel (zest) and squeeze 1/4 cup juice. In a big mixing bowl, combine lentils, peppers, parsley, lemon juice and peel, oil, garlic powder, liquid aminos, and pepper. Serve warm or chilled.

• **F Y I**

Lentils

Lentils are an excellent source of protein, calcium, magnesium, phosphorus, potassium, zinc, and folic acid. These nutrients benefit nearly every organ and system in the body. The organic green lentil is the classic one to use for soups as it "melts" in just 30 minutes, making a thick, smooth base, to which you can add all your favorite vegetables and seasonings. The Beluga are tiny black lentils indigenous to Syria. They look like caviar and are heavenly. They're higher in protein than French, green, or red. Try them in salads or soups. The French lentil, a Persian variety, are tiny gray to green-black ovals. And Crimson (red) lentils are famous for their beauty and flavor and they bring elegance to any dish. Always buy organic lentils.

Spicy Black Bean Salad

Serves 4 to 6

This high-protein dish is great as a snack, side dish, or main meal.

3 cups cooked chilled black beans
1 red or yellow bell pepper, diced
1 large carrot, diced
2 tablespoons chopped fresh cilantro
1/2 fresh lemon, juiced
Dash ground cumin

Dash cayenne pepper or crushed red pepper flakes

Sea salt to taste

Combine everything in a large bowl and serve at room temperature on a bed of crisp lettuce leaves.

VARIATION: Substitute any variety of bean for the black such as navy, garbanzo, pinto, black-eyed, anasazi, lima, butterscotch calypso, azuki (aduki), or kidney, or a combination.

• **F Y I**

Beans, Beans, Beans

Beans are brimming with soluble fiber that helps lower cholesterol and normalize blood sugar levels. They also are an excellent source of protein, iron, and are rich in vitamins and minerals such as potassium and calcium. And here's the bonus. They are very low in fat. Being concentrated sources of protein, they need to be soaked for at least 4 hours before cooking and preferably overnight. If you forget to soak, there is a quick soak method: bring beans to a boil, then let sit for one hour. Either soaking beans overnight and/or cooking with kombu (a sea vegetable aids in the digestibility of beans.

After soaking beans, always pour the soaking water out and add fresh water for cooking. Also, don't add salt until the beans have finished cooking, because salt toughens the beans' skins.

Cucumber–Tofu Salad with Toasted Pecans

Serves 4 to 6

This low calorie, high protein salad is elegant enough for the most discriminating party guests and easy enough to whip up at the last minute.

1 package (12.3 ounces) extra firm silken tofu

5 to 6 large celery stalks, juiced, (save 3/4 cup)

1 small lemon, juiced

1 tablespoon white or yellow miso

$^1/_4$ teaspoon sea salt

7 radishes, thinly sliced

4 large cucumbers, thinly sliced

4 green onions, finely chopped

$^1/_4$ cup finely chopped fresh parsley

$^1/_4$ cup finely chopped fresh mint

$^1/_2$ cup pecans, toasted (dry sauté 4 to 5 minutes
   in a skillet), for garnish

In a food processor or blender, combine the lemon juice, celery juice, tofu, miso, and salt until creamy smooth. In a large salad bowl, combine the rest of the ingredients, except the pecans, with the dressing. Chill for at least one hour. Arrange the salad on individual plates or on a bed of crisp greens and garnish with toasted pecans.

VARIATION: Instead of pecans, substitute toasted coarsely ground almonds, cashews, pine nuts, or sesame seeds.

*If the cucumbers are organic, you don't need to peel them. I like to cut the peeling in wide strips before I slice it so the slices have a pretty, scalloped edge.

• F Y I
Cucumbers
Cucumbers are a dieter's best friend. They are very low in calories and rich in potassium and beta carotene, they are naturally diuretic and laxative, and dissolve the uric acid that causes kidney and bladder stones. They support digestion and regulate blood pressure.

4–Bean Salad
Serves 4 to 6

This tastes best with fresh cut beans, but if you only have canned or frozen, they will work just fine.

$^1/_2$ pound fresh green beans, trimmed and cut in 1$^1/_2$-inch pieces (or
   one 8-ounce can)

$^1/_2$ pound fresh wax beans, trimmed and cut in 1$^1/_2$-inch pieces
   (or one 8-ounce can)

1 cup cooked kidney beans (or one 8-ounce can)

1 cup cooked garbanzo beans (or one 8-ounce can)

1 (8-ounce) can sliced water chestnuts

1 medium red onion, cut in 1/2-inch dice

1/2 cup sliced green onion

1 yellow pepper, cut in 1/2-inch dice

If using fresh beans, steam trimmed in a stockpot for beans about 7 to 8 minutes (you want them to be slightly crunchy/slightly tender). Transfer beans to a large bowl. Add the rest of the ingredients and combine thoroughly. Chill. Toss with the dressing of your choice. (See Chapter 12 for suggestions.)

VARIATION: Substitute asparagus, or broccoli for the green beans.

Sunny Shredded Dill & Toasted Sesame Coleslaw

Serves 6 to 8

This easy-to-make salad provides lots of fiber with very few calories, only 8 calories per 1/2 cup, 16 calories if cooked! Long a staple in Eastern Europe, cabbage is versatile, tasty, filling, and loaded with effective anti-cancer and antioxidant agents. And it retains most of its nutritional goodness even when it's cooked. Drinking cabbage juice is very beneficial for ulcers. If you've only eaten red or green cabbage, it's time to branch out. Look for savoy, or Chinese cabbage—an elongated bundle of leaves with a core, and bok choy—another Asian cabbage with plump white stalks and green floppy leaves.

2 cups shredded red cabbage

2 cups shredded green cabbage

2 carrots, peeled and grated

1 small daikon, peeled and grated

3 stalks bok choy, white parts only, cut in 1/8-inch slices

2 tablespoons toasted sesame seeds

1 tablespoon dill seeds

In a large bowl, combine all the ingredients and toss with the dressing of your choice. I like to use my Lemon-Tahini Dressing (pages 279-280) or one of the vinaigrettes (see Chapter 12).

VARIATION: To add more minerals and variety to this coleslaw, I like to include a package of wakame, a large brown sea vegetable (seaweed). Just soak wakame in scalding water for 15 minutes, then strain. With the tip of a sharp knife, remove the thick membrane and julienne 1/4-inch pieces from the outer leaves. Toss with the rest of the ingredients.

• F Y I
Daikon

If you've never tried this easy-to-grow Japanese radish, rush to the nearest store. It's a pearly white root that's shaped like a carrot and can grow as long as your arm. You don't even need to peel it. Just wash and grate it to use raw in a salad, or to garnish grains, or cook it as you would a carrot in soups or sautéed, simmered, baked, or braised dishes. It contains the digestive enzymes diastase, amylase, and esterase, and contains a substance that inhibits the formation of carcinogens in the body.

Colorful Summer Fruit Combo
Serves 2 to 6

For breakfast, a mid-morning or mid-afternoon snack, or light lunch or dinner, this fresh fruit combo combines the most luscious colors and flavors for a delightful treat. Be creative! Almost any fruit will work in this salad.

1 small or 1/2 medium cantaloupe, sliced and cubed

1/2 medium honeydew melon, sliced and cubed

2 pears, peeled and cubed

2 cups sweet cherries, pitted

1 cup berries of your choice

In a large bowl, combine all the ingredients and chill. If desired, top with one of my fruit dressings (see Chapter 12).

• F Y I

Cherries

Sweet cherries have only 50 calories per 1/2 cup (uncooked). They have a natural laxative effect and are an excellent component of an elimination diet. Being high in iron, they are a natural blood-builder. A 1-cup serving supplies almost 25% of the RDA of vitamin A, along with a moderate amount of fiber. And like most fruits and vegetables, they're virtually free of sodium and fat. For a sweet tooth craving, these usually hit the spot. Keep organic frozen dark sweet cherries on hand to sweeten your smoothies.

Antioxidant Spinach–Sweet Potato Salad

Serves 2 to 6

The colors and sweetness in this salad appeal to children and teens as well as adults. When I make this as my entire meal, I sometimes add tofu, grilled or sautéed, cut in strips, or a few nuts and seeds to increase the protein.

4 cups baby leaf spinach, washed and stemmed

1 small red pepper, diced

1 small yellow pepper, diced

2 cups sweet potatoes, peeled, diced, and steamed

In a large bowl, combine all ingredients and dress with Orange Balsamic, Orange Sesame-Cashew, or Orange Yam Dressing (see Chapter 12).

• F Y I

Spinach

Did you know that spinach has only 6 calories per 1/2 cup when eaten raw and 20 calories when cooked? Not only that, it has the ability to rev up the metabolism and burn more fat. Two big salads a day with lots of greens, including spinach, will do wonders for accelerating fat loss. Spinach is rich in beta carotene, folic acid, potassium, iron, vita-

mins B_6 and C, calcium, and magnesium. An excellent antioxidant, it helps regulate blood pressure, boosts the immune system, and is an anti-cancer food.

• **F Y I**

Sweet Potatoes

Another super health food, sweet potatoes are a root vegetable, not a tuber like white potatoes. They provide calcium, magnesium, potassium, folic acid, vitamins C and E, phosphorus, and loads of beta carotene. Easily digestible and highly nutritious, they are excellent for inflammation of the digestive tract, ulcers, and poor circulation. They are also detoxifying as they bind to heavy metals and help remove them from the body. The National Cancer Institute has indicated that eating a half cup per day of sweet potatoes or those other bright orange vegetables, like carrots and winter squash, can cut the likelihood of lung cancer by as much as 50%.

Sun–Dried Tomato, Hijiki & Romaine Salad

Serves 2 to 6

This very low calorie, mineral-rich salad will fill you up and boost your energy.

2 cups romaine lettuce hearts, torn into bite size pieces

1¹/2 cups combination of arugula and baby leaf spinach, torn into bite size pieces

¹/2 cup cucumber, peeled, seeded, and chopped

¹/2 cup grated daikon

¹/2 cup chopped yellow, orange, purple, or combination bell peppers

6 to 8 sun-dried tomatoes, soaked in water, drained, and chopped

3 tablespoons green onions, finely chopped

1¹/2 tablespoons dried hijiki, soaked in water for 30 minutes, drained and chopped

Fresh parsley sprigs, for garnish

THE DRESSING:

1 tablespoon Bragg liquid aminos

1 tablespoon fresh grapefruit juice

2 teaspoons fresh lemon juice

1$\frac{1}{2}$ tablespoons Barlean's Flax Oil

1 to 2 cloves garlic, pressed

1 teaspoon Dijon mustard

In a large bowl, combine the lettuce and spinach leaves with the cucumber, daikon, bell peppers, tomatoes, green onions, and hijiki. In a separate bowl, combine the dressing ingredients and whisk well. Toss with the salad, garnish with fresh parsley sprigs, and serve.

• F Y I

Hiziki Seaweed

This low-calorie seaweed is the most mineral-rich of all the sea vegetables. It looks like narrow long black ribbons, grows near the low-water mark along the Japanese coast, and is harvested in the winter and spring. It is sun-dried, boiled, and dried again. Its slightly salty flavor and cooling action is a superior kidney food. It also acts as a diuretic, detoxifies the body, supports the thyroid and bones, and stabilizes blood sugar. One cup of cooked hiziki contains more calcium than a cup of milk. It's also a rich source of iron, protein, vitamin A, and B vitamins.

Jicama–Leek & Pepper Salad

Serves 4 to 6

I love the crunchy sweetness of jicama in salads, as part of a raw vegetable or fruit plate, or diced in grains and casseroles.

2 cups diced jicama

2 leeks, finely diced

1 red bell pepper, diced

1 yellow bell pepper, diced

1 large avocado, peeled and diced

1 jalapeño pepper, seeded, white tissue removed, diced (optional)

2 green onions, finely diced

2 stalks celery, finely diced

In a large bowl, combine all the ingredients. Dress with any vinaigrette (see Chapter 12) or my Lemon Tahini Dressing (pages 279-280) or Tahini Salsa Dressing (page 281).

• **F Y I**

Leeks

A sweet cousin of the onion, the leek is a versatile root vegetable that's great in salads, soups, sautéed dishes, pilafs, and casseroles. Many recipes call for cutting off the green tops and only using the white part, but I disagree. I use not only the leek's green leaf but also its many tiny rootlets, which are mineral-dense filaments that add valuable flavor and nutrients. The only parts to discard are the dehydrated end and any large, tough outer leaves. Slice the remaining vegetable in half lengthwise and wash very carefully, making sure to remove any dirt lodged in the leaves.

Leeks are an excellent source of fiber, potassium, vitamins K and A, calcium, folic acid, and the lesser known carotenoids lutein and zeaxanthin. Leeks are cleansing, diuretic, and help eliminate uric acid in gout.

• **F Y I**

Jicama

Pronounced "HEE-kuh-muh," this root vegetable looks like a beige oversize turnip. Peel the skin off and you'll find a crisp, slightly sweet flesh that's similar to water chestnuts—only crunchier. Very low in calories, it's a good source of potassium. It's a nice addition to any vegetable tray because its bland flavor lends itself well to most dips.

Chapter 12

DRESSINGS & SPECIAL TREATS

Many people make the mistake of making or ordering a healthy salad and then drowning it with a creamy, rich, artery-clogging, high fat dressing. When you use dressings on a salad, don't make the mistake of using so much that you can hardly taste the vegetables. Less is always more when it comes to dressings. In addition to dressing salads, I also use many of these dressings over steamed vegetables or grains, or as dips for raw vegetables or artichoke leaves.

Remember, instead of always using a dressing, you can drizzle some fresh lemon juice over your salad, or even fresh grapefruit juice with a couple of drops of tamari or Bragg liquid aminos. Fresh dressing is so much better tasting and better for you than bottled dressings. Get in the habit of making your dressings fresh and using them within 3 days. Look for the freshest cold pressed oils, such as extra virgin olive, which is the best next to Barlean's Flax Oil. Try a variety of vinegars, such as organic balsamic, raspberry, brown rice, raw apple cider, and red wine.

Vitality Vinaigrette

Makes about 3/4 cup

This easy, healthy, and delicious vinaigrette is my favorite dressing that I've used more than any other for years.

1/3 cup fresh lemon juice (juice of 2 medium lemons)

2 tablespoons organic balsamic vinegar

1 teaspoon garlic, pressed (2 to 3 cloves)

1 teaspoon Dijon mustard

1/8 teaspoon sea salt

1/3 cup Barlean's Flax Oil (see the Resource Directory)

Whisk together the lemon juice, vinegar, garlic, mustard, and salt until well blended. Drizzle in a little oil at a time, whisking after each addition until all the oil is thoroughly incorporated. Use within 3 days.

VARIATIONS: You can substitute other vinegars, such as raw apple cider vinegar, raspberry, brown rice, red wine, peach, etc., either for half or all the balsamic vinegar.

• T I P

The Best Way to Juice a Lemon

To get the most juice from a lemon, roll it back and forth on a hard counter for a few seconds, then cut it, and squeeze. Some books tell you to microwave it for a few seconds to make it juicier, but I don't recommend this method because cooking destroys all of the enzymes.

Vitality French Vinaigrette

Makes 2 cups

3/4 cup basic Vitality Vinaigrette (page 273)
1 large ripe tomato, cut into quarters

In a blender or food processor, blend on high speed for 30 seconds. Use within 3 days.

VARIATIONS: Add 1 to 2 teaspoons each of any of the following chopped or minced fresh herbs to the dressings: basil, chervil, chives, cilantro, dill, Herbes de Provence, lemon grass, mint, oregano, parsley, rosemary, tarragon, thyme.

Vitality Thousand Island

Makes 2¹/₂ cups

This dressing is light, colorful, and refreshing on any salad with crisp greens. Try it as a topping on grains, potatoes, and steamed vegetables, as well as over tofu steaks and on soba or other whole grain pasta/noodles.

2 cups Vitality French Vinaigrette (page 274)

6 ounces extra firm lite organic silken tofu

In a blender or food processor, blend vinaigrette and tofu at high speed for 30 seconds. Use within 3 days.

Never–Fail Herb Vinaigrette

Makes about 3/4 cup

This one is quick and easy—great on any green salad or sprinkled over lightly steamed or roasted veggies.

1/4 cup red wine vinegar

1 tablespoon finely chopped fresh parsley leaves

1 tablespoon finely chopped fresh chives

1 teaspoon finely chopped fresh tarragon leaves

1 teaspoon finely chopped fresh chervil

1/2 teaspoon sea salt

1/4 teaspoon coarsely ground fresh black pepper

1/2 cup cold-pressed, extra virgin olive oil

In a small bowl, whisk together all the ingredients except the oil, until thoroughly blended. Whisk in the oil, a little at a time. Cover and refrigerate for up to 3 days if not using right away.

VARIATIONS: Substitute organic balsamic vinegar for the red wine vinegar. For Garlic Vinaigrette: Add 2 to 3 medium garlic cloves, finely minced. For Lemon Vinaigrette: Substitute fresh lemon juice for the red wine vinegar. For Dijon Vinaigrette: Add 1 table-spoon Dijon mustard.

Easy Balsamic Dijon Vinaigrette for Two

Makes about 1/4 cup

With this simple recipe, you'll never need or want to resort to bottled dressings again.

1 tablespoon cold-pressed, extra virgin olive oil

2 tablespoons organic balsamic vinegar

1 medium garlic clove, minced

1/4 teaspoon Dijon mustard

1/8 teaspoon sea salt

1/8 teaspoon coarsely ground fresh black pepper

In a small jar with a tight-fitting lid, combine all the ingredients and shake until thoroughly incorporated. Pour over salad of your choice and toss to coat.

Orange Balsamic Vinaigrette

Makes about 1/2 cup

3 tablespoons cold-pressed, extra virgin olive oil

1 tablespoon fresh orange juice

1 tablespoon organic balsamic vinegar

1 teaspoon honey Dijon mustard

1 teaspoon zest from an organic orange

1/4 teaspoon sea salt

In a blender, jar, or small bowl, thoroughly combine all the ingredients. Just before serving, drizzle over your salad and toss.

Tangerine–Ume Dressing

Makes about 1/2 cup

This refreshing and different dressing is great tossed on your favorite vegetable or noodle salad. Umeboshi in fresh or paste form is available in natural food and Asian food stores.

Juice of 2 medium tangerines

3 tablespoons raw tahini (see Rejuvenative Foods in the Resource Directory)

1 tablespoon cold-pressed sesame oil

1 tablespoon purified water

1 tablespoon fresh lemon juice

2 teaspoons umeboshi paste or minced umeboshi
  (pickled Japanese plums)

1 garlic clove, minced

1 teaspoon chives, for garnish

In a blender or food processor, blend all the ingredients, except the chives, until smooth. Add the chives and chill for 30 minutes before using. Use within 5 days.

VARIATION: Substitute fresh orange or grapefruit juice for the tangerine juice. If using grapefruit juice, add 2 teaspoons brown rice syrup to sweeten the dressing.

Lemon Mustard

Makes about 2 cups

This zesty dressing will jazz up any salad and also works well as a marinade for tofu steaks, drizzled over hot or cold streamed vegetables, or as a topping on all kinds of grains including brown rice, quinoa, kamut, and millet.

6 ounces firm lite organic silken tofu

1/2 cup plain or lemon soy yogurt or Lemonaise Spread (page 239)

1/4 cup purified water

1/4 cup fresh lemon juice (omit if using lemon soy yogurt
  or Lemonaise Spread)

1/4 cup brown rice vinegar

1/4 cup stone ground mustard, low sodium

2 to 3 cloves garlic, minced

1 tablespoon chopped fresh Italian parsley

1 tablespoon chopped fresh tarragon

1 to 2 teaspoons red onion, minced

1/4 teaspoon sea salt

Dash cayenne pepper

In a blender or food processor, blend all ingredients together thoroughly.

Orange Sesame–Cashew Dressing

Makes about 3/4 cup

On a crisp romaine lettuce or baby leaf spinach salad with cucumber, thinly sliced sweet onions, hearts of palm, yellow, red, or orange bell pepper, and toasted sesame seeds, nothing tastes better.

1/4 cup unhulled sesame seeds

10 raw cashews

2 tablespoons mango, peach, raspberry, or other fruit vinegar

2 medium oranges, peeled and diced (or 3 tangerines or jar of unsweetened mandarin orange slices)

1/2 cup fresh orange juice

1/8 teaspoon sea salt

Toast the sesame seeds in a dry, hot skillet for 3 to 4 minutes, stirring occasionally so they don't burn. In a blender or food processor, blend together the orange juice, 1/4 cup orange pieces, cashews, vinegar, and 2 tablespoons of roasted sesame seeds. Next, add the remaining orange pieces (or tangerine) to the salad and toss with the dressing. Sprinkle the extra toasted sesame seeds on the top. Use right away.

Cilantro Thousand Island

Makes about 2 3/4 cups

This is a healthy, low-fat version of Thousand Island dressing for cilantro lovers everywhere.

1/3 cup diced red bell pepper

2 tablespoons chopped fresh cilantro

1/4 cup onion, diced

1 tablespoon chopped green olives

1 tablespoon chopped fresh Italian parsley

4 ounces firm lite silken organic tofu, cut in 1 1/2-inch cubes

2/3 cup organic tomato purée

1/2 cup purified water

1/2 cup plain soy yogurt

1/4 cup brown rice syrup

1/8 teaspoon sea salt

In a food processor, combine red pepper, cilantro, olives, onion, and parsley. Set aside. In a blender, purée the remaining ingredients. Add the purée mixture to the food processor and pulse until desired consistency. If you want to make it creamier, blend on high speed for 15 to 20 seconds. Use within 5 days. Keep refrigerated.

Dill Honey–Mustard

Makes about 3/4 cup

Great on salads, as well as steamed vegetables, especially broccoli or cauliflower florets.

1/2 cup plain soy yogurt

1/4 cup purified water

1 tablespoon honey mustard (Dijon)

1 tablespoon white miso

2 teaspoons dried dill or 1 1/2 tablespoons minced fresh dill

Dash or two of hot sauce

In a small bowl, combine all ingredients and whisk to blend. Use within 5 days. Keep refrigerated.

Lemon Tahini

Makes about 1/2 cup

This is another one of my favorite dressings that is a rich source of protein, calcium, and omega-3's.

The Basic Recipe

1/3 cup purified water

1/4 cup raw or roasted tahini (pour off any oil that has risen to the top of the jar)

2 tablespoons fresh squeezed lemon juice

Sea salt to taste

In a blender or food processor, blend all ingredients until smooth. Add more water if you prefer a thinner consistency. Use within 5 days. Keep refrigerated.

VARIATION: Add some minced garlic, chopped parsley, or a dash of cumin or turmeric and blend.

Deluxe Tahini Recipe
Makes about 2 cups

1$1/2$ cups warm water

8 ounces raw or roasted tahini

3 cloves garlic, minced

Juice of one large lemon

2 tablespoons tamari or liquid aminos

1 tablespoon chopped fresh parsley

2 teaspoons raw cider vinegar

1 teaspoon dried basil

1 teaspoon sea salt

$1/2$ teaspoon ground coriander

$1/4$ teaspoon ground cumin

3 to 4 dashes Tabasco sauce

Pinch freshly ground pepper

In a blender or food processor, combine all ingredients and blend until smooth. Store in a covered jar in the refrigerator. Use within 6 days.

• F Y I

Tahini

Tahini is sesame paste and while it's comparatively high in fat, the nutritional and culinary virtues of it warrant its inclusion in a healthy diet. It provides protein and calcium and gives body and a rich taste to dressings and sauces. Because of its higher caloric content, don't overdo consumption if losing weight is your goal. A few times weekly in small amounts is okay.

Tahini Salsa Dressing

This dressing gives any salad a Tex-Mex flavor and turns the basic tahini dressing into a lower calorie, lycopene-rich topping. Also great on potatoes, steamed vegetables, or as a dip.

1 cup Basic or Deluxe Lemon Tahini (pages 280)
1 cup Sensational Salsa (page 243)

In a medium bowl, combine the dressing and the salsa thoroughly, and serve. Store in the refrigerator for up to 5 days.

Tahini Mint Dressing

Makes about 3/4 cup

This refreshing version of tahini dressing is heavenly—tossed with chickpeas, carrots, diced cucumbers, and red onions on a bed of Boston or romaine lettuce or stuffed into whole grain pita bread.

1 cup loosely packed chopped fresh mint leaves
1/4 cup raw tahini
1/4 cup purified water
3 tablespoons fresh lemon juice
1/2 teaspoon lemon zest from an organic lemon
1/8 teaspoon low-sodium tamari

In a blender or food processor, blend all the ingredients until smooth. Store in the refrigerator. Use within 5 days.

Orange Yam Dressing

Makes about 13/4 cups

This beta carotene-rich dressing adds distinctive flavor and color to any salad. Try it on grilled vegetables, too.

1/2 cup steamed yam
1/2 cup fresh orange juice
2 tablespoons cold-pressed, extra virgin olive oil

1 tablespoon organic balsamic vinegar

2 teaspoons lemon juice

2 teaspoons white or yellow miso

1 teaspoon orange zest from an organic orange

1 teaspoon nutritional yeast

Dash cayenne pepper

Steam yam until soft. Cool, peel, and cut into 1½-inch pieces. Combine all the ingredients in a blender or food processor and blend until smooth. Keep in the refrigerator. Use within five days.

Ginger–Pear Vinaigrette

Makes about ½ cup

The combination of pear and ginger together make this dressing a heavenly treat—especially tossed with Hearts of Palm & Romaine Salad (page 259)

1 pear

2 tablespoons fresh lemon juice

⅛-inch slice ginger, juiced

¼ cup cold-pressed walnut or sesame oil

2 tablespoons brown rice vinegar

Sea salt, to taste

Juice the pear and ginger together. Then, in a small bowl, whisk together the pear-ginger juice with the remaining ingredients.

Zesty Avocado Dressing

Makes about 1½ cups

If you're looking for a terrific topping for your baked potatoes so you won't miss butter and sour cream, this one is perfect.

1 ripe avocado, peeled, pitted, and sliced

½ tomato, diced

1/2 cup celery juice or water

1/4 cup plain soy yogurt

1 clove garlic, minced or pressed

1 tablespoon finely chopped fresh tarragon

2 teaspoons fresh lemon juice

4 basil leaves

Dash sea salt

Dash cayenne pepper

In a blender or food processor, blend all the ingredients until smooth. Keep in the refrigerator. Use within 2 days.

Spicy Soy Dressing

Makes 3 to 4 cups

For a dressing to top udon or soba noodles, whether cold or warm, this spicy dressing will work well.

1 cup unsalted soy nut butter

2 to 3 cups water—depending on the consistency you want

2 cloves garlic, pressed

1 tablespoon fresh ginger, grated

2 teaspoons white or yellow miso

1/2 teaspoon cayenne pepper, to taste

In a blender or food processor, blend all the ingredients until smooth. Keep in the refrigerator. Use within 4 days.

VARIATIONS: Substitute natural, unsalted peanut butter, cashew butter, or almond butter for the soy nut butter.

Miso–Walnut Dressing/Topping

Makes about 2¹/2 cups

Besides being an elegant dressing for salads, try this on top of vegetables or potatoes.

1¼ cups plain soy yogurt

1 cup walnuts

1 tablespoon amber-colored miso

1½ teaspoons fresh lemon juice

½ teaspoon brown rice vinegar

8 basil leaves

Roast the walnuts in a large, heavy skillet over medium heat, stirring constantly for 5 to 6 minutes. In a blender or food processor, blend all the ingredients until chunky. Use within 3 days.

Fabulous Fruit Dressing

Makes about 3 cups

Using this topping over chilled fresh fruit makes a delicious, nutritious breakfast. Top with ground almonds or walnuts to make it a complete, balanced meal.

½ cup pineapple chunks

½ cup blueberries

½ cup strawberries

½ cup seedless grapes

1 ripe banana

¼ cup fresh apple juice

¼ cup fresh orange juice

⅛ teaspoon cinnamon

In a blender or food processor, blend all the ingredients until smooth. Chill in the refrigerator before serving. Pour over fresh fruit of your choice. Use within 2 days.

VARIATION: Triple the recipe and pour the blended fruit mixture into ice cube trays and freeze. Take about 7 to 10 frozen cubes and some fresh juice and blend together to make a delicious fruit slush or a special, healthy dessert.

Fat–Free Italian Raspberry Dressing

Makes about 2$\frac{1}{2}$ cups

No oil is needed because the vegetables emulsify the dressing.

1 small red onion, peeled, cored and cut into quarters

1 medium red pepper, seeded and cut into quarters

1 large yellow pepper, seeded and cut into quarters

$\frac{1}{2}$ cup raspberry vinegar

$\frac{1}{2}$ cup water, or more as needed

$\frac{1}{3}$ cup brown rice syrup

1 tablespoon fresh oregano, finely chopped

2 teaspoons garlic, minced

1 teaspoon finely chopped fresh chervil

1 teaspoon finely chopped fresh tarragon

1 teaspoon fresh lemon juice

Dash sea salt

Place all ingredients in a blender or food processor and blend at high speed for 1 minute. Keep in the refrigerator. Use within 2 days. Mix well before reusing.

Sweet Pepper–Apple–Sun Dressing

Makes about 2 cups

1 cup fresh apple juice

$\frac{1}{2}$ cup chopped apple

$\frac{1}{2}$ cup seeded and chopped red, yellow, or orange bell peppers

$\frac{1}{2}$ cup sunflower seeds, soaked for 8 hours or overnight

1 tablespoon flax seeds, soaked for 8 hours or overnight

1$\frac{1}{2}$ teaspoons dried dill

In a blender or food processor, combine all ingredients and blend until smooth. Serve immediately. Keep in the refrigerator. Use within 2 to 3 days, and be sure to remix before reusing.

Green Goddess Dressing

Makes about 2 cups

Here's another marvelous topping for potatoes, steamed vegetables, or grain dishes or as a dip for vegetables in addition to crisp green salads. It's guaranteed to bring out the goddess in you to get your family to worship and appreciate you!

1 large ripe avocado, peeled, pitted and cut into quarters
1 small red onion, peeled, cored and cut into quarters
2 celery stalks, juiced
1 cucumber, peeled and cut into quarters
1/4 cup fresh parsley
1/4 cup fresh dill
1/4 cup fresh basil
1/4 cup watercress
1/2 cloves garlic, minced
1 to 2 teaspoons fresh lemon juice
1/2 teaspoon lemon zest using an organic lemon
Low sodium tamari, to taste

In a blender or food processor, blend all ingredients together until smooth. Use extra celery juice to reach desired consistency. Keep in the refrigerator. Use within 2 days.

Ranch Dressing

Here's a healthier version of most store-bought ranch dressings that doubles as a vegetable dip or topping on potatoes.

8 ounces firm organic silken lite tofu, cubed
1/4 cup plain soy yogurt or Lemonaise Spread (page 239)
1/4 cup purified water
3 scallions, finely chopped
2 tablespoons fresh lemon juice
1 to 2 cloves garlic, minced
1 tablespoon chopped fresh parsley

2 teaspoons chopped fresh dill

1 teaspoon chopped fresh oregano

1 teaspoon ground cumin

1 teaspoon sea salt

In a blender or food processor, combine all ingredients and blend until smooth. Keep in the refrigerator. Use within 4 to 5 days.

Pear Cashew Cream Dressing

Makes about 3 cups

This is a superb dressing for fruit or other desserts. It also makes a delicious dip for strawberries or apple quarters.

2 pears

2 cups water

1 cup raw cashews

1/8 teaspoon cinnamon

Peel and dice pears. In a blender or food processor blend together all ingredients until smooth. Chill.

Other Fat–Free Dressing Suggestions

Check out the dressing aisle in your natural health food store and see what you can find that appeals to you in the nonfat and low fat categories. While bottled dressings aren't as fresh as home-made, they'll do when you're pressed for time or don't have any supplies on hand. My favorite bottled dressings are made by Spectrum Naturals. I especially like their nonfat and low-fat Sweet Onion, Creamy Garlic, Toasted Sesame, Zesty Italian, and Dijon. They also double as excellent marinades on grilled vegetables and tofu steaks.

Have you ever used a marinara or other pasta sauce as a salad dressing? It's different and quick. Make sure you get fat-free, low sodium brands from your natural food store if you don't have time to make them yourself. With tomato-based sauces, you get an extra bonus of lycopene, the phytonutrient that may help reduce the risk of cancer and heart disease.

Roasted Garlic

This simple-to-make treat is so delicious and nutritious. A couple times a week, you can smell garlic roasting in my home. Slowly baked, the garlic becomes mild and so soft you can spread it on bread like butter. Bake several heads at a time and keep them in the fridge, then warm up in the microwave for a few seconds before using. I often squeeze all the soft cloves from their skins and put them in a small bowl to use in a variety of dishes such as roasted garlic mashed potatoes, in soups, sprinkled on salads, and in dips, spreads, sauces, and marinades.

THE QUICK & EASY WAY:

6 heads garlic

1/2 teaspoon dried thyme

1/2 teaspoon sea salt

Nonstick cooking spray

Water

Preheat oven to 300°F. Slice 1/2 inch off the top of each garlic head (not the bottom or root end). Rub off as much lose garlic skin as possible without separating the cloves. Lightly spray a small baking dish with nonstick spray. Place the skinned garlic heads, cut-side up, clustered together in the baking dish. Sprinkle the top of each head with a dash each of salt and thyme. Add 1/4 to 1/3 cup purified water in the baking pan surrounding the garlic clusters. Cover and bake until the garlic cloves are tender (when pierced with knife) and begin to pop out, about 1 1/2 to 2 hours. Serve hot or cooled to room temperature.

I serve a whole head of garlic to my guests to squeeze out the soft cloves from their skins to spread on baguette toast, or any variety of whole grain breads instead of using butter or margarine.

VARIATIONS: Instead of salt, drizzle some tamari or Bragg liquid aminos over the top of each head. It gives it a nice flavor and darker color. Or, substitute other herbs such as oregano, rosemary, basil, dill, cilantro, chives, or cumin for the thyme.

ANOTHER VARIATION: Take 3 to 5 heads of garlic, separate all the cloves and peel away all the skin. Discard any cloves that are small and not worth it. In a small saucepan, combine the garlic cloves with 1/2 cup vegetable broth. Bring to a high simmer, cover, reduce heat to a gentle simmer and cook until the cloves are tender but not mushy, about 20 minutes. Check periodically to make sure the broth has not evaporated. If low, add some more. When cooked, they are as soft as butter, easy to use, and will last 2 to 3 days in the refrigerator.

• F Y I

Garlic, Superfood

Garlic is a superfood that has been studied worldwide for its medicinal properties. It's packed with antioxidants known to fend off cancer, heart disease, high blood pressure, and all-over aging. It is also available in a supplemental form called Kyolic, which is not detectable on your breath. This is the best garlic supplement on the market. Please refer to the garlic section in Chapter 6 and to the Resource Directory.

Roasted Onions

Like roasted garlic, roasted onions are easy to make and wonderfully delicious and versatile. Even kids love their mild taste. I make several roasted onions at a time to have on hand or to freeze. Use them as a spread, in mashed potatoes, in dips, soups, sauces, on sandwiches, or wherever a recipe calls for onion.

CONVENTIONAL OVEN:
Preheat oven to 400°F. Select onions of similar size, red, white or yellow, and place whole and unpeeled on a baking sheet. Bake until tender and soft to the touch, usually about 25 to 30 minutes. Set aside to cool. With a sharp knife, cut off the root end and squeeze out the soft interior. Depending on the size, one medium onion yields about 1 to 1¼ cups diced roasted onion.

MICROWAVE OVEN:
Place onion in the oven on high or full power for about 5 minutes, or until soft to the touch. Set aside to cool. Cut off root end and squeeze out the soft interior.

• F Y I

Onions

With only 27 calories per ½ cup of uncooked onions, these flavorful, aromatic, inexpensive health foods are one of the few foods that actually help boost the beneficial HDL cholesterol, and also help lower total blood cholesterol, thin the blood, retard blood clotting, kill bacteria, and may even have some value in counteracting allergic reactions. When purchasing, make sure the onions are firm, dry, and well shaped. If soft or acrid-smelling, don't get them. Store in a cool, dry place with good ventilation. Like most kids, I am very fond of the sweeter onions such as the Vidalia (Georgia), Maui (Hawaii), Sweet Texas, or Walla Walla (Washington) varieties.

Roasted Peppers

Roasting peppers is easy and brings out their natural sweetness. Select any color: red, yellow, orange, purple, or green.

Place each pepper directly on a gas stove-top burner, over a charcoal fire, or under a preheated broiler. Using tongs to turn, cook pepper on all sides until the skin blackens and blisters. Transfer to a heavy duty plastic (zip top) or paper bag, seal, and let steam for about 5 minutes. When cool, peel away the charred skin with your fingers. Don't rinse them under water as that will wash away some of the flavor. Cut away any black spots with a small knife. Then cut in half, remove seeds and ribs, and slice thinly.

• F Y I

Bell Peppers

The red bell pepper is the sweetest but who can resist the luscious colors and refreshing taste of the yellow, orange, or purple bell peppers? Because cooking makes the flesh of the purple peppers turn gray, it's best to eat them raw. The banana pepper is usually bright yellow, long and tapered, but can also be found in orange-red and green. Also called a Hungarian pepper, the banana pepper is great raw or cooked. I don't recommend eating raw green bell peppers as they are an unripened red pepper, but they still roast well if you need a green color in a recipe.

Plain Croutons

1 day-old baguette, cut in to ³⁄₈-inch dice

Preheat oven to 375°F. Arrange diced baguette on a baking sheet and bake for about 10 minutes, or until golden brown. Midway through baking, mix and toss the bread pieces. Cool.

Using a Misto or Misto-style spray pump bottle (see the Resource Directory), lightly mist the diced bread with tamari or shoyu before baking. If you use shoyu instead of tamari, mist the bread dice about 4 minutes before they're done instead of before the baking process. This will give your croutons a slightly salty flavor without too much sodium. I also dilute sea salt with a little purified water and mist the bread with this. To add color, juice any produce with the desired color you want and add some of this juice (strained carefully so you have only liquid) and mist onto the bread before baking. You can also spray an herbed olive oil from the Misto or Misto-style spray pump bottle during the second toss.

I'm fortunate to live a few blocks from a marvelous bakery that makes whole grain, nonfat baguettes. Try finding them instead of using white flour baguettes. Try to avoid all white flour products as they're void of nutritional value and unfavorable when weight loss is a goal.

Herbed Croutons

2 tablespoons minced fresh parsley

1 tablespoon minced fresh thyme

1 teaspoon minced fresh basil

1 teaspoon minced fresh chives

1 teaspoon minced fresh oregano

1 teaspoon paprika

1 teaspoon onion powder

1 teaspoon garlic powder

Dash cayenne pepper

1/3 cup vegetable broth

2 tablespoons cold-pressed, extra virgin olive oil

1 tablespoon Bragg liquid aminos or low sodium tamari

12 slices day old whole grain bread

Preheat oven to 375°F. In a small bowl, mix together all the herbs. In another small bowl, whisk together Bragg or tamari, oil, and broth. Combine the herbs with the liquid and mix well. Add enough extra broth to make the mixture brushable. Brush mixture on both sides of the bread. Cut into 3/8-inch dice and spread on a baking sheet. Bake until golden brown, about 10 minutes, toss and mix thoroughly half way through the baking process.

• **T I P**

Freezing Croutons

I make large batches monthly and freeze for later use on salads, in soups, to use for bread crumbs, or as a garnish in a variety of recipes. They thaw in minutes by placing on a plate at room temperature.

• **F Y I**

Parsley

A relative of celery, parsley is the world's most popular herb. Because of its rich supply of chlorophyll, the green coloring in the plant, parsley is a superb blood purifier and over-all body rejuvenator, which acts as a diuretic, and even freshens breath: by eating a sprig of it. Parsley has three times as much vitamin C as oranges, and twice as much iron as spinach. It's also a good source of vitamin A, copper, and manganese. And because it's an alkaline food, it helps eliminate acidic wastes from the body.

Peeled Tomatoes

Peeling tomatoes is a breeze to do and, in many recipes, gives a more elegant result.

Tomatoes

Bowl of ice cold water

In a medium saucepan, bring enough purified water to a boil so you can immerse a tomato in it for about 1 minute. With a slotted spoon, remove the tomato and immediately plunge it into a bowl of ice cold water. Drain and peel the tomato. If the recipe calls for a peeled and seeded tomato, then cut the peeled tomato in half through the middle (the belly) and gently squeeze each half over a bowl to remove the seeds.

• F Y I

Tomatoes

Tomatoes are one of the very best sources of the antioxidant lycopene. Lycopene reduces the risk of cancer by 40%—notably prostate, lung, and stomach cancer—and increases cancer survival according to studies. In addition, research discloses that tomato eaters function better mentally in old age and suffer half as much heart disease. Concentrated tomato sauces (such as pasta sauces) have 5 times more lycopene than fresh tomatoes. Canned tomatoes have 3 times more than fresh!

Organic Gomasio (Sesame Seed Salt)

Also referred to as sesame salt, I use this often because of the rich minerals it provides. It's delicious sprinkled on salads, noodles, soups, potatoes, grains, and cooked vegetables.

1 cup organic unhulled sesame seeds
1 teaspoon sea salt (Celtic Sea Salt is the best)

Wash the sesame seeds and drain well. In a dry skillet, over medium heat, toast the sesame seeds for about 3 to 4 minutes, stirring constantly, until the seeds start to pop. Reduce the heat and continue to stir and toast just until the seeds turn a shade darker, for about another minute. Set aside to cool. Transfer the toasted seeds to a blender, add the salt, and grind in several on-off pulses until about 80% of the seeds are ground, being careful not to grind into a paste, which will happen if you grind even a few seconds too long! Transfer to a small, covered container. It stores well at room temperature for about 3 to 4 months. I use a tiny wooden spoon for serving and keep the spoon in the container.

VARIATIONS: To add more trace minerals and a different flavor, I make the recipe above and add 1/4 ounce of dulse, wakame, or other sea vegetable. To use these sea vegetables, put the sea vegetables on a baking sheet and bake in a 350°-preheated oven for about 10 minutes, or until they start to brown. Cool. Blend until almost pulverized, about 12 to 15 seconds. Add to the blender with the salt and sesame seeds.

Instead of sea vegetables, try other variations of ground toasted cumin, cardamom, cinnamon, fennel, fenugreek, mustard seeds, or black sesame seeds for a different color.

• F Y I

Sesame Seeds

Sesame seeds provide protein, calcium, iron, vitamins A, B_1, B_2, B_6, and niacin (B_3). Black sesame seeds have more flavor than white sesame seeds and are popular in Asian cooking as a garnish and also as an ingredient in many dishes.

Cheesy Sesame Seasoning Salt

Try this for a delicious cheese-like flavor on popcorn, potatoes, noodles, grains, salads, and soups.

1/3 cup sesame salt (page 293)
1 1/2 tablespoons nutritional yeast flakes

Stir the sesame salt and yeast flakes together and store in a small airtight container. This will keep about 3 months, if you can keep it around that long!

• F Y I

Nutritional Yeast

Nutritional yeast provides an impressive array of B vitamins and is also rich in protein content. Look in your natural foods store for a brand that's organic and natural and has some fortification with other nutrients. It lends a cheese-like flavor to many dishes without the negative effects of dairy. This is not recommended for those individuals with weak or yeast-infected digestive systems.

Garam Masala

This aromatic spice mix is used often in Indian dishes and in Ayurvedic medicine, and is known to help digestion and warm the body.

1 cinnamon stick (3 inches) broken into pieces

1/2 cup coriander seeds

1 cup cumin seeds

1/4 cup fennel seeds

1 tablespoon unhulled sesame seeds

2 tablespoons black peppercorns

2 tablespoons black cardamom seeds

2 tablespoons whole cloves

2 teaspoons sea salt

In a large, heavy skillet over low heat, toast all the seeds and spices (except the sea salt), stirring often, for about 12 to 15 minutes, or until their aroma is released. Set aside to cool. (Your kitchen and home will smell heavenly.) Transfer to a spice mill or blender. Add the salt and grind into a fine powder. Sift through a fine sieve. Store in an airtight container and store in a cool, dry place for up to 4 to 5 months.

• F Y I

Cumin

A member of the carrot family, cumin has a pungent flavor that loses its essence quickly to become bitter tasting in most store bought brands. Look for the whole cumin seeds and take the time to grind them fresh. It's beneficial for the digestive system, improves liver function, promotes the assimilation of other foods, and helps relieve headaches and abdominal distention due to gas.

• F Y I

Pepper and Peppercorns

As for peppercorns, it's always best to grind them fresh, too, for the taste and to prevent rancidity. Once ground, add pepper at the end of cooking to prevent the pungent flavor from becoming bitter. Pepper is a good source of chromium and acts as an anti-inflammatory and parasite inhibitor. Black peppercorns are picked when mature but still green in color. Their flavor is hot with a hint of spice and sweetness. Green peppercorns are picked when mature but still green, and are packed in brine or dried. Red peppercorns have rose hips added for a color change and different taste. They're sweet and only mildly pungent. Because much of pepper's pungency is in its red skin, which is removed when soaked in brine, white pepper's fragrance excels over that of black pepper.

Herbed Garbanzo Flatbread

Makes light 5-inch flatbreads

I use these for a pizza shell, to accompany soup, or as a base for different spreads such as hummus and guacamole. Garbanzo flour can be found in most natural food stores or made at home by grinding dried garbanzo beans in your food processor.

1 1/2 cups garbanzo flour

3 tablespoons sesame salt (page 293)

2 teaspoons freshly ground flax seed meal

1/2 teaspoon dried dill

1/2 teaspoon dried rosemary

1/2 teaspoon dried cilantro

Dash cayenne

1/3 cup organic vegetable broth

In a bowl, thoroughly combine the garbanzo flour, sesame salt, flax meal, herbs, and cayenne. Stir in just enough vegetable broth to form a dough ball. If you need extra liquid, use more broth or purified water, adding only a little at a time. Knead the dough with your hands for about 30 to 45 seconds, then divide the dough into 8 chunks and roll each into balls. Place each ball, one at a time, between 2 pieces of plastic wrap and roll out from the center with a rolling pin or press out with your hands. In a nonstick skillet, over medium heat, cook each one for about 2 minutes on each side, or until brown spots appear.

VARIATIONS: For a sweet dough, instead of broth, use water and substitute 1 teaspoon cinnamon for the herbs. On top of this use applesauce or other fruit spread. For a heavier dough, substitute oat flour for the garbanzo flour.

• **F Y I**

Garbanzo Beans

Garbanzo beans or chick peas have only one mature pea per pod and have a wrinkled round surface. The high-protein flour is more easily digested and the whole beans have nearly double the amount of iron (soy excepted) and more vitamin C than most other legumes. They're beneficial for the heart, spleen, pancreas, and stomach. In addition to including them in salads and making them into hummus, I also use them whole or mashed in soups, in vegetable and grain dishes, or eaten just plain: simmer until tender, with garlic and some toasted cumin seeds.

Chapter 13

SOUPS

Whether hot, cold, as an appetizer, snack, or main meal, if made with healthy ingredients, soups are a great way to provide a nutrient-rich, satisfying food without too many calories. Like a green salad, if you have a cup or bowl of soup before your main course, it will fill you up so you don't overeat. And as the main course, it can be a delicious entrée that won't leave you with that stuffed feeling.

Soups are a much better on-the-go meal than anything from a fast food restaurant. Just fill up a thermos and take some with you to work, doing errands in your car, to school, or to watch the sunset or sunrise. You can make fruit or vegetable soups and even dessert soups: The sky's the limit! Most soups freeze beautifully so they're a practical way to always have something healthy and delicious on hand.

Vegetable Broth

This quick, easy versatile broth can be used in so many ways: by itself or as the liquid for grains, dressings, dips, and sauces. Any recipe that calls for chicken broth can be made successfully with vegetable broth. When you cut the vegetables into small pieces, about 1/2 inch or smaller, their flavor will saturate the liquid in only 20 minutes. I usually triple the recipe and freeze it in 1-cup containers or in freezer-quality zipper top bags so I always have it on hand. By making your own, you can ensure that only the highest-quality organic vegetables are used, and also keep the sodium level down.

1 red onion, diced
1 yellow onion, diced

3 carrots, peeled and diced

4 stalks celery, diced

2 cups sliced shiitake mushrooms

2 parsnips, peeled and diced

1 turnip, peeled and diced

1 leek, white and pale green parts only, diced

3 large garlic cloves, minced

1 strip kombu, approximately 4 inches in length
  (kombu is a sea vegetable)

6 sprigs fresh thyme (you can substitute 1 tablespoon
  dried thyme, but fresh is far better)

1 bay leaf

6 sprigs parsley

3 whole cloves

1 teaspoon whole coriander seed

In a large pot, combine all the ingredients, bring to a boil (remove the kombu just before the water boils), lower heat, and simmer for 20 minutes, uncovered. Strain through a fine sieve or double thickness of cheesecloth.

VARIATION: Create a bouquet garni with the fresh herbs by filling a celery or fennel stalk with sprigs of fresh herbs such as thyme, oregano, tarragon, rosemary, basil, chervil, parsley, etc., and tying it with a cotton thread or string. Leave a long tail so you can remove it easily before serving.

• **F Y I**

Thyme

Thyme's aromatic oil contains two chemicals: thymol and carvacol. Both chemicals have preservative, antibacterial, and antifungal properties. They also have expectorant properties (phlegm-loosener) and may be useful as digestive aids. As an antiseptic, thyme fights several disease-causing bacteria and fungi. Pregnant women may use thyme as a culinary spice, but they should avoid large amounts and should not use the herb's oil.

Potassium–Powered Broth

This delicious alkaline broth is a natural diuretic that I use as a soup base, beverage, or the liquid when cooking grains or casseroles.

10 cups purified water

2 1/2 pounds white, red, and Yukon Gold potatoes,
    washed and cut in 1/2-inch chunks

2 cups chopped green cabbage

1 1/2 cups chopped broccoli, stalks and florets

5 large carrots, diced

2 red onions, diced

1 yellow onion, diced

1 bunch celery, corded and chopped, including the leaves

2 cloves garlic, minced

Fresh bouquet garni (see page 299) (I usually use sprigs of fresh parsley, rosemary, thyme, and 2 bay leaves.)

In a large pot, combine all ingredients and bring to a boil. Reduce heat and simmer for 1 1/2 hours, uncovered. Strain through a fine sieve. Keeps in refrigerator for 3 to 5 days or freeze in 1 to 2 cup containers for future use.

• F Y I

Potassium

Potassium is involved in healthy, steady functioning of the nervous system and supports the heart, muscles, kidneys, and blood. Besides potatoes and broccoli, other sources of potassium include cantaloupe, citrus fruit, lima beans, bananas, avocados, parsnips, mushrooms, and dried apricots.

Shiitake Consommé with Greens

Serves 4 to 6

This simple, rejuvenating, immune-boosting soup is always a winner, especially if you're under extra stress or need an energy enhancer.

7 cups Vegetable Broth (see recipe, pages 298-299)

1 cup thinly sliced fresh shiitake mushrooms (or 2/3 cup dried)

1 tablespoon unrefined sesame oil (optional)

2 cloves garlic, minced

1 pound chopped greens (such as chard, kale, collard, mustard)

1 tablespoon white miso

2 teaspoons lemon juice

1 teaspoon lime juice

In a large stockpot, heat the vegetable broth. While the broth is heating, sauté the garlic and mushrooms with the oil in a skillet until slightly tender, 3 to 4 minutes. Add sauté mixture to the stockpot. Then add the greens and simmer for about 12-15 minutes. Place 1/2 cup of the soup stock in a small bowl. Dissolve the lime and lemon juices and miso into this warm stock. Mix back into the soup but don't boil. Serve hot.

• F Y I

Shiitake Mushrooms

The shiitake mushrooms have long been used in Chinese and Japanese cooking and are known for their medicinal properties of strengthening the immune system and restoring youthful vitality. Their chewy, firm texture and woodsy taste make them particularly satisfying in meatless cooking. I add them to soups, vegetable stews, stir-fries, veggie burgers, and pasta sauces. When buying fresh, look for firm ones with a nice aroma and refrigerate them in a single layer on a small tray, covered with a dampened towel so they'll keep a few days. Dried shiitake must be softened first in water: hot for half an hour, or cold for several hours. Make sure to use the flavorful soaking water, too.

Fresh Tomato Basil Soup

Serves 3 to 6

This easy-to-prepare soup freezes well and is good hot or cold. Make it in the summer, when tomato season is at its height.

4 pounds fresh ripe tomatoes, peeled, seeded,
  and coarsely chopped

1/2 cup vegetable broth

1/4 cup diced onion

1 clove garlic, pressed

Sea salt to taste

1/3 cup finely chopped fresh basil, for garnish

In a medium nonreactive saucepan, combine tomatoes, broth, onion, garlic, and salt to taste. Bring to a boil, reduce heat to medium-low, and cook just until the onions are tender, about 12 to 15 minutes. Serve garnished with the chopped basil.

VARIATIONS: Use other freshly chopped herbs such as cilantro, oregano, Italian parsley, chives, or mint, and if you like garlic, try adding 2 to 3 large cloves, minced. To increase protein and enhance the basil flavor, blend 3 ounces silken lite tofu with 3 tablespoons vegetable broth and 1/4 cup extra basil. Add to the soup during the last 5 minutes of cooking so it's heated throughout. If serving cold, add a few cubed pieces of silken tofu. Top with homemade croutons (page 291) and a dollop of plain soy yogurt or soy sour cream.

• T I P

Peeling & Seeding Tomatoes

Here's an easy way to peel and seed tomatoes. Bring a large pot of water to a boil. In the rounded end of each tomato, cut a shallow "X" and place in the boiling water for about 30 seconds (longer if they are not quite ripe and less if they are very ripe). Then transfer them to a bowl of ice water to stop cooking. When cool, lift them out and peel back the skin from the "X." Cut in half, core, and gently squeeze to remove the seeds, using your fingers to pry the seeds out of their cavities. Never cook tomatoes in aluminum or cast iron. The acid in the tomatoes binds with these metals, and this imparts a metallic flavor to the tomatoes.

Sweet Squash & Parsnip Soup

Serves 2 to 4

*You'll become an instant lover of squash and parsnips
with this great-tasting, easy-to-prepare soup.*

5 crookneck squash, chopped

4 medium zucchini, chopped

6 parsnips, chopped

1/3 to 1/2 cup purified water, vegetable broth, or soy beverage

1/3 cup fresh parsley, chopped

1/4 cup fresh orange juice

1 tablespoon rice syrup

1/2 tablespoon Bragg liquid aminos

Dash ground cardamom

In separate pans, steam the squash and parsnips until tender (they
take different lengths of time to steam). In a blender or food processor, purée the squash and parsnips with the ingredients and enough
liquid to create the desired consistency. Reheat and garnish with
fresh parsley.

VARIATIONS: Substitute cinnamon for cardamom. For added protein and a creamier soup, blend in 3 ounces of organic silken tofu
with some of the liquid and stir into the soup, heating through.

Simple Fresh Corn & Avocado Soup

Serves 2

*This light, uncooked soup would make a perfect meal
for a summer evening.*

1 cup vegetable juice (I like to use a combination of carrot,
    celery, romaine lettuce, and 1 to 2 green onions)

1 large ear of fresh corn, cut off the cob

1 small avocado

Sea salt to taste

Fresh chopped cilantro, parsley, or chives as garnish

In a blender or food processor, blend all the ingredients. Serve chilled, at room temperature, or warmed. Garnish with fresh herbs.

- **F Y I**

Corn, Wonderful Corn

Corn offers so many nutrients, including iron, zinc, and potassium, not to mention lots of fiber. We think of it as a vegetable, but it's really a grain. Mixed with legumes, it provides a complete protein. When cooking the kernels, never add salt to the water because it toughens them. My favorite way of eating corn is freshly picked, right off the cob, or the raw kernels cut right into my salad for added color, flavor, crunchiness, and nutrition. And it has only 75 calories per ear or 1/2 cup (raw) or 90 calories (cooked).

Papaya Gazpacho

Serves 3 to 6

Everything about this chilled soup—the color, the taste, and the easy preparation—make this unique dish a wonderful appetizer, snack, or meal.

2 cups (2 pounds) ripe papayas, cut into chunks and chilled

2/3 cup freshly squeezed orange juice

1/2 to 1 teaspoon fresh habañero chile, if available*,
    seeded and minced, or 1 to 2 teaspoons fresh red
    Fresno chile, seeded and minced

2/3 cup vegetable broth

1/3 cup fresh lime juice

2 teaspoons fresh lemon juice

1/4 cup chopped green onions

3/4 cup ripe (but still firm) avocado, peeled
    and diced in 1/2-inch pieces

1/3 cup green papaya, peeled, seeded and diced in 1/4-inch pieces

3 tablespoons chopped fresh cilantro or parsley, for garnish

Sea salt to taste

*Habañero chiles are among the hottest peppers. Always wear latex gloves when handling them.

First set aside about 1/2 cup of the papaya cut into 1/2-inch dice for garnish. In a blender or food processor, combine the remaining papaya chunks, orange juice, and chile, and blend until smooth. Transfer this mixture into a bowl. Add the vegetable broth, lime and lemon juices, and green onions and stir to combine. Add salt to taste. Chill in the refrigerator for 4 to 8 hours. To serve, pour or ladle the liquid into individual serving bowls. In each bowl, add equal portions of the green and ripe papaya and the avocado. Sprinkle with fresh herbs and adjust salt to taste.

Meal–in–a–Bowl White Bean Soup
Serves 3 to 6

1 cup uncooked dry navy beans

2 teaspoons cold-pressed, extra virgin olive oil

1 large red onion, diced

3 large garlic cloves, minced

3 to 4 large Yukon Gold or your favorite potatoes,
    cut in 1/2-inch dice

3 medium carrots, cut in 1/4-inch slices

2 medium stalks celery, cut in 1/4-inch slices

1 1/2 cups shredded red/green cabbage
    (combined to make 1 1/2 cups)

3 cups vegetable broth

3 cups purified water

1 large bay leaf

In a medium bowl, cover the beans with 2 inches extra water and soak for 2 hours. Drain and rinse. Discard the soaking water. In a large stockpot, heat oil over a medium heat. Add the onion and sauté until tender, about 5 to 7 minutes. Add garlic and sauté for another minute or two, stirring constantly. Add the remaining ingredients and bring to a boil. Reduce heat to low and simmer for about 60 to 70 minutes, or until the beans are tender. Add more water to create the desired consistency.

VARIATION: For added minerals and flavor, add a 4-inch strip of the sea vegetable kombu when simmering, and remove before serving.

• F Y I

Beans

If consumed regularly, beans can lower cholesterol and are a good source of plant protein. They are also an excellent insoluble fiber. They're so easy to add to many soups, salads, or to simply eat as a snack, side dish, or dip. If you're worried about flatulence or abdominal discomfort, you should know that most research shows that the body adjusts to beans fairly rapidly. If you eat them every day, in about a week, they should no longer be a problem, especially if you soak your beans well before cooking them and don't use the soaking water, or rinse cooked canned beans first before eating them. If you're still experiencing problems, try using Beano. It's made of a naturally-occurring enzyme and is the answer for the occasional bean-eater.

Mango–Butternut Squash Soup

Serves 3 to 5

The delightful combination of mangoes and butternut squash gives this raw soup an especially rich and beautiful color and packs it with vitamin A.

3 cups butternut squash, peeled, seeded and chopped
  (I use it raw, but you can lightly steam it if you prefer)

1 large mango, seeded and cubed

3¼ cups fresh orange juice

³⁄4 cups fresh apple juice

¹⁄3 cup (about 3 to 4) pitted dates

1 tablespoon fresh lime juice

2 teaspoons curry powder

1 teaspoon lemon zest from an organic lemon

Sprigs of mint, diced mango, fresh chopped parsley
  or minced jalapeño pepper, for garnish

In a blender or food processor, combine all the ingredients and blend until creamy smooth. Serve immediately. Garnish with your favorites. I like mint and diced mango.

• F Y I

Mangos

One of my favorite tropical fruits, the juicy mango is perhaps best eaten in the shower, alone or with someone special. They contain more than a full day's supply of vitamin A in the form of beta carotene, as well as lots of vitamin C. Their fat content is barely detectable and there are only 130 calories per 7 ounces. The versatile mango makes a great snack, for breakfast combined with papaya and kiwi, or added to smoothies.

Potato Leek Soup

Serves 2 to 4

Hot or chilled, here's a delicious way to add health-promoting leeks to your diet. Double the batch and freeze in 1^1/2 cup containers.

2 teaspoons cold-pressed, extra virgin olive oil

4 large leek stalks, sliced

1 medium red onion, diced

1 clove garlic, minced

2 cups water

2 cups vegetable broth

4 large Yukon Gold or your favorite variety of potatoes, diced

1^1/2 teaspoons tamari

1/4 cup fresh tarragon, minced

In a large stockpot, heat the oil and sauté garlic, onion, and leeks over medium heat for about 6 to 7 minutes. Add the broth, water, potatoes, and tamari. Simmer for 15 minutes or until the potatoes and leeks are soft. Transfer 3/4 cup of the mixture to a blender or food processor and blend until smooth. Return to the pot. Add the tarragon and stir well. Serve as is or you can purée the soup with a hand blender for a creamy smooth texture. Serve warm or chilled.

Hot 'n Spicy Miso Tofu Soup

Serves 4 to 6

This Asian-style soup uses the wonderfood soy in three ways: miso, tofu, and tamari. It's a little saltier than most of my soups (miso and tamari are naturally salty from fermentation), but it packs a real protein punch.

1/2 cup vegetable broth

1 large onion, thinly sliced

4 slices (1/4-inch) ginger

2 cloves garlic, minced

8 cups water

1/2 pound firm tofu (2/3 cup), cubed

2 tablespoons tamari

2 tablespoons rice vinegar

3 medium carrots sliced diagonally

1 strip kombu, about 6 inches

3 tablespoons red miso

1/2 teaspoon freshly ground black pepper

Dash cayenne

In a large stockpot, steam-sauté the onions, garlic, and ginger in the vegetable broth, until the onions are translucent. Add the water, tofu, carrots, kombu, tamari, and vinegar. Gently simmer until the kombu is soft, about 15 to 20 minutes. Take out the kombu, cut it into thin strips, and return them to the pot. Right before serving, scoop out 1 cup of the broth and dissolve the miso in the broth, then return to the pot. Add the pepper and the cayenne and stir well. Serve hot.

• F Y I

Miso

Fresh miso is a paste made from soybeans that can be used as a stock base for risotto, soups, and sauces. It provides potent anti-cancer properties without any of the chemicals often found in stock cubes and powders. The lighter color misos, like white or yellow, are more mellow in flavor than the darker ones, such as amber.

Zesty Roasted Yellow Pepper & Orange Soup

Serves 2 to 4

3 yellow bell peppers, roasted (see page 290), peeled and chopped

1 yellow onion, chopped

1/2 cup fresh orange juice

1³/4 cups vegetable broth

Grated rind of one organic orange

1 jalapeño pepper, seeded and white tissue removed, minced

Dash of nutmeg

Sea salt to taste

Garnish with fresh chopped parsley or chives

In a medium pan, sauté the onion in 2 tablespoons of the orange juice until onions are tender, about 5 minutes, stirring often. In a blender or food processor, combine the roasted peppers, sautéed onion, remaining orange juice, half the orange rind, the vegetable broth, and jalapeño pepper. Blend until smooth. Add the nutmeg. Season to taste with salt. Heat until warm through, about 2 to 3 minutes. Garnish with the fresh herbs and serve right away.

Savory Ginger–Winter Squash Soup

Serves 3 to 4

Ginger gives this winter soup its extra zip and wonderful warming properties.

1 large winter squash, peeled, seeded and cut in 1-inch pieces

1 cup plain soy milk

4 cloves garlic, chopped

1¹/4-inch piece fresh ginger, peeled and juiced

1/2 teaspoon sea salt

2 cups vegetable broth

3 tablespoons minced fresh chives

In a large pot, combine the squash, soy milk, vegetable broth, ginger, and garlic. Bring to a boil. Reduce heat and simmer until squash is tender. Add salt to taste. Mix well. Let soup cool slightly, then transfer to a blender or food processor and purée until smooth. Pour into individual soup bowls and garnish with fresh chives. This is equally good warm or chilled.

• **F Y I**

Squash

Squash is a wonderful low-calorie and highly nutritious food. Rich in calcium, magnesium, potassium, beta carotene, and vitamin C, squash helps to relieve acidosis because of its alkalinity.

Black Bean Stew/Soup

Serves 6 to 8

With its lemon grass and cilantro accents, this black bean soup has a distinctly Southeast Asian flavor.

2 cups dry black beans or 6 cups cooked black beans

1 large onion, chopped

1 cup chopped carrots (2 to 3 carrots)

1 cup chopped celery (2 to 3 stalks)

2 to 3 large garlic cloves, pressed

1 teaspoon cold-pressed, extra virgin olive oil

4 cups vegetable broth

3 tablespoons fresh cilantro, chopped

1 tablespoon fresh lemon grass, chopped

1 tablespoon fresh thyme, chopped

1 teaspoon sea salt

Dash cayenne pepper

If using dry beans, soak 2 cupfuls overnight. Drain, rinse, cook until tender in water to cover. If using canned beans, drain and rinse 6 cups and set aside. In a large stockpot, sauté onion, carrots, celery, and garlic in the olive oil and 1 tablespoon of the vegetable broth.

Add 1 cup broth along with the 6 cups cooked beans and combine everything thoroughly. Simmer 10 minutes, covered, stirring occasionally. Add the herbs, salt, and dash of cayenne pepper, and simmer 10 more minutes. You can stop here, as this makes a delicious black bean stew. For a soup consistency, add the rest of the broth and simmer 10 minutes more.

Serve with whole grain bread and a salad of organic greens with a balsamic vinaigrette for a hearty, satisfying meal, on a cold winter day or evening. If you don't make the broth yourself, keep some organic vegetable (or mushroom) broth on hand. You should be able to find it at the health food store in the soup aisle.

VARIATIONS: For a creamy soup, blend 6 ounces of organic silken tofu with 3 ladles full (about 2 cups) of the soup mixture (liquid, beans, and veggies) until smooth. Return mixture to the stockpot and simmer a few more minutes. For an even creamier version, blend the entire soup mixture with 9 ounces of tofu. Return to the stockpot and simmer a few minutes more.

Cream of Asparagus

Serves 4 to 6

Asparagus fans rejoice: This fabulous soup takes fewer than 30 minutes to make!

4 cups vegetable broth

2 cups chopped fresh asparagus

1/3 cup chopped Maui or any sweet onion

1 cup plain soy yogurt

Sea salt

Fresh chopped cilantro, parsley, or chives, for garnish

In a medium saucepan, heat the broth. Add the onion and asparagus and cook over medium heat until soft, about 10 minutes. Cool slightly. In a food processor or blender, purée the soup in 3 to 4 batches. Return to the saucepan, add the soy yogurt, and gently reheat. Salt to taste and garnish with fresh herbs. Serve immediately.

VARIATIONS: Substitute broccoli, carrots, Brussels sprouts, or cauliflower for the asparagus.

• F Y I
Asparagus

Four spears of asparagus have only 13 calories! And it's chock full of iron, protein, potassium, calcium, magnesium, selenium, beta carotene, and vitamins A and K. One of nature's most complete vegetables, this gourmet delight also contains asparagine, which stimulates the kidneys. It is the asparagine that gives asparagus its diuretic qualities and gives certain people's urine a characteristic odor just minutes after eating (these folks lack the gene needed to break asparagine down, but there's no harm in that). Studies at the University of California and Mount Sinai School of Medicine in New York have linked regular asparagus consumption to dramatically lower rates of cancer and heart disease. According to the National Cancer Institute, it is the food highest in glutathione, an important anti-carcinogen. A note of caution: Asparagus contains purine, so avoid it if you suffer from gout.

Chilled Cantaloupe–Lime Soup

Serves 3 to 6

This raw and refreshing soup is perfect on a hot summer day!

2 ripe cantaloupe, cut into chunks
1 cup fresh orange juice (or tangerine or combination)
1/3 cup fresh lime juice
1 teaspoon grated fresh ginger root
1/2 organic lime, thinly sliced
4 to 6 fresh mint sprigs

In a food processor or blender, purée the melon, orange juice, lime juice, and ginger. Pour into serving bowls and chill in the bowl. Garnish each serving with a slice of lime and a sprig of mint.

VARIATIONS: Substitute honeydew or Crenshaw melon for cantaloupe and fresh apple, peach, nectarine, or strawberry juice for the orange juice.

• F Y I

Melons

Melons have one of the highest fiber contents of any food. Add to this large amounts of vitamins A and C plus more than 800 milligrams of potassium in half a cantaloupe. One day a week try eating just melon for a great and easy cleanse and rejuvenator. When buying cantaloupe, look for fine, even netting even if the melon requires a few days to ripen. The finer the netting, the sweeter the flesh but with only about 50 calories per cup, melon is your friend.

Curried Split Pea Soup

Serves 6 to 10

6 cups vegetable broth

6 cups purified water

1 pound organic split peas

3 medium carrots, diced

3 stalks celery, diced

1 large Maui or sweet red onion, diced

2 garlic cloves, minced

2 large bay leaves

2 teaspoons curry powder

2 teaspoons sea salt (optional)

Rinse peas well in a strainer and make sure to discard any stones. In a large stockpot, bring the broth and water to a boil. Add the peas, return to a boil, reduce heat, simmer and cover, stirring occasionally, for about 30 minutes. Skim off any foam that accumulates on the top. Add onion, celery, carrots, garlic, bay leaves, curry powder, and salt. Continue to simmer for 45 to 50 minutes, stirring occasionally. Adjust seasonings to taste and serve.

VARIATION: Substitute yellow split peas or lentils for the green split peas.

Cauliflower–Carrot Soup with Tarragon

Serves 4 to 6

3 cups vegetable broth

1 large onion, finely diced

1 to 2 cloves garlic, finely minced

$2^{1}/4$ cups ($1^{1}/2$ pounds) carrots, peeled and cut in $1/2$-inch dice

$1^{1}/3$ cups ($3/4$ pound) Yukon Gold potatoes (if you can't find them, russet will do), peeled and cut in $1/2$-inch dice

2 green onions, finely chopped

$1^{1}/4$ cups purified water

2 cups (1 pound) cauliflower, in small florets

$1/3$ cup (2 ounces) silken lite tofu

1 tablespoon chopped fresh tarragon

In a stockpot, combine $1/4$ cup of the vegetable broth, onion, and garlic. Cover and simmer over medium heat until onion is translucent, about 5 to 7 minutes. Add the carrots, potatoes, green onions, remaining vegetable broth, and water. Bring to a boil. Lower the heat and simmer about 5 minutes. Add the cauliflower, cover and simmer about 15 more minutes, or until all vegetables are tender. Cool slightly, then transfer to a blender and purée with the tofu. Return to the stockpot. Add the tarragon. Stir about 1 to 2 more minutes over low heat. If desired, thin with water. Season to taste and serve.

VARIATION: Substitute broccoflower, a pale green cauliflower-broccoli hybrid for the cauliflower to make a lovely color and delicious soup.

• F Y I

Cauliflower

This extremely low-calorie member of the cabbage family has virtually no fat or sodium, so you can eat as much of it as you want. One cup serving provides 100 percent of the RDA for vitamin C, and it's also rich in phosphorus. The National Academy of Sciences singled out cauliflower as one of the best cancer-preventing foods.

• **F Y I**

Tarragon

Like many culinary herbs, the oil in tarragon fights disease-causing bacteria. For garden first aid, press some fresh crushed tarragon leaves onto wounds on the way to washing and bandaging them. The oil contains an anesthetic chemical, eugenol, which is the major constituent of anesthetic clove oil, supporting its age-old use for toothache.

Chapter 14

VEGETABLE ENTRÉES

Vegetable meals are becoming more and more popular these days as the research pours in supporting the salutary effects of eating more plant-based foods as a way to heal the body and promote radiant health and youthful vitality.

The U.S. Department of Agriculture and the National Cancer Institute recommend a diet with at least 5 to 7 servings of fruits and vegetables every day to maintain good health. I suggest that you increase that amount to 7 to 12 servings daily. By incorporating the salads, smoothies, snacks, and soups found in previous chapters, you're well on your way. Add the vegetable entrées you'll find in this chapter, and you'll be doing your body a favor. In addition to fruits and vegetables, you'll find recipes with foods rich in phytochemicals (the disease preventing, health enhancing properties), such as legumes, whole grains, nuts, and seeds.

Simple & Super Marinara Spaghetti Squash

Serves 2

This low-calorie, low-fat treat is easy to make and really delicious.

1 spaghetti squash, cut in half
1 1/2 cups fat-free organic marinara sauce
1/2 cup mushrooms, sliced

Cover each half of the spaghetti squash with plastic wrap. In a microwave oven, cook until tender, about 12 to 15 minutes (about 40 minutes in a preheated 350° oven). While the squash is cooking, add the sliced mushrooms to the marinara sauce and heat through. When the squash is done, scrape out the strands with a fork. (When scraped, spaghetti squash dislodges in strands much like spaghetti, hence the name.) Arrange them on a warmed plate and top with the sauce.

VARIATION: Substitute portabello or shiitake mushrooms for the regular mushrooms.

Grilled or Oven–Roasted Vegetable Packets

Serves 4 to 6

Combine your favorite vegetables in foil and place them on the grill or in the oven and voilá: You have a scrumptious and very nutritious meal in minutes!

3 cups broccoli florets

1 cup cauliflower florets

1 medium onion, thinly sliced

1 medium yellow squash or zucchini, sliced diagonally

1 red bell pepper, sliced

1 teaspoon dried basil

1 teaspoon dried oregano

1 teaspoon garlic powder

1 teaspoon tamari

1 teaspoon cold-pressed, extra virgin olive oil

3 ice cubes

1 sheet (18 x 24 inches) heavy duty aluminum foil)

Preheat the oven to 450°F or the grill to medium-high. Place the vegetables on the center of the foil. Sprinkle with the seasonings and top with the ice cubes (to produce a steaming effect). Close up the foil by bringing the ends in to seal but leave room inside for the air to circulate. Bake on a baking sheet for 20 to 25 minutes or grill for 15 to 20 minutes. When serving, open the foil in front of your guests and wait for the compliments. Serve with a favorite grain such as millet, quinoa, or brown rice.

VARIATIONS: Substitute any combination of your favorite herbs for the oregano and basil and add several whole cloves of garlic.

Instead of drizzling the tamari and oil, I combine these in a spray pump bottle and spray lightly over the vegetables before cooking. This way you use less oil and distribute the oil and tamari more evenly.

Try adding several diced red potatoes to the packet, and if you like hot and spicy, add some jalapeño peppers along with a dash of cayenne pepper and/or chili powder.

Nori Veggie Burritos

Nori are the sheets of seaweed used to wrap sushi. They make a delicious and mineral-rich "tortilla" that will hold just about any-thing you put into them. These little cross-cultural vegetable packets make a great portable meal. You can purchase toasted nori sheets, but you can also toast them yourself. Simply toast them in a large dry skillet over medium heat for a few seconds on each side. They will turn a light green color.

1 pack nori sheets, toasted

Sprouts of choice such as alfalfa, red clover,
    sunflower, mixed

Steamed vegetables of choice such as carrot sticks,
    sliced mushrooms, bell pepper sticks, etc.

Sliced avocado

Favorite sauce or dressing (try Tangerine-Ume Dressing,
    page 276, or Spectrum Natural's Toasted Sesame)

Arrange a small amount of the vegetables, sprouts, and avocado slices on each sheet of nori. Top with the dressing. Roll up like a burrito or cone style. Seal the edge with a few drops of water. Eat whole or cut into strips. (It may drip, so have napkins available or wrap with a napkin or foil and roll it down.) I also add cucumber strips and sushi ginger (if sushi ginger is unavailable in the Asian foods aisle of your supermarket, Asian market, or health food store, see the Grain & Salt Society in the Resource Directory).

• F Y I
Sea Vegetables

Sea vegetables, such as nori, increase the blood's alkalinity, which helps eliminate wastes and may also lower cholesterol, ward off certain cancers, control blood sugar in people with diabetes, prevent obesity, prevent constipation, and fight hemorrhoids and diverticular disease. They are a potent source of iodine, a key factor in the control and prevention of many endocrine deficiency conditions such as breast and uterine fibroids, tumors, prostate inflammation, adrenal exhaustion, and toxic liver and kidney states. Sea vegetables have no equals when it comes to major mineral and trace mineral content. Nori's subtle flavor makes it a great choice for those just beginning to experiment with sea vegetables. You can purchase it in sheets dried naturally or already toasted, and in flakes you can add to noodle dishes, soups, stir-fries, and salads.

Roasted Herbed Asparagus & Potatoes

Serves 3 to 4

There's nothing like the smell of roasting potatoes to make your kitchen smell warm and homey. Roasting the asparagus brings out a deep, nutty flavor.

1 pound small red potatoes

2 teaspoons cold-pressed, extra virgin olive oil

2 teaspoons tamari or Bragg liquid aminos

2 cups asparagus, bottoms cut off and sliced diagonally in 1-inch pieces (I prefer using the top half)

1 tablespoon finely chopped fresh basil

1 tablespoon finely chopped fresh rosemary

1 teaspoon freshly ground red peppercorns

Freshly chopped basil for garnish

Preheat oven to 400°F. In a large bowl or zip-top bag, combine the potatoes, oil, and tamari. Toss well so the potatoes are evenly coated. Transfer to a shallow roasting pan that's been lightly sprayed with a nonstick spray. Bake 40 minutes, stirring 3 or 4 times after the first 10 minutes of cooking. Add the asparagus, herbs, and pepper and bake an additional 15 minutes, or until the vegetables are tender. Sprinkle with the basil and serve with your favorite grain and/or beans and a crisp green vegetable salad.

Broiled Vegetables

Almost any vegetable can be used in this recipe.

1 cup zucchini, cut in 1/2-inch slices
1 cup eggplant, cut in 1/2-inch slices
1 cup mushrooms, cut in 1/2-inch slices
1 cup bell peppers, cut in 1/2-inch slices
1 tablespoon Bragg liquid aminos or tamari
Dash cayenne (optional)
1 teaspoon extra virgin olive oil (optional)

Preheat the oven to 550°F. Place the oven rack at its highest position. Combine the Bragg, cayenne, and oil, and brush lightly over the vegetables. Arrange the veggies on a lightly sprayed baking sheet and set on the top rack in the oven. Watch carefully so they don't burn. Cooking time will range from 4 to 10 minutes depending on the vegetables you're using. Thin veggies (such as bell peppers, squash, or mushrooms) might brown faster than they cook, so lower the baking sheet one level. Check for doneness by color and tenderness.

VARIATIONS: Add herbs to the vegetables, such as dried rosemary, thyme, or basil, or for some added zing, add minced garlic and minced ginger to the mixture.

Ginger Broccoli & Shiitake Steam–Fry

Serves 4

Using broth instead of oil to "steam fry," you cut the fat and calories in this vitality-promoting dish.

1 orange, cut in pieces

3 tablespoons vegetable broth

1 tablespoon tamari or shoyu*

2 teaspoons minced garlic

2 teaspoons minced ginger

1 small onion, minced

2$\frac{1}{2}$ cups broccoli florets, cut in 1$\frac{1}{2}$-inch pieces

1 cup shiitake mushrooms, cut in 1$\frac{1}{2}$-inch pieces

1 tablespoon fresh orange zest from an organic orange

3 tablespoons fresh orange juice

Grate the zest off the orange. Then cut off the rest of the peel and white pith and cut the orange in 1-inch pieces. In a large nonstick skillet or wok, heat the vegetable broth and tamari on medium high. Add the garlic, ginger, and onion and cook for about 2 minutes, stirring occasionally. Add the broccoli, mushrooms, and orange zest and cook for 3 more minutes, stirring occasionally. When the broth has reduced by $\frac{1}{4}$, add the orange juice and orange pieces. Partially cover and simmer for 2 to 3 minutes, or until the broccoli is just crisp-tender.

*If you use shoyu instead of tamari, add it in the last 3 minutes of cooking only, not at the beginning because extended heat diminishes its flavor and nutritional value.

• F Y I

Broccoli

Part of the cabbage family, like cauliflower, nutritionally broccoli is prize-worthy. It's slightly diuretic, contains twice the vitamin C of an orange and almost as much calcium as whole milk, and its calcium is better absorbed. Broccoli also contains selenium, vitamins A and E, and is rich in chlorophyll, which is an excellent detoxifier and rejuvenator of the body. It's also considered the number one cancer-fighting vegetable. With almost no fat and just 12 calories per $\frac{1}{2}$ cup (raw), 23 calories (cooked), and loads of fiber, it is a perfect diet food. Lightly steam up a large batch to keep refrigerated to eat as a snack by itself, to dip, or to slice on salads.

Rainbow Stuffed Peppers

Serves 4

*I love to make these peppers for company. The variety
of colors is just a knockout.*

4 large sweet bell peppers in all colors

1 cup finely diced celery

3 ripe tomatoes, chopped

3 scallions, finely diced

1 large ripe avocado, mashed

1 carrot, grated

1 cup mixed sprouts

1/4 cup diced jicama

1/4 cup finely chopped green onions

1 tablespoon sesame salt (see page 293)

Butter lettuce

Fresh parsley sprigs for garnish

Cut off the top of each pepper, remove the seeds and ribs and wash
and dry with a paper towel. In a bowl, combine all other ingredients. Spoon the filling into the peppers. Serve on a bed of lettuce
and garnish with fresh parsley sprigs.

VARIATIONS: When you're in the mood for something a little
spicy, drizzle the stuffed peppers with a little salsa or add a chopped
jalapeño pepper. Try adding some fresh corn kernels cut off the cob
or fresh peas. To add some extra protein, include some diced silken
or grilled tofu to the mixture or a dollop or two of soy yogurt.
Squeeze a little lemon over the top for a clean, lively flavor.

• F Y I

Bell Peppers

*Sweet or bell peppers are among the most nutrient-dense foods avail-
able. They supply impressive amounts of fiber and vitamins C and A,
as well as silicon, an element that promotes beautiful hair, skin, nails,
and teeth. With only 12 calories per 1/2 cup raw, they can be enjoyed*

raw, roasted, juiced, or added to a variety of recipes. They are definitely a superfood.

Lettuce & Vegetable Sandwich

Serves 2

While any lettuce will do, iceberg gives the most support.
I don't usually recommend iceberg—it has virtually no nutritional
value—but for this purpose, it works best.

6 lettuce leaves, washed and separated

2 tablespoons hummus

1 carrot, grated

1 medium ripe tomato, sliced

1 sweet onion, sliced

1/2 cup red clover or alfalfa sprouts

1/2 ripe avocado, sliced

8 cucumber slices

6 roasted garlic cloves, mashed

8 roasted bell pepper slices

Dash of sea salt

Remove the outer lettuce leaves carefully so you don't tear them. Use 2 pieces of lettuce for the bottom to give your sandwich more strength. Spread the hummus or other favorite spread on the bottom 2 leaves. Distribute half of the remaining ingredients on top of the hummus. (Avocado helps to hold the vegetables together.) Fold the leaves over the veggies and wrap the third leaf over the top and around the bottom leaves. Repeat with the next sandwich. Use two hands and enjoy!

• **F Y I**

Lettuce

Lettuce is one of those excellent nutrient-dense foods that has virtually no fat and very few calories, but supplies your body with the necessary elements to keep it healthy and detoxified. Lettuce is alkaliniz-

ing, cleansing, slightly diuretic, and contains the sedative lactucarium, which relaxes the nerves. It's also a superlative source of magnesium, and along with bell peppers, contains the highest amount of silicon, which not only beautifies the skin, hair, nails, and teeth, but also supports pancreatic function. When you eat fresh fruits, I encourage you to also eat a fresh lettuce leaf, which adds fiber and helps neutralize the sugar content in the fruit and slows down the digestion.

Chopped Brussels Sprouts Stir–Fry

Serves 4 to 6

Here's a delicious and different way to serve one of everyone's favorite vegetable (kids included): Brussels sprouts.

2 teaspoons extra virgin olive oil

1 medium red onion, finely chopped

1 large carrot, finely chopped

2 garlic cloves, minced

1 teaspoon minced fresh ginger

$2^{1}/2$ cups (1 pound) chopped young (small) Brussels sprouts

$1/2$ cup finely chopped jicama

1 yellow or orange bell pepper, seeds removed
    and finely chopped

1 cup corn kernels, cut fresh off the cob

$1/2$ cup vegetable broth

2 teaspoons Dijon mustard

Sea salt to taste

Freshly ground pepper to taste

In a large skillet, heat oil over medium heat. Sauté the onions until tender, about 3 to 4 minutes. Add the garlic, ginger, carrot, Brussels sprouts, and jicama and sauté for another minute, stirring often. Add the bell pepper, corn, and vegetable broth, and simmer about 4 to 5 more minutes, or until the liquid evaporates, stirring often. Add the salt and pepper and cook for 1 to 2 more minutes. Serve on top of a bed of brown rice, quinoa, couscous, or millet alongside a fresh salad.

• F Y I

Brussels Sprouts

As the name implies, Brussels sprouts originated in Brussels, Belgium, and are really baby cabbages. Try them in stir-fries, soups, braised, in baked dishes, or added chilled in salads (steamed first). You can even juice them. Like broccoli and cauliflower, Brussels sprouts are at the pinnacle of phytochemical research showing them to be full of anti-cancer nutrients. They are rich in fiber, iron, protein, chlorophyll, calcium, and vitamins C and E, as well as being a superior source of vitamin U, an ulcer remedy. With only 30 calories per 1/2 cup, they are a nutrient-dense food that's perfect when fat loss and vitality are your goals.

Roasted Vegetable Wraps with Hummus Spread

Serves 6

The combination of the roasted vegetables and the hummus spread makes this an equally easy and delicious meal for family gatherings, parties, or picnics.

1 medium red bell pepper, cut in 3/4-inch pieces

1 medium red onion, cut in 1/2-inch pieces

1 medium zucchini, cut in half lengthwise and
  then cut crosswise in 1/4-inch slices

11/2 cups mushrooms, cut in quarters

1/2 cup yellow squash, cut in 1/4-inch slices

2 tablespoons cold-pressed, extra virgin olive oil

2 teaspoons Bragg liquid aminos or tamari

1/2 teaspoon dried basil

1/2 teaspoon dried oregano

1/2 cup hummus (see page 246)

1 ripe avocado, diced

6 (8-inch) whole wheat, fat-free tortillas, warmed

11/2 cups shredded romaine lettuce

Preheat over to 450°F. In a large bowl, toss together the vegetables, oil, Bragg, and herbs, then arrange in a shallow, nonstick roasting pan. Bake 12 to 15 minutes or until crisp-tender. While the vegetables are roasting, make up a batch of your favorite hummus and spread about 1 tablespoon on each warmed tortilla. Place about 1/2 cup of the vegetable mixture in the center of each tortilla. Top with lettuce and diced avocado. Fold one end of each up about 1 inch over the filling. Fold sides, overlapping over the folded end.

Vegetable, Rice & Lentil Casserole

Serves 4 to 6

3 cups cooked short grain brown rice

1 1/4 cups frozen corn

2 cups diced carrots

1 cup cooked red lentils

1 cup frozen peas

1 cup chopped green beans

1/3 cup chopped green onions

1 sweet red bell pepper, diced

2 cups vegetable broth

2 tablespoons Cheesy Sesame Salt (see page 294)

Preheat oven to 350°F. In a bowl, thoroughly combine all the vegetables and seasonings. Transfer to a covered loaf pan or casserole dish. Pour the broth over the mixture until it just covers. Bake for about 20 minutes, or until it's heated through and the carrots are tender.

Chilled Roasted Vegetable Salad

Serves 4

Roasting the garlic, peppers, and onions brings out their rich nuttiness. They also give a wonderful visual and texture contrast to the crisp, fresh veggies in this summer salad.

2 cups shredded romaine lettuce

1 cup grated daikon

1 cup shredded red cabbage

1 head garlic, roasted and squeezed out

1 large onion, roasted and squeezed out

4 sweet red and/or yellow/orange bell peppers,
    roasted and sliced into strips

2 ripe tomatoes, cut into quarters

Vinaigrette dressing of your choice

2 tablespoons toasted sesame seeds (see page 293)

1 lemon, cut into quarters

In a large bowl, combine the lettuce, daikon, and cabbage. Arrange on individual serving plates. Add garlic, onion, and then criss-cross the pepper slices over the top. Arrange the tomato wedges around the edge. Spoon on a small amount of dressing and sprinkle with toasted seeds. Garnish each plate with a lemon wedge.

Red Cabbage with Apples & Pistachios

Serves 4 to 6

Over a bed of couscous or quinoa, this sweet and sour treat will wake up your taste buds.

3 green apples, cored and sliced

1 medium-large head of red cabbage, sliced thinly

1 onion, chopped

1/3 cup raisins

2 tablespoons fresh lemon juice

1 tablespoon brown rice syrup

1 tablespoon balsamic vinegar

1/4 teaspoon sea salt

1/4 teaspoon dried tarragon

1/4 teaspoon dried basil

1/4 teaspoon celery seeds

In a large saucepan, combine all ingredients and cook for 25 to 30 minutes, covered, stirring from time to time. Serve with a salad of crisp greens and 3 to 4 more vegetables.

Vegetable Noodle Delight
Serves 4

2 large carrots, juiced

2 stalks celery, juiced

6 cups purified water

1/4 cup vegetable broth

1 medium onion, thinly sliced

1 large garlic clove, minced

1 large yellow, orange, or red bell pepper, chopped

1 teaspoon dried basil

1/2 teaspoon dried dill

1/8 teaspoon sea salt

1 package (12.3 ounces) firm or extra firm organic silken tofu

2 tablespoons yellow or light miso

Pinch of red chili powder

12 ounces soba noodles

Juice the carrots and celery and reserve 1/2 cup. (Drink any extra!) In a large saucepan or stockpot, bring the water and sea salt to a boil.

In a large skillet, heat the broth over medium heat. Add the onion and sauté until tender, about 4 minutes. Add the garlic and sauté 1 more minute. Add the pepper and herbs, and sauté another 4 minutes—just until the peppers are tender.

Meanwhile, in a blender or food processor, blend the carrot/celery juice, tofu, miso, and chili powder until smooth. Add to the sautéed vegetables and mix well.

When the pasta water comes to a boil, add the noodles and cook until al dente. (Check the directions on the package.) Drain but do not rinse. When you rinse soba or pasta, you lose some of the flavor as well as the sticky coating that enables the sauce to cling to the noodles. Transfer to warm plates. Top with the colorful sauce and serve.

Pacific Rim Vegetable Stew

Serves 4 to 6

As you savor this mixture of textures and flavors, you'll think you're across the world in a corner of paradise.

1 small red onion, chopped

1 cup vegetable broth

3 green onions, chopped

2 cloves garlic, minced

2 teaspoons minced fresh ginger

3 ears of corn, kernels cut off the cob

2 carrots, sliced

1½ cups organic frozen edamame (fresh soy beans can be purchased already shelled)

1 pound squash, such as yellow crookneck, sliced

1 large zucchini, sliced

½ pound cherry tomatoes, cut in half

⅓ cup lite coconut milk

1 teaspoon dried thyme

Shoyu to taste

Sea salt to taste

Cayenne to taste

In a large skillet over medium-high heat, steam-fry the onion with a dash of sea salt and ⅓ cup of the broth until the onions are tender, about 4 minutes. Add ginger, garlic, and green onions and sauté another 1 to 2 minutes, stirring constantly. Add the rest of the vegetables and the remaining broth and the coconut milk, reduce the heat to medium, cover, and cook, stirring occasionally, for 12 to 15 minutes, until the squash and carrots are tender. A few minutes before the stew is done, add a teaspoon of shoyu along with a dash of cayenne to taste. Serve hot alongside couscous or jasmine or basmati rice.

Stir–Fry Hearts of Palm & Artichoke with Shiitake Mushrooms

Serves 4

This delicious, exotic combination can be pulled together anytime, especially if you keep a few cans of hearts of palm and a few packages of frozen artichoke hearts on hand.

2 teaspoons extra virgin olive oil

2 cans organic hearts of palm drained, rinsed, and each stem cut into 3 pieces

1 package (8 ounces) frozen artichoke hearts, thawed and cut in half

1 cup fresh pea pods

1/4 cup dried shiitake mushrooms, rehydrated in hot water, drained, and sliced

1/4 cup vegetable broth

1 1/2 teaspoons arrowroot or kuzu

1 tablespoon tamari

1 tablespoon dry sherry

1 teaspoon minced garlic

1/2 teaspoon minced ginger root

In a skillet over medium heat, stir-fry the hearts of palm, artichoke hearts, pea pods, and mushrooms in the oil for 1 minute. Add the broth, lower the heat, and simmer, covered, about 1 minute or until the vegetables are tender. In a bowl, combine the arrowroot/kuzu with the tamari, sherry, garlic, and ginger. Add to the vegetables. Stir-fry until clear. Serve by itself or on top of a bed of couscous, quinoa, millet, or a combination of brown and wild rice.

• F Y I

Hearts of Palm

Hearts of Palm are truly international delicacies and favorites of chefs the world over. They make a delightful appetizer, or a side dish when sautéed, and they may also be enjoyed straight from the can as a low-calorie snack, or sliced and served as a wonderful addition to any salad. They are actually the undeveloped leaves of the palm that have

*yet to differentiate and emerge from their casing within the stalk. The
wild palm stalks, once harvested, fully regenerate themselves. My
favorite brand, Native Forest Organic Hearts of Palm, is grown ecologically in Guyana, South America, on the Barima River—a project
that has brought a higher standard of living to the region, while maintaining respect for its culture and its vast natural resources.*

Roasted Cauliflower, Edamame & Bell Peppers

Serves 4

*Once again, roasting the vegetables brings out a wonderful
sweet nuttiness.*

2 pounds cauliflower florets

2 cups frozen shelled edamame (fresh soybeans),
thawed, or lima beans

1 medium red bell pepper, cut in 1-inch strips

1 medium yellow bell pepper, cut in 1-inch strips

1 teaspoon minced garlic

1/4 cup sesame salt (gomasio) or Cheesy Sesame Salt
(see page 293-294)

Preheat oven to 450°F. Place vegetables in a shallow, nonstick pan
and sprinkle with the garlic. Spray lightly with a nonstick spray.
Bake 20 to 25 minutes, stirring a couple times, or until you begin to
see a tinge of brown. Place in a serving dish and sprinkle with
sesame salt. Serve with a salad and grain dish.

• F Y I
Cauliflower

*The National Academy of Sciences has singled out cauliflower as one
of the best cancer-preventing foods. A cruciferous vegetable, it's also
a great source of folic acid, vitamin C, and fiber. With only about 15
calories per 1/2 cup and virtually no fat or sodium, it's a good friend to
those desiring to lose weight. Because of its high phosphorus content,
it can cause flatulence. Make sure to chew well, especially when eat-*

ing it raw, and give your digestive system 2 to 3 weeks to adjust. Lightly steamed, it's great served with fresh lemon juice and some fresh herbs such as dill, tarragon, basil, or parsley.

Vegetable Pita Pizza

Serves 4 to 8

These low-fat pizzas are fun for the whole family to make together.

4 (8-inch) whole wheat pita breads, cut in half (around the edge) with a scissors or knife, to make 8 pizza shells

2 heads of roasted garlic, squeezed out

1/3 cup loosely packed fresh oregano

2 cups baby leaf spinach

24 cherry tomatoes, sliced in half

1 cup sliced mushrooms

1 yellow squash or zucchini, sliced

1 carrot, grated

1 package frozen artichoke hearts, thawed and chopped

1 sweet bell pepper, chopped

3 tablespoons cold-pressed, extra virgin olive oil

1 teaspoon Bragg liquid aminos

1 1/2 cups fat-free soy mozzarella, shredded

Preheat oven to 400°F. In a blender or food processor, purée the roasted garlic and oregano. Brush over the 8 pita shells. Arrange on a baking sheet and bake in the middle oven rack about 5 to 6 minutes or until golden brown and crispy. Layer the shells with spinach, followed by the remaining vegetables. Cover with the cheese and bake 8 to 10 minutes or until all the cheese is melted.

VARIATIONS: Some other great toppings are black beans (whole or mashed), sun dried tomatoes, roasted onion and eggplant, imported sliced olives, roasted peppers, jalapeño peppers, lentils, and tofu.

Yukon Potatoes, Corn & Pea Roast

Serves 4 to 6

This roast is colorful, delicious, and so good for you!

2 pounds Yukon or Finnish potatoes,
    cut in 1¼-inch dice, unpeeled

1½ cups frozen peas

1½ cups frozen sweet corn

6 green onions chopped

2 tablespoons tamari

2 teaspoons cold-pressed, extra virgin olive oil

2 teaspoons organic balsamic vinegar

2 to 3 cloves garlic, minced

2 teaspoons dried oregano

2 teaspoons dried rosemary

1 teaspoon minced ginger root

Preheat oven to 400°F. In a medium saucepan, parboil the potatoes for 5 minutes. Drain. In a small bowl, whisk together the tamari, balsamic vinegar, oil, garlic, ginger, and herbs. In a shallow, non-stick roasting pan, mix together potatoes, peas, corn, and green onions with the liquid mixture. Roast for 15 minutes, or until the potatoes are tender, stirring a couple of times.

Soy Thai Vegetable Sauté

Serves 4

If you like Thai food, you're in for a special treat. Serve this sauté over brown jasmine or basmati rice, a wild rice mixture, couscous, or quinoa.

1 medium onion, sliced

¼ cup vegetable broth

1-2 teaspoons minced garlic

Juice of 1 lemon

1 teaspoon tamari

2 red bell peppers, sliced

12 medium mushrooms, sliced

1 1/2 cups thinly sliced broccoli stems

1 cup snap peas

1/2 cup sliced water chestnuts

1 cup (8 ounces) firm tofu, diced

1 (15-ounce) can baby corn

1/2 cup lite coconut milk

1/4 cup soy nut or peanut butter

1 teaspoon shoyu

2 teaspoons minced fresh ginger root

Dash of cayenne and red chili flakes

Vegetable broth to thin

In a large nonstick skillet or wok, combine the onion and the broth. Sauté for 4 minutes or until slightly tender. Add garlic, tamari, and lemon juice, and sauté 2 minutes longer. Add the remaining vegetables and the tofu, and sauté, stirring often, until tender-crisp.

In a blender or food processor, purée the coconut milk, nut butter, shoyu, ginger, and chili flakes. Use extra broth to adjust thickness. Pour over the vegetables, stir to coat, and heat through. Serve hot.

Shiitake Mushrooms, Tofu, Carrots & Eggplant Sauté

Serves 6 to 8

16 dry shiitake mushrooms, rehydrated in hot water
   and cut into strips

2 cups broccoli florets, cut in bite-size pieces

2 cups baby carrots, cut in half

2 cups eggplant, cut in bite-size pieces

12 ounces firm tofu, diced

2 to 3 large garlic cloves, sliced finely

2 teaspoons fresh ginger root, minced

2 cups vegetable broth

1 tablespoon cold-pressed, extra virgin olive oil

1$^1\!/_2$ tablespoons shoyu or tamari

1 tablespoon chopped fresh thyme

1 tablespoon chopped fresh basil

1 tablespoon chopped fresh parsley

1 tablespoon kuzu or arrowroot

4 tablespoons purified water

$^1\!/_2$ cup slivered almonds, or coarsely ground cashews, toasted

In a large nonstick skillet or wok, heat the oil over medium heat. Sauté the garlic and ginger, stirring constantly for 1 minute. Add the mushrooms, broccoli, carrots, eggplant, and tofu, along with $^1\!/_4$ cup of vegetable broth and sauté for 5 minutes. Add enough water to the broth to make 1$^1\!/_4$ cups, and add to the vegetable mixture. Add the thyme, basil, and parsley. Cook until tender-crisp, about 5 to 6 more minutes.

Meanwhile, dissolve the kuzu in 3 tablespoons water and add the shoyu/tamari. Add this sauce to the vegetable mixture and stir, until the sauce thickens. Serve over a bed of brown and wild rice, couscous, or quinoa. Sprinkle with the toasted nuts.

Chapter 15

GRAIN & BEAN RECIPES

Grains and beans are two of the best superfoods you can eat. Dried beans, peas, lentils, and chickpeas are collectively known as legumes. They have the most protein with the least fat of any known food, and they're high in potassium and low in sodium. A pot of beans, peas, or lentils is warm and filling, and when added to soups, stews, chilis, casseroles, or salads, beans and legumes strengthen the kidneys and adrenals glands and offer a great source of protein without adding cholesterol, saturated fat, or the toxic nitrogen byproducts found in meat protein. In fact, most legumes and beans range from 17 to 25% protein, higher than that of eggs and most meats. Soybeans rate exceptionally high, with 38% protein. When you combine *any* bean with *any* grain you get a complete, top quality protein.

In the Middle East, people mix chickpeas (or garbanzo beans) or lentils with wheat or barley; in Asia, soybeans are mixed with rice or noodles (wheat or buckwheat); in South and North America, corn is often combined with black, kidney, or pinto beans; in Africa, the mixture of millet and peanuts is popular; and in Italy, it's pasta (wheat) and white beans. And here's my easy suggestion: I make short grain brown rice for 1 or 2 people, and then I add three extra tablespoons of water with 1 to 1^{1}/$_{2}$ tablespoons red lentils to the rice mixture, just on top. Bring this to a boil, cover, and reduce to simmer. When the rice is done, so are the lentils and the red adds a lovely color to the rice. You get a complete protein and a delicious, simple dish all in one.

Legumes are also rich in potassium, calcium, iron, zinc, and several B vitamins, including folic acid, as well as the phytochemical diogenin, which appears to inhibit cancer cells from multiplying. Their insoluble fiber makes them very beneficial for reducing the levels of serum cholesterol, thus offering protection from heart disease. Their fiber and superior carbohydrate make legumes/beans one of the best foods for people with diabetes or blood sugar imbalances, because they are digested slowly and cause only a gradual rise in blood sugar levels. Cultivated for thousands of years, yet they're not washed, parched, polished, gassed, colored, or preserved. And if you purchase organically grown legumes, their richness and earthy good taste make them a winner.

The most common complaint about beans is that they cause gas, but there are things you can do to make them more digestible. Make sure you rinse your beans thoroughly in cool water first. Then soak them until they are uniformly soft, which can take anywhere from 2 to 24 hours depending on the variety. If you soak them longer than 8 hours, refrigerate them to prevent the beans from souring, and after 8 hours, change the soaking water. Soaking softens beans by leaching out their indigestible sugars (trisaccharides) and by activating enzymes that break down complex carbohydrates into simpler, easier to digest starches. Soaking also eliminates the phytic acid in the beans, thus making their minerals more bioavailable. After soaking, throw away the water and use fresh water for cooking.

If you are pressed for time, here's a quicker method that may be helpful (although, if you have the time, go with the longer method because the boiling water prematurely kills beneficial enzymes): After rinsing the beans, put them in a pot and cover them with boiling water. Let them soak in that water for 4 hours or longer. Remove any beans that float to the top. Then drain and cook in fresh water, filling the pot until you have about 2 inches of water over the top of the beans. Cooking time varies from 1 to 3 hours, depending on the type of bean. I recommend adding a 2- to 3-inch strip of kombu (which you can remove before serving) and 1/4 teaspoon of sea salt for each cup of dried beans. These work as softening agents and flavor enhancers. (Unlike regular table salt, sea salt has a variety of trace minerals that soften the beans and add nutrients.) Of course, you can add your own favorite spices, too.

You can also sprout beans, peas, and lentils. I highly recommend sprouting, because you retain all the enzymes and actually increase nutritional value. Sprouts can be tossed in salads, made into sprouted bread, mixed with grains, and processed into patties, pâtés, and all sorts of treats.

Grains, as members of the grass family, are the most complex and highly evolved plant species and cover more of the earth's surface than any other, writes Rebecca Wood in her terrific cookbook, *The Splendid Grain*. Unlike most other plants, which have a separate fruit and seed, the fruit and seed walls of a grain unite in a single unit. Three seeds that are not members of the grass family and are still commonly considered along with grains (because their use is similar), are quinoa, amaranth, and buckwheat.

Throughout this book, I emphasize eating foods as close to the way Mother Nature made them as possible and staying away from refined foods. This is certainly true when it comes to grains. Whole grains are a top-quality energy food. They are complex carbohydrates rich in the B-complex group of vitamins: B_1, B_2, B_3, B_5, B_6, B_9 (folic acid), and biotin. When combined with a legume (within a 48-hour period), they provide a complete protein, which means you get all the essential amino acids. When grains are sprouted, their energy quotient is increased many times, as the enzyme action involved in the sprouting process increases the nutrient value.

So much is being written these days about avoiding grains and other complex carbohydrates if you want to lose weight. But there's a big difference between whole food complex carbohydrates and refined carbohydrates. Whole foods lose much of their nutritional benefits when refined (many of the vitamins and minerals are destroyed and the healthy fiber is removed) and wreak havoc on the body's ability to manage blood sugar. This can create mood swings, depression, lethargy, weight gain, and irritability. Even a diet too high in unrefined complex carbohydrates can upset this delicate balance, causing wild fluctuations in blood sugar. That's why it's so important to balance all carbohydrates with lots of fiber (especially greens), protein, and a little healthy fat.

For optimum health, white flour products should be avoided as much as possible. Why? Because when carbohydrates are consumed, digested, and absorbed into the blood stream, hormones trigger the pancreas to release insulin to help transport glucose across the individual cell membranes. If the level of sugar (glucose) in the blood stream is in excess of what the body requires, the surplus is sent to the liver to be stored until needed. If the blood sugar level rises too rapidly, as it does when you veer away from whole foods and eat refined carbohydrates, i.e., sweets, candy, sodas, cakes, pastries, white flour pasta, white flour bread, etc., the pancreas responds by releasing a large dose of insulin. This causes the highs and lows that many people experience after eating a sweet snack.

For example, after eating a candy bar, donut, or piece of cake, you might feel an initial burst of energy, but within a short space of time, you'll probably feel more lethargic than you did to start with. This pancreatic reaction is known as 'reactive hypoglycemia.' A diet high in refined carbohydrates consumed over an extended period can lead to adult onset diabetes. The release of insulin from the pancreas is initiated by vitamin B_3 (niacin) and the mineral chromium, which work together. Chromium is often deficient in those who suffer from reactive hypoglycemia and those with poor diets, as the pancreas becomes overworked and exhausted. Finally, this stress from consuming too many refined foods leads to an increase of insulin, promoting weight gain and even obesity.

So eat whole grains, but don't overdo them. And always combine them with other foods such as greens in salads, beans, in soups, or with vegetables as a way to stabilize blood sugar and insulin. Pre-soaking and light toasting enhance the flavor and digestibility of all grains and even shortens the cooking time of longer-cooking grains, such as wheat, wild rice, rye, barley, and long grain brown rice.

Enjoy several servings of beans and grains weekly and see how your vitality blossoms.

Sweet Lentil–Parsley Salad

Serves 5 to 6

This salad makes a nice change from tabbouleh and is terrific by itself or spooned into warmed whole wheat pita triangles.

1 1/2 cups dry lentils

3/4 cup vegetable broth

1 bay leaf

2-inch strip of kombu

1 1/2 cups finely chopped, loosely packed, fresh Italian parsley

1 medium sweet onion, thinly sliced

2 red and/or orange bell peppers, roasted (see page 290), peeled and cut in 1/2-inch strips

2 teaspoons lemon zest

1/4 cup freshly squeezed lemon juice

1/3 cup minced fresh mint

1/4 cup cold-pressed, extra virgin olive oil
or Barlean's Flax Oil

1 teaspoon sea salt

1/4 teaspoon coarsely ground black pepper

1/4 teaspoon allspice

5 to 6 large purple or green cabbage leaves,
as a shell for the salad

Rinse the lentils carefully and remove any small stones. In a large saucepan, combine the lentils, bay leaf, vegetable broth, kombu, and enough water to cover the lentils by 2½ inches. Bring to a boil. Reduce heat to medium-low and cover. Simmer 20 minutes, just until the lentils are tender.

Place the onion slices in a colander and drain lentils over the onion to give them a natural softness. Discard the bay leaf and kombu or you can cut it into small pieces and add it to the salad if you want. Transfer the lentils to a bowl. Add the lemon zest and juice, parsley, roasted peppers, mint, oil, allspice, salt, and pepper to the lentils. Place a washed and dried cabbage leaf shell on each plate and heap several spoonfuls of the lentils on each leaf. Serve warm or chilled. Garnish with thin lemon wedges and warmed whole wheat pita triangles.

• F Y I

Lentils

If you say you don't have time to properly cook beans, lentils are your answer. They don't need to be presoaked, take only minutes to cook, and have no sulfur so they don't produce gas. Like other legumes, they provide a complete protein when combined with any grain. Since Biblical times, they have been a dietary staple and their versatility makes them terrific in salads, soups, casseroles, stews, or as a side dish. A cup of cooked lentils packs 16 grams of protein, where as a 3-ounce patty of lean ground beef has only 15. And when you consider that lentils are very low in fat and that a burger has 18 grams or 162 calories of fat, you will see why lentils are becoming more and more popular. They are also rich in iron, zinc, phosphorus, folic acid, calcium, potassium, and magnesium. This makes them a good source for nearly every organ of the body and they also help to neutralize acids. They help to reduce blood cholesterol, to control insulin and blood sugar, and to lower blood pressure. There are varieties of different colors to choose from, either whole or split and husked.

White Bean & Tomato Casserole

Serves 6

1 can (28 ounces) organic whole tomatoes, drained
(reserve 1/2 cup) and chopped

2 (15-ounce) cans of cooked white beans, drained and rinsed

1 1/2 cups coarse fresh whole wheat breadcrumbs

2 red onions, finely chopped

2 large garlic cloves, minced

2 tablespoons cold-pressed, extra virgin olive oil

2 teaspoons minced fresh parsley

1 1/2 teaspoons minced fresh tarragon

1/2 teaspoon chili powder

1/4 teaspoon sea salt

1/4 teaspoon fresh lemon juice

In a small bowl, mix the breadcrumbs, 1 tablespoon of the oil, dash of salt, and the lemon juice and set aside.

In a large skillet, heat the remaining oil, add the onions and sauté over medium heat until onions are tender, about 3 to 4 minutes. Add garlic and sauté 1 more minute. Stir in tomatoes, tomato juice, beans, tarragon, parsley, and salt. Bring to a boil. Lower the heat and simmer for about 5 minutes, or until juice thickens.

Preheat broiler. Transfer the bean mixture to an 8-inch baking dish. Sprinkle breadcrumb mixture over the top of the beans. Broil for 3 minutes in the middle rack, or until the crumbs turn a golden brown. Be careful not to burn the top. Let it sit for 5 minutes, then serve.

VARIATIONS: Instead of tarragon and parsley, you can change the flavor by substituting other favorite fresh herbs such as basil, oregano, cilantro, chervil, cumin, or lemon grass, or you can give it a Tex-Mex twist by adding jalapeño pepper, chili powder, cayenne, and/or salsa.

• TIP

Breadcrumbs

To make the coarse breadcrumbs, simply tear whole grain bread into large chunks, then pulse until the bread pieces are about the size of a pea.

Garlicky Quinoa with Chestnuts & Toasted Pine Nuts

Serves 4 to 5

Revered by the Incas as their mother grain, quinoa is a high-energy grain that's easy to digest, and an ideal endurance and fitness food.

2 cups water or vegetable broth or a mixture

1 tablespoon lime juice

1 cup canned chestnuts, sliced and cut in half

1/2 medium red onion, chopped

3 cloves garlic, minced

1 1/3 cups quinoa, washed 3x and rinsed until the
    water is almost clear

1 tablespoon minced fresh cilantro

3 tablespoons pine nuts, toasted in a dry skillet

Sea salt to taste

In a medium saucepan, steam-fry the chestnuts and onion with lime juice and 1 tablespoon of the vegetable broth, until tender. Add the garlic and cook 1 more minute. Add the rest of the water or broth and bring to a boil. Add the washed quinoa and return to a boil. Cover. Lower the heat and simmer about 12 minutes. Add the cilantro, pine nuts, and salt to taste. Stir. Cover and remove from heat. Let stand 5 more minutes. Fluff with a fork and serve warm or chilled.

• F Y I

Chestnuts

Chestnuts roasting on an open fire, as the song goes, are as fun to eat as they are nutritionally beneficial. They are more like a grain or bean than a nut because of their high carbohydrate content and their low oil content, making them the most easily digested nut. Available fresh, dried, fresh-frozen, bottled; or canned, either whole or puréed, they add a nice crunchiness to any dish. You can boil them, roast them, mash them like potatoes, sweeten, or purée them. I like them sliced or diced in salads, dressings, and stir-fries, or grated and added to green beans, mushrooms, and peas. One of their virtues is that they stay crisp after cooking.

Chestnuts are sweet like a fruit, but, unlike fruit, they build and warm, rather than cool and cleanse. They help strengthen tendons, nourish the stomach, spleen, liver, and pancreas. They have virtually no fat, so keep a few cans in your pantry.

Coconut Rice Almondine

10/26/02 ok — but not necessary to make again

Serves 4

1/4 cup broth and dash of tamari or Bragg liquid aminos

1 cup chopped onion

2 cloves garlic, minced

2 1/4 cups water

1 cup lite coconut milk

1 tablespoon fresh lemon juice

1 1/2 cups short grain brown rice

1/2 cup chopped mushrooms

3 green onions, chopped

1/3 cup chopped red bell pepper

3 tablespoons slivered almonds, toasted in a dry skillet
    for 3 to 4 minutes

1 teaspoon dried dill

1/2 teaspoon dried parsley

In a saucepan, steam-fry the onion with broth and tamari for about 4 minutes. Add the garlic and cook for 1 more minute. Add the water, coconut milk, lemon juice and rice and bring to a boil. Lower the heat, cover, and simmer about 35 minutes, until all the liquid is absorbed. Add remaining ingredients, stir well, remove from the heat and let it stand, covered, for 5 more minutes. Fluff with a fork and serve.

• **F Y I**

Brown Rice

One cup of brown rice provides 5 grams of protein and only 230 calories. To get that much protein from steak, you'd need to consume a whopping 500 calories, which has lots of saturated fat as well.

Calming to the nervous system and an impressive energy food, brown rice is rich in calcium, iron, magnesium, phosphorus, potassium, zinc, manganese, vitamins B_3, B_5, B_6, and folic acid. Keep in mind that brown rice is far superior to white rice because it retains its nutrition-laden, fiber-rich outer cover, which is better for stabilizing blood sugar and insulin levels.

Millet–Tofu Salad with Toasted Pecans

Serves 4

2 cups cooked millet

1 cup firm or extra firm tofu, cubed and marinated in your favorite nonfat dressing

3 green onions, finely chopped

1 jalapeño pepper, roasted and minced

1 small garlic clove, minced

1/2 lime, juiced

1/2 lemon, juiced

2 tablespoons chopped pecans, toasted in a dry skillet

2 teaspoons finely chopped fresh cilantro

1 teaspoon minced fresh ginger root

In a large bowl, toss all the ingredients together and chill. Serve on a bed of crisp greens.

• **F Y I**

Millet

With only 50 calories in 1/2 cup, millet has the richest amino acid pro-tein profile and the highest iron content of all the true cereal grains. It is also very rich in phosphorus, magnesium, and potassium. Unlike wheat, it is gluten-free, and due to its high alkaline ash content, it's the easiest grain to digest and helps eliminate acidic wastes from the body. Great hot, warm, or chilled, this high-fiber, low-allergenic grain lends itself well to breakfast, lunch, dinner, or snack meals. Toasting it for about 5 minutes, or until it begins to pop, brings out a nutty flavor.

Zesty Couscous with Black Beans & Carrots

Serves 3 to 4

1 1/4 cups vegetable broth

1 cup whole grain couscous

1 (15-ounce) can black beans, drained and rinsed

1 cup carrots, finely diced

1/4 cup minced fresh parsley

1/2 teaspoon ground cumin

1/8 teaspoon ground nutmeg

In a large saucepan, combine seasonings and broth. Bring to a boil, then remove from heat. Stir in the couscous, followed by the beans and carrots. Remove from heat and let sit, covered for about 10 minutes. Serve with salad with lots of crisp greens.

• **F Y I**

Couscous

Couscous is a delectable feather-light form of semolina wheat. Indige-nous to North Africa, it is essentially a minuscule pasta that only takes 5 to 10 minutes to prepare. While not as nutritionally rich as other grains, it does provide fiber, some B vitamins, protein, and trace min-erals such as zinc, iron, copper, and manganese. You can purchase it in bulk but if you've never prepared it before, start with a package and follow the directions. Most packages contain too much sodium and seasonings for me, but it's a good way to learn how to make it. For best results, cook couscous in a wide pan. Both whole grain and refined couscous are available, but. I, of course, prefer the whole grain variety for the extra fiber and nutrition.

Barley–Lentil–Cashew Stew
Serves 3 to 4

1 cup vegetable broth

1 cup water

3/4 cup whole lentils

1/3 cup cashew pieces, toasted in a dry skillet

1/4 cup barley

1 medium onion, chopped

6 large mushrooms, sliced

2 cloves, garlic, minced

1 teaspoon lemon zest from an organic lemon

1 teaspoon ground cumin

1/2 teaspoon fresh lemon juice

Sea salt to taste

In a medium nonstick saucepan, sauté the onion in 3 tablespoons of the broth. Add garlic and mushrooms and sauté 1 more minute. Add all the remaining ingredients, stir well, cover, and simmer over low heat for about 50 to 60 minutes. Check periodically to see if extra boiling water is needed to make it the right consistency for stew.

• F Y I

Barley and Wheat

Barley and wheat are the world's oldest cereal crops. Whole barley is a tan-colored grain, larger and plumper than all other grains except corn. While the bulk of barley is consumed in a malted form, otherwise known as beer, it is also known as a favorite in soup and stews. With only 200 calories per 1/2 cup, barley is a complex carbohydrate energy food that has respectable levels of fiber and protein and low levels of fat. Whole barley is the most acidic of the grains but can be made more alkaline and flavorful by roasting it a shade darker prior to cooking. Pearl barley has had its bran polished off, has lost all of its fiber and half of its protein, fat, and minerals, such as potassium, calcium, and iron. So pick the whole barley and reap the benefits. Studies reveal that whole barley lowers cholesterol and has powerful anti-cancer agents. It's also an excellent laxative.

Roasted Garlic Risotto with Sun–Dried Tomatoes & Artichoke Hearts

Serves 4 to 6

Risotto is elegant, rich, fragrant, and soothing. Most risotto recipes call for quite a bit of fat in the form of butter. This risotto is low in fat without any sacrifice in flavor.

4 cups vegetable broth

1 medium onion, minced

2 teaspoons coconut oil

1/2 cup chopped artichoke hearts (you can find them frozen at the supermarket)

1/2 cup chopped sun-dried tomatoes (not packed in oil)

1 cup arborio (short grain) rice

1 head garlic, roasted, cloves squeezed out, and sliced in half

1/2 cup dry sherry

3 tablespoons fresh oregano, chopped

Sea salt to taste

Freshly ground pepper to taste

In a medium saucepan, bring the broth to a boil, then reduce the heat, cover the pan and simmer gently.

In separate saucepan, heat the oil, 2 tablespoons water, and add the onion, artichoke hearts, and sun-dried tomatoes and sauté until the onion is tender, about 3 minutes. Add the rice and garlic and stir for 2 minutes. Add the sherry and cook, stirring constantly until most of the sherry evaporates, about 2 minutes.

Add 1/2 cup of the hot broth at a time to the rice, stirring constantly, until most of the liquid is absorbed. Continue adding the broth until it is absorbed and the rice is al dente and creamy, about 20 minutes. Stir in the oregano, salt and pepper. Serve hot.

• F Y I
Coconut Oil

For years, the fatty acids pressed from coconut meat were falsely accused of raising blood cholesterol levels. While it is a highly satu-rated fat, which means that it's solid at room temperature, it's been found to be an exceptionally healthy fat for vegetarians and people with low fat/cholesterol consumption. Coconut oil and palm oil are the only two unrefined vegetarian fats that are not denatured when heated above 240 degrees. Purchase only unrefined coconut oil which is free of the toxic trans-fatty acids found in hydrogenated and refined oils. It's over 50% medium-chain fatty acids, the kind that are not stored as fat. In fact, the body readily metabolizes medium-chain fatty acids into energy. This makes coconut oil a favorite food of dieters and athletes. Perhaps the best feature of coconut oil is that it's an excellent source of lauric acid, which is a medium-chain fatty acid found in human milk that enhances brain function and the immune system.

Baked Jasmine or Basmati Rice with Chickpeas

Serves 5 to 6

I usually double this recipe and freeze one casserole for a later date. Its buttery aroma and nutty flavor will make it a popular dish with family and friends. Of course, if you can't find jasmine or basmati rice at your natural food store, brown rice will do just fine.

2 1/2 cups cooked jasmine or basmati rice

3/4 cup cooked garbanzo beans (chickpeas), if canned, drain and rinse

1 small onion, chopped

1/3 cup sliced green onions

1/3 cup plus 2 tablespoons vegetable broth

2 cloves garlic, chopped

1¹/₂ tablespoons nutritional yeast

1 teaspoon coconut oil

1 tablespoon tamari

¹/₄ teaspoon paprika

¹/₈ teaspoon ground cumin

¹/₄ teaspoon dried oregano

Preheat oven to 350°F.

In a skillet, steam-fry the onion with 2 tablespoons broth and a few drops of tamari for about 4 minutes. Add the garlic and cook for 1 minute. Transfer to a large bowl. Add the rest of the ingredients and transfer to a nonstick casserole dish. Bake uncovered for about 40 minutes. Serve with a salad.

Grain Burgers

Serves 6 to 8

These freeze very well so consider tripling the recipe so you'll have lots on hand when you need them for burgers or to add to pasta sauces, on pizzas, or chopped into soups and stews.

2 cups cooked millet

1 cup cooked short grain brown rice

1 cup cooked quinoa

1 medium carrot, grated

2 cloves garlic, minced

¹/₂ cup grated zucchini

¹/₂ cup finely chopped red onion

¹/₄ cup minced fresh parsley

1 tablespoon Cheesy Sesame Salt (see page 294)

2 teaspoons unrefined coconut oil

¹/₄ teaspoon dried thyme

¹/₂ teaspoon dried basil

¹/₈ teaspoon ground cumin

Bragg liquid aminos or tamari to taste

Preheat oven to 350°F.

In a large bowl, mix all the ingredients together using your hands. Form into 6 to 8 patties and place on a nonstick baking sheet. Bake for 15 minutes. Serve on whole grain buns or on a bed of greens with all your favorite condiments.

Portabello Mushroom Chili

Serves 6 to 8

The wonderful, almost meaty flavor of portabellos stands up well to the strong spicing of chili. Serve this cozy stew on a cold night.

1 pound pinto beans, soaked overnight, drained and rinsed

3 cups water

3 cups vegetable broth

4 small carrots, grated

3 large portabello mushrooms, finely chopped

1 (6-ounce) can organic tomato paste

1 large onion, finely diced

1 red pepper, seeded and diced

1 (2-inch) strip of kombu (remove before serving)

2 tablespoons chili powder

2 teaspoons ground cumin

1 bay leaf

1 teaspoon sea salt

1 teaspoon unrefined coconut oil or cold-pressed, extra virgin olive oil

1/2 teaspoon ground celery seeds

1/8 teaspoon ground coriander

Cayenne pepper to taste (optional)

In a large pot, heat oil and sauté onion for 3 minutes. Add carrots and sauté 3 more minutes, stirring often. Add the remaining ingredients and cook, uncovered, over medium heat. Keep stirring to prevent sticking. Add extra boiling water or vegetable broth if the chili gets too dry. This chili should be thick and rich.

VARIATIONS: Instead of portabello mushrooms, try 1/4 pound of shiitake mushrooms, and if you like it really hot and spicy, add extra cayenne or chili powder.

• **F Y I**

Portabello Mushrooms

Portabello mushrooms are just a super-large version of the white button mushrooms you find in any supermarket. When they grow to this size, their flavor tends to intensify, becoming earthier and richer. They are fantastic grilled or sautéed and are a great substitute for beef or chicken in sandwiches, topped with lettuce, tomato, onion, and a couple slices of avocado, or a favorite spread such as hummus, Dijon, or lemonaise.

Millet with Garbanzo Beans & Vegetables

9/15/02

Serves 6

1 cup millet, rinsed and drained

2 cups water

1/2 cup vegetable broth

1 small onion, diced

1/2 cup thawed frozen corn

1/2 cup thawed frozen peas

1/2 cup diced carrots

1/2 cup cooked garbanzo beans, if canned, drain and rinse

2 green onions, thinly sliced

1/2 teaspoon sea salt

After rinsing and draining the millet, dry sauté it in a saucepan over medium heat, stirring constantly for about 4 minutes or until the millet starts to pop. Toasting will give it a nutty, full-bodied flavor.

Add the water, broth, and salt to the millet and bring to a boil. Lower the heat and simmer 10 minutes, covered. Add the corn, peas, onion, carrots, and garbanzo beans, cover and simmer 10 minutes.

Remove from heat, add the green onions, cover and let sit for 1 to 2 minutes before serving.

VARIATIONS: Instead of garbanzo beans, substitute edamame, black beans, kidney beans, pinto beans, Northern beans, lima beans, sliced chestnuts, hearts of palm, or artichoke hearts.

• F Y I
Millet

A study at the University of Minnesota suggested that middle-aged women who ate slightly more than 1 whole grain food per day had a 15% lower death rate than women eating lots of refined processed grains. Millet is a whole grain rich in fiber and protein, is easy to digest, and highly alkaline. This healthy "fast food" cooks in minutes.

Sushi Rice Salad

Serves 6

THE SALAD:
1 cup vegetable broth
2 cups water
1 1/2 cups short grain brown rice
2 medium carrots, diced
1/3 cup daikon, diced
4 nori sheets, toasted, and torn into small pieces
1/8 teaspoon sea salt

THE DRESSING:
1/4 cup black sesame seeds
1/4 cup cold-pressed sesame seed oil
2 tablespoons brown rice vinegar
2 tablespoons brown rice syrup
1 teaspoon Dijon mustard
1/4 teaspoon sea salt

In a saucepan, bring broth and water to a boil. Add the rice and salt and cover the pan with a lid. Simmer over low heat 40 to 45 minutes, or until all the liquid is absorbed. Uncover and let rice cool. Transfer the mixture to a large bowl and add daikon, carrots, and nori.

In a small bowl, whisk together all of the dressing ingredients. Pour over the rice. Serve on a bed of crisp greens.

You can toast the nori sheets yourself over a gas stove flame. Turn the flame on high. Use tongs and hold the dull side down about 1 inch from the flame. Fan it quickly over the flame until it turns from black to green. You can also toast the sheets in a skillet over high heat until the sheets turn color.

• T I P

Vegetable Broth

You'll notice that I often recommend vegetable broth as the liquid when cooking grains because it adds flavor and nutrients. You can find organic vegetable or mushroom broth in your health food store or make it yourself in large batches and freeze it in plastic containers or zip-lock bags (see pages 298-299). Of course, if you don't have any vegetable broth on hand, you can always use water.

Marinated Baked Tofu Slices

Serves 4

This high-protein recipe is great by itself or added to a variety of dishes. Try serving it with your favorite grain or to accompany a salad.

1 pound firm tofu (silken is too soft)

1/4 cup shoyu

1/4 cup vegetable broth

1 tablespoon Dijon mustard

1 tablespoon nutritional yeast

2 teaspoons brown rice syrup

1 teaspoon minced garlic

Chili pepper to taste (optional)

Preheat oven to 400°F.

Cut tofu into 1/2-inch slices and place in a baking dish.

In a small bowl, mix together all other ingredients and pour the marinade over the tofu slices. Bake for 20 minutes, or until the liquid is dissolved and the tofu is crispy brown.

VARIATIONS: If you're in a hurry, cut the tofu into 1/4-inch slices, top it with a few drops of tamari or shoyu, and dry fry it in a non-stick skillet for 1 or 2 minutes on each side. You can add some lemon pepper, garlic power, cayenne, or any favorite herb.

Sweet & Sour Black–Eyed Pea Salad
Serves 4 to 6

2 1/2 tablespoons apple cider vinegar

1 1/2 teaspoons balsamic vinegar

1 tablespoon brown rice syrup

1 tablespoon fresh lemon juice

2 teaspoons grainy mustard

1/4 teaspoon hot pepper sauce

1 tablespoon Barlean's Flax Oil

2 (15 ounces each) cans black-eyed peas, drained and rinsed

2 cups yellow cherry tomatoes, cut in half

1 medium sweet or red onion, chopped

1 medium red bell pepper, chopped

1/2 teaspoon sea salt

In a bowl, whisk together the vinegars, brown rice syrup, mustard, hot pepper sauce, lemon juice, and salt. Slowly whisk in the flax seed oil. Add the peas, tomatoes, onion, and red pepper. Toss well to combine. Serve on a platter garnished with a ring of sliced red and yellow tomatoes around the edges.

Mexican Black Beans

Serves 4 to 6

Once you get in the habit of soaking beans, recipes like this one are a snap.

1 cup dry black beans, soaked overnight, drained and rinsed
1¹/2 cups vegetable broth
1¹/2 cups water
2 tablespoons tamari
¹/2 teaspoon chili powder
¹/4 teaspoon ground cumin
¹/8 teaspoon ground chile pepper
Dash cayenne

In a large saucepan, combine all the ingredients and bring to a boil. Lower the heat and cook until beans are tender, about 1¹/2 hours. Serve with a green salad.

• **F Y I**

Black Beans

One of my favorite legumes, the black bean, also referred to as the black turtle bean, may be interchanged with the pinto bean in any recipe. But keep in mind that they will color the other ingredients they are cooked with. They have a sweet, spicy taste and are delicious in soups, mashed in dips, or sprinkled on top of salads to add more fiber, protein, calcium, potassium, iron, zinc, and many B vitamins, including folic acid. Black beans are an excellent kidney support.

• **T I P**

Freezing Beans

Consider making large batches of beans once a month and then freezing them for later use. It's much cheaper than buying canned beans and they freeze well for up to 4 months. When you purchase canned beans, try to find organic (they are readily available in natural food stores) and always drain and rinse in water to help prevent digestive problems and flatulence.

Quinoa with Soybeans, Dried Cherries & Toasted Almonds

Serves 5 to 6

1 1/3 cups quinoa, washed 3x and rinsed until the water
    runs almost clear, then toasted for 3 minutes

1 1/8 cups vegetable broth

1 cup water

1/2 cup cooked soybeans, or canned beans drained and rinsed

1/3 cup chopped dried cherries

1/3 cup chopped almonds, toasted in a dry skillet

3 tablespoons fresh orange juice

2 tablespoons Barlean's Flax Oil

1 garlic clove, minced

1 teaspoon lemon zest from an organic lemon

1 tablespoon fresh parsley, minced

1 tablespoon fresh mint, minced

1/4 teaspoon sea salt

In a medium saucepan, bring the broth and water to a boil. Add the toasted quinoa and return to a boil. Lower the heat, cover the pan, and simmer about 12 minutes, or until all the liquid is absorbed. Fluff with a fork, then stir in the soybeans, cherries, and almonds. Set aside for 5 to 6 minutes, uncovered.

While the quinoa is cooking, in a small bowl, whisk together the orange juice, oil, garlic, and zest. Then add half the parsley, half the mint, and the salt.

Toss the dressing into the cooked quinoa. Transfer to a serving bowl or individual plates and top with the remaining parsley and mint. Serve warm, hot, or chilled.

VARIATIONS: Instead of soybeans, substitute lima beans or leave out the beans entirely. Try toasted sunflower seeds, hazelnuts, pumpkin seeds, or cashews.

Instead of water or broth, use lite coconut milk or 1/2 soy milk, or use cold-pressed unrefined coconut oil in place of the flax oil and to sweeten the dish a bit.

- F Y I

Quinoa

Quinoa contains more calcium than milk and is high in the amino acid lysine, which is scarce in the vegetable diet. It's also a balanced source of other nutrients such as iron, phosphorus, B vitamins, and vitamin E and can be substituted in recipes for rice, millet, or cous-cous. It's great by itself as a side dish or as an ingredient in soups, casseroles, stews, pilafs, and even puddings. The flour can be used in breads, cookies, and other treats in place of wheat flour for those people with allergies. It also comes in a black color, which has a nut-tier flavor than the lighter colors.

Spicy Lemon Grass Tabbouleh with Toasted Walnuts

Serves 4 to 6

The Thai flavors in this salad lend an exotic twist to familiar tabblouleh.

2 cups boiling water
1$^{1}/_{2}$ cups bulgur (cracked wheat)
3 stalks lemon grass or 1 tablespoon fresh lemon zest
1$^{1}/_{2}$ cups loosely packed finely chopped fresh parsley sprigs
$^{1}/_{2}$ cup loosely packed finely chopped fresh cilantro sprigs
$^{1}/_{2}$ cup loosely packed finely chopped fresh mint leaves
1 to 2 garlic cloves, minced
1 small red or sweet onion, finely chopped
1 large organic ripe tomato, chopped
$^{1}/_{3}$ cup coarsely ground walnuts, toasted in a dry skillet
$^{1}/_{4}$ cup cold-pressed, extra virgin olive oil
$^{1}/_{4}$ cup fresh lemon juice
$^{1}/_{2}$ teaspoon ground coriander
$^{1}/_{4}$ teaspoon cardamom
$^{1}/_{8}$ teaspoon cayenne (optional)
$^{1}/_{2}$ teaspoon sea salt
Mint sprigs for garnish

In a large bowl, combine the bulgur with 2 cups boiling water. Set aside for about 40 to 45 minutes, until all the liquid is absorbed.

Trim the lemon grass to 5-inch-long stalks, peel away outer layers, and coarsely chop the tender inside stalks.

In a separate bowl, combine the lemon grass, parsley, cilantro, mint, and garlic. (I use a food processor with a knife blade to chop the herbs.)

Add the chopped herbs to the bulgur (after all the water is absorbed) and combine thoroughly. Add the remaining ingredients. Cover and refrigerate for 1 hour before serving. Garnish with mint sprigs and serve with warmed whole wheat pita triangles, with some hummus, shredded carrots, and alfalfa or red clover sprouts.

• F Y I
Walnuts

The most popular and widely used nut around the world, the walnut is rich in omega-3 fatty acids, which help to reduce inflammation and alleviate pain. Being a nut, it is fatty (over 60%) but it's still a healthy fat, mostly mono-unsaturated and omega-3. It also provides protein, zinc, calcium, and potassium. Studies at Harvard University have found that eating more than 5 ounces of nuts a week (not daily) cut heart attack deaths in women by 40% and helped prevent deadly irregular heart-beats in men. Walnuts may also help lower blood cholesterol. Like seeds, nuts are best eaten unsalted and raw. And if you want to lose lots of weight as quickly and healthfully as possible, limit your nuts and seeds to only 1 ounce daily or 3 to 4 ounces weekly, spread out.

Mexican Wild Rice with Olives
Serves 2 to 3

Black, green, red, yellow—this brightly colored salad is a quick and beautiful dish worthy of guests.

1 cup cooked wild rice
1/2 cup cooked brown rice

¼ cup diced orange or yellow bell pepper

1 large ripe tomato, diced

⅓ cup chopped fresh cilantro

¼ cup pitted and chopped black cured olives

2 teaspoons cold-pressed, extra virgin olive oil

1 teaspoon chili powder

Juice of 1 small lemon

Sea salt to taste

In a large bowl, combine all the ingredients and refrigerate for one hour. Serve on a bed of lettuce. If you serve it with warmed whole wheat pita halves, serve at room temperature.

VARIATION: I prefer to make this recipe with just the wild rice and instead of cooking it, I sprout it and create a raw "living foods" nutritious meal that's wrapped in double butter lettuce leaves and eaten with both hands.

• **F Y I**

Olives & Olive Oil

Olive oil is a major part of the Mediterranean diet. Researcher Ancel Keys declared olive oil the main dietary reason for remarkably low mortality rates among Mediterranean populations. Unlike other vegetable oils, olive oil is high in antioxidant activity. For the freshest and healthiest, select organic cold-pressed, extra virgin olive oil.

Olives acquired a bad reputation because of their high salt and fat content (up to 20%), but don't let that scare you away. You don't need to eat them by the handful, but a few added weekly to your favorite recipes is fine. They provide calcium, iron, and beta carotene, and are beneficial for the liver and gall bladder, and stimulate peristalsis.

Green olives are picked unripe and soaked in a lye solution and then cured in a salt solution. Ripe or black olives are cured directly in salt or in a salt brine. In the past, the best olives came from the Mediterranean. Now California produces excellent olives. Black olives mixed with your favorite spices make a great spread when puréed.

• F Y I

Wild Rice

Wild rice has a nutty sweet flavor with a hint of spice. It's richer in protein, minerals, and B vitamins, and higher in carbohydrates than wheat, barley, rye, or oats. It's a warming food that's great for strengthening the kidneys.

Lima Bean Sauté

Serves 4

Even lima bean resistors will ask for seconds of this recipe.

1 small onion, chopped

1 large ripe tomato, chopped

2 tablespoons red wine vinegar

1 tablespoon cold-pressed, extra virgin olive oil

2 teaspoons tamari

3 garlic cloves, minced

2 cups frozen lima beans

1 tablespoon chopped fresh cilantro and parsley
   (combined to make 1 tablespoon)

In a skillet, sauté the onion in vinegar, tamari, and oil for 3 minutes. Add the garlic and sauté 1 minute. Add the tomato and sauté 1 minute. Add the lima beans and sauté until heated through, about 3 to 4 minutes.

Just before serving, toss in the chopped herbs and season to taste.

• F Y I

Lima Beans

As you probably guessed, the lima bean gets its name from Lima, Peru, where the bean originated. The flavor is similar to chestnuts, with a sweet and starchy taste, and they are used often in succotash, soups, casseroles, and as a side dish. I mash them like potatoes and use them in dips and spreads. They're beneficial to the liver and lungs, neutralize acidic conditions, and have less fat than most other beans.

Cardamom & Parsley Basmati Rice

Serves 4 to 6

The rich yellow color of this recipe, with flecks of green, make it a feast for the eyes. The rich, lemony, aromatic flavor will get you breathing deeply and naturally, just to take in its essence.

1¹/2 cups basmati rice

6 cups water

¹/3 cup chopped loosely packed fresh parsley

4 to 5 cardamom seeds

¹/2 teaspoon turmeric, ground

2-inch strip kombu (remove before serving)

2 bay leaves

1-inch cinnamon stick

Wash the rice in a bowl of water and rinse until the water runs clear. Drain. Then soak the rice in 4 cups of water for 30 to 35 minutes. Drain. In a stockpot, combine the rice with 2 cups of the water and add all the remaining ingredients. Bring to a boil. Cover tightly, reduce heat to very low, and gently simmer for 15 minutes, or until all the water is absorbed. Turn off the heat and let the rice rest for 10 minutes covered.

Remove the kombu, cinnamon stick, and seeds. Serve as a side dish or along with some beans and a salad.

• F Y I

Cardamom

Cardamom is a spice with a lemon zest and eucalyptus flavor that aids digestion. It's commonly used in Indian and Middle Eastern cuisines, especially in curries, desserts, and pilafs. I recommend purchasing cardamom in small green pods that have been air dried. Fresh seeds are plump and a uniform dark brown in color. Grind it yourself only in the amount needed because the flavor quickly becomes camphorous.

• F Y I

Turmeric

Also referred to as Indian Saffron or Yellow Ginger, the rhizome, or root of turmeric, is bright orange, but otherwise it has the shape and skin of its relative, ginger. It has the highest known source of beta carotene and is known to relieve inflammation, strengthen the immune system, and enhance digestion. As an essential ingredient in curry, turmeric may be used to add color and flavor to any vegetable or grain dish. Buy in small amounts and store in a tightly covered dark glass jar since light quickly reduces the color, flavor, and aroma.

Garbanzo, Carrot & Tomato Salad

Serves 2 to 4

I like to make a double batch of this recipe to have on hand when I feel like a quick yummy snack or to add to my salads or grains for a boost of protein, beta carotene, folic acid, calcium, fiber, and omega-3s.

2 (15-ounces each) cans organic garbanzo beans,
  drained and rinsed

2 organic carrots, chopped

1 pint cherry tomatoes, sliced in half

1/2 medium sweet onion, chopped

1 tablespoon finely chopped fresh parsley

2 teaspoons Barlean's Flax Oil

2 teaspoons organic balsamic vinegar

1 teaspoon finely chopped fresh dill

Sea salt to taste

In a large bowl, combine all ingredients and refrigerate for one hour before serving.

Spicy Southwestern Black Bean Patties

Serves 4 to 8

I like to serve these "burgers" with salsa on a bed of greens or with a whole grain bun topped with salsa.

2 (15-ounces each) cans black beans, drained and rinsed

1/4 cup organic cornmeal, or extra if needed

2 tablespoons unrefined coconut oil

1/4 cup vegetable broth

2 tablespoons lime juice

1 to 2 garlic cloves, minced

1 small jalapeño pepper, seeded, tissue removed, and minced

2 teaspoons chili powder

1 teaspoon tamari

1/8 teaspoon cayenne

3 tablespoons fresh cilantro, minced

1 tablespoon Cheesy Sesame Salt (see page 294)

1 tablespoon extra virgin olive oil

In a large bowl, mash the black beans with a potato masher. In a small bowl, combine cornmeal, coconut oil, broth, garlic, chili, tamari, lime juice, cayenne, and cilantro. Add the liquid mixture to the mashed beans and purée. Stir in the sesame salt and add enough cornmeal so you can shape it into 8 patties, each about 3 inches in diameter.

In a nonstick large skillet, heat the olive oil and cook the patties over medium heat until they turn a slightly darker shade, about 4 to 5 minutes on each side. You may want to add a little extra oil to cook the other side.

Toasted Herb Rice with Shiitake Mushrooms

Serves 6

3 cups short grain brown rice

3¹/4 cups water

1³/4 cups plus ¹/4 cup vegetable broth

3 cups fresh shiitake mushrooms, sliced (or 1 cup dried, rehydrated in hot water)

1 teaspoon dried dill

1 teaspoon dried sage

1 teaspoon dried marjoram

1 teaspoon dried rosemary

¹/2 cup sunflower seeds, toasted in a dry skillet

1 to 2 cloves garlic, minced (optional)

Bragg liquid aminos or tamari to taste

In a large saucepan, bring the water and broth (except ¹/4 cup to a boil. In a small bowl, combine the dill, sage, marjoram, and rosemary.

In a large heavy skillet, toast the rice and ¹/2 herbs over medium-high heat, stirring constantly, until the rice is a shade darker, about 5 minutes.

When the liquid is boiling, add the toasted sunflower seeds and the toasted rice and herb mixture. Cover, lower the heat, and simmer until all the liquid is absorbed, about 40 minutes. Remove from the heat and let stand covered for 10 minutes.

Steam-fry the mushrooms in the remaining herbs, the reserved ¹/4 cup broth, garlic, and Bragg for 7 to 10 minutes, or until the mushrooms are tender and heated through. Add to the cooked rice, stir and serve immediately.

• F Y I

Shiitake Mushrooms

The second most widely produced edible mushroom, the shiitake has a rich woodsy flavor and meaty texture when cooked. Studies reveal *it contains substances that enhance the well-being of the whole body because they are rich in vitamins D, B_2, and B_{12} (rarely found in plant-based foods). You'll find them fresh and dried. To reconstitute, soak in warm water for 2 or 3 hours, preferably overnight. Use the soaking water for stock. Cut off the tough stem portion. Use shiitake mushrooms in stir-fries, entrées, side dishes, pasta sauces, or grill them with marinade.*

Tomato Couscous with Cashews & Raisins

Serves 3 to 4

2 cups fresh tomato juice (or organic bottled)

1 cup whole wheat couscous

1/2 cup vegetable broth or water

3 tablespoons chopped sun-dried tomatoes

1 to 2 cloves garlic, minced (optional)

1/3 cup raisins

1/3 cup chopped cashews, toasted in a dry skillet

2 1/2 tablespoons minced fresh parsley

1/4 teaspoon sea salt

In a saucepan, bring the tomato juice, broth, and salt to a boil. Add the rest of the ingredients, except for the 1 tablespoon parsley for garnish. Stir well. Cover, remove from the heat, and let stand 6 to 7 minutes. Fluff with a fork. Spoon into serving bowls or a platter and garnish with reserved parsley.

Citrus Basmati Rice Pilaf & Mushrooms

Serves 5 to 6

1 cup basmati brown rice

1 cup water

1 cup fresh orange juice

2 green onions, finely chopped

1 stalk celery, finely chopped

2 tablespoons chopped favorite fresh herbs, such as dill, oregano, tarragon, chervil, thyme, marjoram, sage, parsley, or basil

2 teaspoons unrefined coconut oil or cold-pressed sesame oil

6 shiitake mushrooms, (if you can't find them, use button), sliced (to equal one cup)

2 teaspoons fresh lemon juice

1 teaspoon orange zest

1 teaspoon lemon zest

Sea salt to taste

In a large saucepan, combine rice, water, and orange juice and bring to a boil. Then lower heat, cover, and simmer 40 to 45 minutes, until all liquid is absorbed. Add all the remaining ingredients and mix well. Let stand, uncovered, for 5 minutes. Fluff with a fork and serve.

• T I P

Cooking Rice

The age of the rice determines how much water is needed to cook it: The older the rice, the more water it will take. I use short grain brown rice for stuffing, loaves, vegetarian sushi, and molds because it is stickier. I use long grain brown rice when I want a fluffier rice.

Chilled Grain Salad with Sweet Corn

Serves 4 to 6

This salad mixes 4 grains and wonderful, sweet corn for a mouthful of interesting textures and flavors.

3/4 cup cooked millet

3/4 cup cooked short grain brown rice

3/4 cup cooked wild rice

3/4 cup cooked quinoa

1 1/2 cups frozen sweet corn, thawed

1 medium red bell pepper, finely diced

1/3 cup minced green onions (about 2)

1/4 cup chopped cured black olives

1/4 cup chopped fresh parsley

2 tablespoons fresh lemon juice

2 tablespoons Barlean's Flax Oil

Sea salt to taste

Freshly ground pepper to taste

In a large bowl, combine all the ingredients. Refrigerate for at least 1 hour before serving. Arrange on a bed of greens and garnish with lemon wedges and sprigs of fresh parsley.

VARIATIONS: Instead of all the grains combined, use a combination of just one or two, such as brown and wild rice or quinoa and millet or millet and couscous.

• T I P

Buying Olives

Look for olives that are organic and cured in fresh water and are unrefined (still raw). Two of my favorites are Aragon black olives from Spain with a hint of thyme and Manzanilla olives that are cured for almost 1 year in fresh water, unrefined sea salt, thyme, fennel, garlic, and lemon. No vinegar, caustic acids, or dyes are used. Or try Garum Organic Black Olive Paste from Spain made from minced organic olives, olive oil, herbs, and unrefined sea salt. It's great on whole grain bread or crackers, in salads, and on pasta/noodle dishes. All these products are available through Gold Mine (see Resource Directory).

Vegetable Lentil–Sweet Potato Cakes

Serves 6 to 8

Serve these veggie cakes on a bed of lettuce greens or with a whole grain bun.

3 cups water

2 cups vegetable broth

2 cups yams, peeled and diced

1 cup dried lentils

1/2 cup uncooked short grain brown rice

1/2 cup cornmeal

1/2 cup minced celery

1/3 cup grated carrots

1/3 cup diced zucchini

1/3 cup diced red or yellow bell pepper

1/8 teaspoon ground cumin

In a large stockpot, combine all the ingredients. Bring to a boil. Lower the heat to medium and simmer 45 minutes, stirring occasionally, until lentils and rice are soft. Using your hands, form into 6 to 8 patties. In a nonstick pan, brown on each side, about 5 minutes each. You can also broil them.

Asian Rice

Serves 3 to 4

I love the Asian flavors in this easy rice dish.

1 cup water

3/4 cup vegetable broth

3/4 cup brown basmati rice

1 (15-ounce) can French-cut green beans, drained and chopped

1 (8-ounce) can sliced water chestnuts, drained

1/2 cup plain soy milk

3-inch strip of kombu (remove before serving)

11/2 tablespoons Thai green chili sauce

2 green onions, thinly sliced, for garnish

1 tablespoon black sesame seeds, toasted in dry skillet, for garnish

In a medium saucepan, bring the water and broth to a boil. Stir in the rice, lower the heat, cover, and gently simmer for about 25 minutes, or until all the liquid is absorbed.

Meanwhile, in a skillet over medium-high heat, combine the green beans, water chestnuts, soy milk, and Thai sauce. Stir frequently while cooking, about 6 to 7 minutes. Serve over the hot rice. Sprinkle with the green onions and toasted sesame seeds.

• F Y I

Whole Grains

In a study conducted at the University of Minnesota, 36,000 healthy Iowa women, aged 55 to 69, were given a questionnaire in 1986. After six years, 1,141 of the women were diagnosed with diabetes. Those who consumed the most whole grains (average: 3 servings a day) had a 21% lower risk of diabetes than those who consumed the least (average: once a week). Those who consumed the most fiber (average: 10 grams a day) from whole grain breads, cereals, and other grains had a 29% lower risk than those who consumed the least (average: 3 grams a day). And those who consumed the most magnesium, a mineral found in whole grains, had a 24% lower risk than those who consumed the least. So eat your whole grains regularly and combine them over a two-day period with beans to get the best protein value.

Chapter 16

SIDE DISHES & SNACKS

Whether fat loss is your goal or you just want to feel more energetic and look more youthful, it's best to stay away from huge meals except for big green salads. As I explained in Chapter 5, eating frequent, small meals throughout the day, as opposed to three large ones, revs metabolism, stabilizes blood sugar and mood, and helps prevent overeating.

The Best Apple Berry Sauce

Serves 6 to 8

I keep lots of this yummy sauce on hand to eat as a snack between meals. You can also use it in baked goods. It reduces the need for oil and other fats and keeps cakes and breads nice and moist.

6 to 8 apples, your favorite variety

1 1/2 cups freshly squeezed apple juice (or water or both)

1 cup blueberries, strawberries, or raspberries or combination

4 teaspoons concentrated fruit sweetener, such as apple,
    berry, or black cherry

1 teaspoon cinnamon

1/4 teaspoon lemon zest

1/4 teaspoon orange zest

2 dates, pitted and chopped

Core and chop the apples (if they're not organic, peel them first). In a large saucepan, bring the juice (or water) to a boil and add the apples. Cover and return to a boil, then lower the heat and simmer for about 10 minutes. Drain. Set aside to cool. Place cooked apples in a food processor, along with the berries and purée. Add the dates and the spices and pulse until you get the consistency you like best.

Keep refrigerated in an airtight container. Try this applesauce over fresh fruit, on whole grain pancakes, oatmeal, or spread on whole grain toast.

VARIATIONS: For a fruitier taste, blend in 1/2 cup fresh raw strawberries, raspberries, or blueberries, or for a tropical fare, blend in 1/2 cup mango, pineapple, or papaya and garnish with unsweetened coconut. Kids love this special homemade treat.

• **F Y I**

Apples

Apples are the perfect health and diet food. They elevate your blood glucose level safely and gently, and then keep it up for a longer period of time than apple juice or sweeter fruits, such as bananas or grapes, so you feel fuller longer. Apples have abundant soluble fiber, which helps stabilize blood sugar levels and guards against sudden drops or swings. They have virtually no sodium, saturated fat, or cholesterol. In fact, according to studies at Yale University, apples help to reduce the level of cholesterol in your blood and also lower blood pressure. I guess the old saying is true: An apple a day really does keep the doctor away!

Kale Chips

Serves 3 to 6

Most people think of kale as a slow-cooked green that goes in soups and stews. Try this easy, fat-free, and wonderfully tasty way to eat kale and increase the calcium in your diet. Even kids love this special crunchy treat.

10 kale leaves
Spice of your choice

Preheat broiler. While the broiler is heating, wash the kale leaves well and shake, then pat dry with a paper towel. Lay them out on a broiling pan or baking sheet. Do not overlap them. Sprinkle leaves with your favorite spice/seasoning such as onion or garlic powder, cayenne, sea salt, ground cumin or other herbal blend seasoning.

Broil for 5 to 10 minutes, turning a couple of times, and enjoy warm or cool. Kale burns easily, so watch them carefully. I like to use a Misto or Misto-style spray pump bottle and lightly mist the kale with tamari before broiling. Serve warm or at room temperature.

• F Y I
Kale

Kale is a member of the cruciferous or cabbage family. The leaves are slightly curled and crimped (the word for kale in French translates as "curly cabbage") and strongly flavored. It can be streamed, sautéed, added to soups, stews, and stir-fries, or eaten raw in salads. Remove the stems and center veins and tear into small pieces for salads. It's an abundant source of calcium and chlorophyll and one of the best vitality and rejuvenating foods you can eat.

Edamame

Serves 3 to 6

Pronounced "ed-a-ma-may," this is one of the most popular snacks in Asia and a favorite appetizer in Japanese restaurants. These delicious young soybeans in the pod offer a powerhouse of nutrients and are as fun to eat as they are simple to make.

8 to 10 cups water

1 pound frozen edamame (check the vegetable freezer
    section of your market or health store)

Seasoning to taste

In a large saucepan, bring water to a boil. Place the edamame in the boiling water and continue to boil. Cook 5 minutes over medium heat uncovered. Drain. Lightly sprinkle with sea salt, spray with tamari, or use any combination of your favorite seasonings. I like them just plain.

• T I P
Eating Edamame

Traditionally served in the pod, edamame need to be husked before eating. Just pinch the pods, aim for your mouth, and enjoy. You can buy edamame out of the pods, too. Add these young soybeans to soups, salads, casseroles, and grains for added protein, calcium, iron, and omega-3 essential fatty acids.

Yukon Gold Potato Salad

Serves 4 to 6

These special potatoes gives this potato salad a delicious richness. There's no mayonnaise, so it's low in calories but high in fiber and lots of nutrients.

2 pounds Yukon Gold or new red potatoes (about 7 small potatoes) cut in 1-inch cubes, unpeeled

3 cups water

1¼ cups vegetable broth

3 celery stalks, diced

1 red, yellow, orange, purple, or combination bell pepper, diced

⅓ cup diced green onions

¼ cup chopped fresh chives

¼ cup pitted and sliced black olives

¼ cup plain soy yogurt

¼ cup red wine vinegar

1 tablespoon chopped fresh dill

1 tablespoon chopped fresh tarragon

⅛ teaspoon sea salt

Place the potatoes in a stockpot, add the broth and water to cover. Bring to a boil and cook until tender, about 20 minutes. Drain. Transfer the potatoes to a mixing bowl and set aside to cool. In a large separate bowl, combine the celery, bell peppers, green onions, chives, and olives.

In a separate bowl, blend yogurt, red wine vinegar, dill, and tarragon. Add this dressing to potatoes and veggies and combine everything thoroughly. Refrigerate for 1 hour before serving. Arrange on a bed of crisp lettuce and garnish with fresh parsley.

Broccoli Cole Slaw with Toasted Sesame Seeds

Serves 4 to 6

This unique colorful slaw is an antioxidant, anti-cancer, immune-boosting, delicious treat.

3 cups broccoli stalks, grated

1/2 cup carrots, grated

1/2 cup purple cabbage, grated

Favorite fat-free dressing

2 tablespoons sesame seeds, toasted in a dry skillet

In a large bowl, combine everything except the sesame seeds. Divide the salad into individual serving bowls and sprinkle with the toasted sesame seeds.

VARIATIONS: Combine with red and yellow bell pepper, onions, and mushrooms, sauté, and wrap up in a whole grain chapati or tortilla.

Cashew–Raisin Balls

These freeze beautifully, so double or triple the batch to keep on hand as the perfect treat or snack to satisfy a sweet tooth. And they're much better for you than M&M's!

1 cup raisins, soaked overnight in water, drained, and dried

1 pound whole raw cashews (or almonds or walnuts)

1/4 cup rolled oats

12 dates, pitted

3 tablespoons raw tahini (I use Rejuvenative Foods Raw Tahini; see the Resource Directory)

2 tablespoons shredded coconut

1 teaspoon cinnamon

1 teaspoon pure vanilla extract

In a blender or food processor, finely grind cashews and oats together. Transfer to a bowl. In a blender, combine the dates, tahini, coconut, cinnamon, and vanilla. Add the raisins and blend again. Transfer mixture to a bowl, then using your fingers, roll into balls. They can be as small as 1 inch or as large as 2 inches in diameter. Store in the refrigerator or freeze for later use.

• F Y I
Cashews

Cashews are higher in calories than many other plant foods, but they are lower in fat than most other nuts, and are rich in calcium, magnesium, iron, zinc, and folic acid.

No Oil Chips & Salsa

1 dozen corn tortillas

Sensational Salsa (see page 243) or Black Bean Dip (see page 245) or Guacamole (see pages 244-245)

Preheat the oven to 375°F. Toast whole tortillas directly on the oven rack for 10 to 15 minutes or until crisp. Cut or break apart into four (quarters) and serve with salsa or other side dishes or dips.

Sweet & Spicy Organic Baby Carrots
Serves 4 to 6

4 cups organic baby carrots

1/4 cup rice syrup

1/4 cup maple syrup

1/4 teaspoon cinnamon

1/4 teaspoon nutmeg

1/8 teaspoon cayenne

1 teaspoon chili powder

1/2 cup purified boiling water

Dash sea salt

Preheat oven to 350°F. Arrange the carrots in a casserole dish. In a small bowl, combine the syrups and spices. Add the boiling water and mix until well blended. Pour over the carrots. Cover and bake for 1 hour.

• **F Y I**

Carrots

Rich in calcium, magnesium, potassium, and beta carotene, carrots are a terrific detoxifier and an excellent food for the digestive tract, eyes, liver, kidneys, and immunity.

Colorful Cumin Spiced Apple–Cabbage with Toasted Walnuts

Serves 4

1$\frac{1}{4}$ cups plus 1 tablespoon vegetable broth

2 cloves garlic, minced

2 tablespoons apple cider vinegar

2 apples, peeled, cored, sliced into 8 pieces, then cut in half (16 chunks)

$\frac{1}{2}$ small head green cabbage, cored and sliced $\frac{1}{2}$ inch

$\frac{1}{2}$ small head purple cabbage, cored and sliced $\frac{1}{2}$ inch

2 tablespoons chopped fresh parsley

1 tablespoon tamari or Bragg liquid aminos

1$\frac{1}{4}$ teaspoons ground cumin

1 teaspoon chili powder

Dash cayenne

$\frac{1}{3}$ cup walnuts toasted in a dry skillet, for garnish

In a large pot, combine the vegetable broth, garlic, and vinegar and bring to a boil over medium-high heat. Add the apples and cabbage and stir to combine. Cover, lower the heat, and simmer until tender, about 8 to 12 minutes, stirring occasionally. In a small bowl, combine the parsley, Bragg, 1 tablespoon broth, cumin, chili, and cayenne. Transfer cabbage mixture to a warmed serving bowl, toss with the spice mixture, and serve hot. Garnish with the toasted walnuts.

• F Y I

Cumin Seed

Cumin is part of the parsley family and enhances testosterone, the hormone that increases libido and muscle strength, among other things.

Roasted Garlic & Dill Stuffed Mushrooms

Serves 3 to 5

My tasters rave about these stuffed mushrooms. They're easy to make, pretty to look at, good for you, and who can resist the sweet and mellow taste of roasted garlic?

15 large mushrooms, washed, stems removed

4 cups water

1 tablespoon fresh lime juice

1 tablespoon fresh lemon juice

1 teaspoon lemon zest

1/4 cup finely chopped red onion

3 tablespoons plain soy yogurt

1 tablespoon shoyu

1 tablespoon roasted garlic (see pages 288-289)

1 1/2 teaspoons dried dill

1 teaspoon Dijon mustard

In a saucepan, combine the water with the lemon and lime juices, and bring to a boil. Add the mushroom caps and cook until tender, reducing heat to medium, about 10 minutes, or until tender. Scoop out the caps with a slotted spoon and immediately plunge into a bowl of ice water to stop the cooking. Drain, pat dry, and arrange on a tray or platter.

In a small bowl, combine the rest of the ingredients. Stuff the mushroom caps with the filling and refrigerate. Serve on a bed of whole Bibb (Butter) lettuce leaves.

• **F Y I**

Dill

Dill has been used in herbal healing since the dawn of Egyptian civilization. In addition to its preservative action, dill is an infection fighter and soothing digestive aid. The oil from the dill seed inhibits the growth of bacteria that attack the intestinal tract and helps relax the smooth muscles. It also helps alleviate intestinal gas.

• **F Y I**

Garlic

Garlic was recommended by Hippocrates for infections, wounds, cancer, leprosy, and digestive problems. Thousands of studies have been done on the salutary effects of garlic. As a natural antibiotic or penicillin, nothing compares. And no standard medications come close to garlic when it comes to acting on so many cardiovascular risk factors at the same time: Some drugs reduce blood pressure; others decrease cholesterol; and some reduce the likelihood of internal blood clots, which trigger heart attacks and some strokes. But garlic does all these things, thanks to allicin and another chemical in the herb called ajoene.

Stuffed Endive

Serves 4 to 8

3 to 4 large Belgian endives

1 large carrot, grated

1 red bell pepper, diced

1 Maui or other sweet onion, diced

1 small rutabaga, diced

1/2 cup cured pitted black olives

2/3 cup raw tahini

1/4 cup fennel, diced

1 to 2 cloves garlic, minced

2 teaspoons Dijon mustard

2 teaspoons fresh lemon juice

Dash cayenne (optional)

Cut off the stems of the endive and separate the leaves, rinse well, and dry thoroughly. Arrange on a platter in a sunburst design. In a blender or food processor, combine the remaining ingredients and purée. Stuff the leaves and refrigerate before serving.

VARIATIONS: I love Belgian endive! Try spreading some hummus on the leaves and top with a little salsa.

Fennel–Dill Slaw

Serves 4 to 6

3 stalks celery, chopped

2 heads fennel, bottom core, tough parts, and leafy tops removed, finely sliced

1 small head purple cabbage, shredded

1 large carrot, diced

6 green onions, finely chopped

1/4 cup fresh dill, finely chopped or 1 tablespoon dried dill

Lemon Tahini or Vitality Vinaigrette Dressing (see Chapter 12)

In a large bowl, combine all the ingredients and serve with or without some of your favorite dressing.

• F Y I

Fennel

Fennel has been used medicinally for thousands of years. In the 3rd century BC, Hippocrates recommended it to treat infant colic. Four hundred years later, Dioscorides called it an appetite suppressant. The Roman naturalist Pliny recommended fennel in 22 remedies, including to help eye problems. These days this aromatic herb is used as a digestive aid to help expel gas, treat diarrhea, and soothe the entire digestive tract (antispasmodic). It's also effective for women's health because of its mild estrogenic effect.

Fancy Potato Skins with Salsa

Serves 4 to 8

If you like Mexican flavors, you'll love these zesty double-baked potatoes

4 large baking potatoes, thoroughly scrubbed
1 small tomato, chopped
1/2 cup black beans, drained and rinsed
3 tablespoons chopped green onions
2 tablespoons roasted garlic (see page 288)
1/2 teaspoon ground cumin
1/2 cup grated soy cheddar cheese
Sea salt
Freshly ground pepper

Preheat oven to 425°F. Bake potatoes until tender, about 1 hour. Set aside to cool. When potatoes are cool enough to handle (about 20 minutes), cut them into quarters lengthwise. Scoop out the flesh, leaving about 1/4 inch and the skins intact.

Place the 16 skins on a baking sheet and sprinkle with Celtic Sea Salt and pepper to taste. If you like it hotter, also sprinkle with some cayenne pepper and/or chili powder.

In a small bowl, combine the tomato, beans, onions, roasted garlic, and cumin. Spoon this mixture evenly on the skins, return to the oven, and bake for about 3 minutes. Sprinkle with the soy cheese and bake until the cheese melts, about 1 to 2 minutes. Don't over-bake or the potatoes will become dry and brittle. Serve with some salsa, guacamole, and soy yogurt.

Tomatoes & Zucchini with Cilantro

Serves 4 to 6

This recipe makes a great topping for grains such as brown rice, millet, or quinoa, or for potatoes.

2 (141/2-ounces each) cans diced tomatoes

1 pound zucchini, sliced on the diagonal

2 tablespoons vegetable broth

2 teaspoons cold-pressed, extra virgin olive oil

2 cloves garlic, minced

1/4 cup diced red onion

1/2 cup fresh cilantro, chopped

1/4 cup chopped fresh spearmint or 1 tablespoon dried

In a large skillet, heat the oil and broth and sauté the garlic and onion until translucent. Add the tomatoes and sauté until tender, 2 to 3 minutes. Add the zucchini, cilantro, and mint, and lower the heat and simmer, covered, for 10 minutes.

• F Y I

Cilantro

Cilantro, the Spanish name for fresh coriander, looks like parsley but has a stronger flavor and is used widely in Mexican, Chinese, Thai, and Indian cooking. It's easy to find in most supermarkets, and remember, a little goes a long way. If the pungent flavor is too strong for you, you may substitute regular parsley for cilantro in any of these recipes.

Stuffed Cucumbers

Serves 3 to 6

This makes a refreshing appetizer, and a terrific snack or a delicious lunch served on a bed of greens.

3 large cucumbers

1 cup minced celery

1/2 cup chopped orange bell pepper

1/2 cup chopped yellow bell pepper

1/4 cup chopped green onions

1/2 cup raw tahini

2 tablespoons minced fresh parsley (or cilantro)

1 tablespoon fresh lemon juice

1 clove garlic, minced

Bragg liquid aminos to taste

Peel the cucumbers, then cut them in half lengthwise and remove the seeds with a spoon. Place the remaining ingredients, except the parsley, in a food processor or blender and blend everything together. Arrange the cucumber shells on a tray or platter. Stuff the cucumbers with the filling and refrigerate. Garnish with the parsley before serving. You can make it smooth or slightly chunky, depending on blender time. I prefer slightly chunky.

Creamy Spicy Herbed Corn

Serves 4

I like to serve this corn dish with a grain such as quinoa or millet, along with a side of black beans, for a complete protein.

3 cups fresh corn kernels

1/2 cup plain organic soy milk

3 tablespoons vegetable broth

1/3 cup diced red bell pepper

1/3 cup diced orange bell pepper

1/4 cup diced red onion

1 jalapeño pepper, minced (remove seeds and membranes
    if you don't want it super hot)

1/2 medium potato cut in to chunks and juiced

1 to 2 cloves garlic, minced

1 teaspoon ground cumin

1/2 teaspoon dried tarragon

1/2 teaspoon dried dill

1/4 teaspoon sea salt

Dash of cayenne pepper

In a large saucepan, combine the corn, soy milk, vegetable broth, bell peppers, onion, jalapeño pepper, garlic, and spices. Bring to a boil, stirring constantly. Cover, lower the heat and simmer gently until the corn is tender, about 3 to 5 minutes, stirring occasionally. Add the potato juice and continue to cook over medium heat, until the sauce thickens, about 1 to 2 minutes.

Cauliflower–Broccoli Curry

Serves 4 to 6

Raw, crunchy, and satisfying, this curried snack is rich in antioxidants and vitamin C.

2 cups broccoli florets, cut in bite-size pieces
1/2 head cauliflower, cut in bite-size florets
1/3 cup cashew pieces
1 large Maui or other sweet onion, diced
1/4 cup purified water
2 tablespoons Barlean's Flax Oil
1 teaspoon minced ginger
1/2 teaspoon ground cumin
1/2 teaspoon turmeric
1/2 teaspoon shoyu

In a large bowl, combine the broccoli, cauliflower, onion, and cashews. In a small bowl, whisk together the water, oil, ginger, cumin, turmeric, water, and shoyu. Pour over the vegetables and toss to combine.

Fruit/Vegetables & Nut/Seed Butters

Simply spread your favorite fruits and vegetables with your favorite nut or seed butters for nutritious, quick, energy boosting snacks.

For fruits, select from apples, pears, bananas, or other favorites that lend themselves to top with a spread.

For vegetables, celery is the best as you can spread the nut/seed butter into the center. Belgian endive, romaine lettuce, and bell pepper quarters work, too.

If you have a juicer, you can make your own seed or nut butters. If not, you can buy them from the natural food store. I recommend those made by Rejuvenative Foods (see the Resource Directory) as they are all raw. The chocolate flavors even work well in the neutral celery when you feel like a splurge.

Mixed Vegetables & Dip

For quick snacks whenever you need them, always keep a platter of mixed vegetables and a few favorite dips in your refrigerator.

Besides fresh fruit, raw vegetables are the healthiest snack you can have. Don't limit yourself to celery, carrots, and cherry tomatoes. Reach out to green onions, bell pepper, cauliflower, broccoli, jicama, mushrooms, sweet onion, Belgian endive—anything that you can dip. Keep most of the vegetables raw or lightly steam a few—such as the broccoli and cauliflower—if you'll enjoy them more that way, but make sure they're still crisp.

For the dips, refer to Chapter 10 or simply buy a variety of nonfat dressings at your health food store. And don't forget about pickled and fermented vegetables that are still raw and alive with enzymes that are great for the digestive tract (see Resource Directory).

Autumn Puree

Serves 3-4

This colorful, antioxidant-rich, skin-beautifying snack or side dish is always a winner with everyone, from toddlers to seniors, and is fabulous served hot, warm, or cold.

1 medium butternut squash
1 medium yam
3-4 medium carrots
Celtic Sea Salt to taste

Cook vegetables (bake or steam) until tender and peel. They can be cooked with or without the skins—your choice. Cut into approximately 2-inch pieces. Puree the vegetables and season to taste.

This healthy dish makes a perfect snack that lends itself well for lunch boxes or eating-on-the-go. A few bites supplies a treasure-trove of nutrients. I usually double or triple the recipe and keep it on hand. It also makes a great spread for whole grain toast and wraps, or a scrumptious dip for raw vegetables.

VARIATIONS: If you want it sweeter, use more yams. As you vary the vegetable amounts, you'll change the flavor slightly. Sprinkle on some cinnamon, nutmeg, or powdered ginger before serving, or garnish it with fresh chopped chives or mint.

Chapter 17

MEALS KIDS LOVE

Although this chapter is geared toward great foods to serve kids, you don't have to be a little one to enjoy them. Experiment and add your own special touches to make them work even better for your entire family.

Sweet Potato Home Fries

Serves 2 to 4

Here's a sweet, healthy, baked treat kids love. But let me warn you: You'll run out of these fast so you might consider quadrupling the recipe.

2 large sweet potatoes/yams, scrubbed and cut
    into 1 x 3-inch "fries"*

2 tablespoons cold-pressed, extra virgin olive oil

Sea salt to taste

*My local market even sells them already precut
    to make into fries.

Preheat oven to 450°F.

Arrange sweet potatoes on a baking sheet and drizzle oil all over them to coat. Sprinkle with salt. Bake for 15 minutes, then broil for about 10 minutes, gently turning over after 5 minutes.

VARIATIONS: If you have a spray pump bottle, try spritzing the potato fries with olive oil mixed with tamari instead of using the salt. The light mist gives you a more evenly applied coating with less fat.

Use cinnamon and maple syrup instead of oil for really sweet, sweet potatoes.

Try sprinkling on your favorite herbs such as rosemary or chives, or use garlic or onion powder. For an earthier treat, try cinnamon, nutmeg, and allspice.

Dip each sliced potato into a bowl of broth and bake, or use 2/3 cup lite coconut milk and 1/3 cup water.

Multicolored Corn

Serves 4 to 6

What kid doesn't love corn? For this festive and colorful vegetable dish, all you need to do is some chopping; the rest comes together in minutes.

2 1/2 cups fresh whole corn kernels
1/3 cup finely chopped red bell pepper
1/3 cup finely chopped orange bell pepper
1/3 cup finely chopped yellow bell pepper
1/3 cup finely chopped purple bell pepper
1/2 cup minced sweet onion (Vidalia, Maui, etc.)
1/3 cup finely chopped green onions
1 clove garlic, minced
1 teaspoon cold-pressed, extra virgin olive oil
1/2 teaspoon ground cumin
Sea salt

In a nonstick skillet, heat the oil, then add sweet and green onions and the garlic, and sauté for 2 minutes. Add all the remaining ingredients and stir briefly. Add salt to taste, if desired, cover, and cook over low heat about 3 to 4 minutes, stirring often.

Flavorful Rice Pilaf

Serves 4 to 6

Don't let the long list of ingredients daunt you. If you have every-thing on hand, this comes together with little effort.

1¹/₂ cups purified water

¹/₂ cup lite coconut milk

1 cup uncooked basmati rice

1 cup grated carrots

¹/₂ cup unsweetened shredded coconut

¹/₂ cup frozen green peas, thawed

¹/₃ cup frozen sweet corn, thawed

2 tablespoons sesame seeds

4 tablespoons slivered almonds

2 tablespoons raisins or currants

2 tablespoons pitted dates, chopped

1 tablespoon cold-pressed sesame oil

5 whole cloves

4 cardamom pods

1 teaspoon sea salt

¹/₄ teaspoon ground cinnamon

Unsalted roasted pistachio nuts

In a large saucepan, heat the water and coconut milk. In a skillet over medium heat, heat the oil and sauté the shredded coconut, sesame seeds, almonds, cardamom pods, cloves, and cinnamon just until the coconut begins to turn light brown.

Rinse the rice and drain. Add rice to the skillet mixture and stir constantly for 3 to 5 minutes.

Bring the water and coconut milk to a boil and add the rice mixture, carrots, raisins, dates, and salt. Stir and return to a boil. Cover, lower the heat and simmer for 25 minutes or until all the liquid is absorbed. Turn off the heat and let the rice sit for 10 minutes. Remove the cloves (they rise to the top). Add the corn and peas just before serving. Coarsely chop the pistachio nuts and sprinkle on top as a garnish.

• F Y I

Basmati Rice

Basmati is a long-grain delicious rice that has a buttery aroma, nutty flavor, and a fluffy texture. Available in both whole grain (brown) and refined white, when cooked, each grain almost doubles in length with little change in thickness. As with all rice, the whole grain is far superior in nutritional value to the refined white version.

Pizza Pizzazz

This is a great way to get the whole family involved in making the meal. You won't miss the dairy or meat toppings on this sensational pizza.

1 or 2 per person whole wheat fat-free chapatis, tortillas, or split whole grain pita

2 tablespoons grated jalapeño soy cheese (soy mozzarella or any soy cheese)

2 zucchinis, cut in half and sliced lengthwise in 1/4-inch-thick strips

1/2 tablespoon per person chopped green onions

2 to 3 strips per person roasted red bell peppers (see page 290)

2 to 3 strips per person roasted yellow bell peppers

1/2 tablespoon per person sliced olives

2 tablespoons per person salsa

2 to 4 slices per person avocado slices or guacamole

Steam zucchinis until slightly tender, about 2 minutes.

On a baking sheet, toast the flat bread until crisp but not brown. You can mist it with a dash of olive oil and tamari if you like. Remove from the oven. Preheat the broiler.

Cover crusts with a thin layer of salsa followed by soy cheese. Then arrange the roasted bell peppers, zucchini, olives, and green onions on the top. Top with more soy cheese.

Broil for 3 to 5 minutes away from the heat, or until the cheese melts. Keep an eye on them so they don't overcook or burn. Remove from the broiler and immediately add a few avocado slices or guacamole. Serve with extra salsa on top.

Potatoes Rose
with Emerald Green Gravy

Serves 4 to 6

The beets turn this potato dish a delightful shade of pink.
The green sauce spooned on top is a hit with the kids.

2 pounds Yukon Gold potatoes, peeled and cut into chunks
1/4 cup plain soy or almond milk
1 small beet
2 teaspoons minced fresh chives or parsley
1 teaspoon sea salt
Emerald Green Sauce (see page 241)

Juice the beet and reserve 3 tablespoons.

In a medium saucepan, cover potatoes with enough water to cover.
Bring to a boil, cover pan with a lid, lower the heat and simmer
for about 15 to 20 minutes or until the potatoes are tender, not
mushy. Drain.

In a small saucepan, warm the milk.

Mash the potatoes, add the 3 tablespoons beet juice, and mash to
combine. Then add enough soy/almond milk to create the desired
consistency. Add salt to taste and garnish with chives or parsley.
Serve immediately with Emerald Green Sauce.

VARIATIONS: Use carrot juice for an orange color or add half
yams or sweet potatoes for half of the Yukon Golds. If your family
loves garlic, add roasted garlic when mashing.

Sensational Spaghetti Squash

Serves 3 to 4

This squash goes well with a mixture of steamed vegetables
and a crisp green salad.

1/2 spaghetti squash, seeded
1/2 cup grated soy cheese
Dash paprika

Place the squash in a large skillet with just enough water to steam without covering the squash. Steam until tender, about 45 minutes. Scoop out the flesh with a fork into spaghetti-like strands and sprinkle with the soy cheese. Season with paprika and serve hot.

VARIATIONS: Add minced garlic, freshly grated nutmeg, ginger, or any of your favorite herbs, and instead of soy cheese, top with your best pasta sauce.

Salad with a Twist of Lemon
Serves 4

1 medium carrot, grated

1 small parsnip, grated

1/2 cup hearts of palm, sliced into 1/4-inch pieces

1/2 cup raisins or currants, rehydrated in hot water
  for a few minutes and drained

1/3 cup walnuts, chopped and toasted

1 tablespoon fresh lemon juice

1/3 cup favorite soy yogurt such as vanilla, lemon, or peach

1 teaspoon maple syrup

Dash cinnamon

In a large bowl combine all the ingredients. Serve with extra cinnamon lightly sprinkled on top.

• F Y I
Soy Yogurt

Soy yogurt is cholesterol- and lactose-free with a fair approximation of the flavor of dairy yogurt. It's available in all natural food stores and most supermarkets in a variety of flavors. It has a comparable nutritional profile to soy milk but has enhanced digestibility because it is fermented.

Fajitas
Serves 4 to 6

You do need to marinate the seitan, so get started on this one early in the day. Once the seitan is marinated, these are quick to prepare

and assemble. I usually serve these with guacamole and salsa or a spicy red chili sauce.

1/2 pound seitan* cut into long strips

11/2 cups chopped tomatoes

2 yellow or orange bell peppers (or both), thinly sliced

2 green chiles, chopped (if you prefer it a bit tamer, be sure to remove the membranes and seeds)

1 onion, thinly sliced

1 to 2 cloves garlic, minced

1/2 cup mushrooms, sliced

1/2 teaspoon cold-pressed, extra virgin olive oil

1/2 cup balsamic vinegar

1/4 cup purified water

2 tablespoons tamari

Whole wheat tortillas

*Seitan, or wheat gluten, is a versatile meat substitute with a hearty flavor and texture.

In a large bowl, combine the vinegar, water, tamari, and garlic. Add the seitan and marinate for 3 hours. In a skillet or wok, heat the oil. Add the onions, peppers, and chiles and sauté 7 to 8 minutes. Add the tomatoes and mushrooms and sauté for 5 minutes. Add the seitan and sauté 7 to 10 minutes.

Warm tortillas in the oven or on a dry skillet, then fill with the seitan mixture and roll them up.

NO–GUILT SWEETS YOU CAN FEED YOUR KIDS

Raw Cherry, Orange, Applesauce Deluxe

Serves 2 to 4

This fruit sauce can be eaten with a spoon or topped on fruit, whole grain bread, or toast, pancakes, waffles, muffins, and crackers. I make double batches weekly, because adults love it as much as kids do.

. 2 apples, cored, chopped (peel if you prefer)

1 orange, peeled and sectioned

1 to 2 dates, pitted

16 bing cherries, pitted and cut in half

2 tablespoons fresh apple juice (or water)

1/2 tablespoon fresh lemon juice

1/4 teaspoon cinnamon

In a blender or food processor, combine all the ingredients and pulse until a sauce texture is created. Refrigerate before serving.

VARIATIONS: When berries are in season (late spring through summer), add your favorites: blueberries, strawberries, blackberries, or strawberries.

Muesli Parfait

Serves 3 to 4

Layered into a parfait glass, this crunchy and refreshing treat looks especially appealing to kids.

1 cup muesli (see recipe on page 225) or granola

1 cup favorite soy yogurt such as blueberry, strawberry, apple, or kiwi lime

1 cup fresh fruit, sliced

1 cup all-fruit preserves or applesauce

Fresh mint

In a parfait glass alternately layer yogurt, sliced fruit, and muesli or granola. Garnish with fresh mint.

Stuffed Dates

Serves 3 to 6

12 to 16 medjool dates

1/2 cup almond, sunflower, or cashew butter

Whole raw pecans, cashews, or almonds, one for each date, to stuff
into the dates

1/2 cup almonds, pecans, or walnuts (or all of them) to grind
into a meal

Split each date with a small, sharp knife, and remove the pit. Press it
as you would a baked potato. Stuff each date with nut butter and a
whole almond, pecan, or cashew. You can make each one different
as you would find in a box of candy. Then close each one up by
pinching with your fingers. In a blender, grind almonds, pecans, or
walnuts into a meal. Transfer to a shallow bowl. Roll each stuffed
date in the nut meal, arrange on a plate or tray, and refrigerate
before serving.

VARIATIONS: Add some flax seed meal to the walnut, almond, or
pecan meal to add more omega-3's. Try any organic chocolate
spread, such as the products made by Rejuvenative Foods (see
Resource Directory).

• F Y I
Dates

*As the date dries, its fructose changes to sucrose, so the drier the
date, the sweeter it is. Dates are 60%-75% sugar so they're not recommended for people with diabetes, obesity, yeast infections, or respiratory infections. However nutritionally, they are rich in fiber and
are good sources of iron, niacin, and potassium.*

*Dates can be used to sweeten baked goods, smoothies, granola, pud-
dings, spreads, and sauces. My favorite soft dates, the medjool, are
allowed to sun dry on the tree and are then hydrated with steam to
plump them back up.*

*Date sugar, made from 100% pitted dehydrated dates that are
coarsely ground, used in moderation, is a quality sweetener, certainly
more natural and unrefined than most. It contains all the nutrients of
dried dates. You can sprinkle it on cereal, on top of yogurt, or add to
baked goods or smoothies.*

*Try to find organic dates to avoid the pesticide residues found on
commercially grown fruits.*

Healthy Candy Balls

For this one, I intentionally omitted any specific measurements so you could have fun experimenting with the ingredients. Kids love to help make them so get the whole family involved and make lots of extra, which you can freeze and pull out any time for unexpected guests, for a quick snack, or when a sweet craving hits. They're even great frozen!

Raw sunflower seeds

Raw sesame seeds

Raisins

Favorite dried fruit such as dates or cherries

Apple butter

Pure maple syrup

Pinch of sea salt

Toasted, shredded coconut

In a food processor, grind together the seeds and dried fruit. Add a little maple syrup, apple butter, and salt. Process until it forms a cohesive ball. (Add more apple butter or syrup if needed.) Section pieces and roll into small balls, about 1½ inch in diameter. Roll these small balls in the shredded coconut.

VARIATIONS: Add in some freshly ground flax seed, cashews, almonds, walnuts, or other favorite nut.

Guilt–Free Banana Split

Makes 1

Here's a way to eat a banana split without all the fat and calories.

1 banana

½ cup low-fat soy yogurt

3 to 4 strawberries, sliced

¼ cup diced fresh pineapple

1 tablespoon chopped pecans and walnuts

1 or 2 fresh pitted cherries

Slice the banana lengthwise and spoon the yogurt between the halves. Top with the strawberries, pineapple, pecans, and walnuts. Top with a fresh cherry or two.

• **F Y I**

Bananas

You might not think of bananas as a diet food but think again. They combat hunger pangs and leave you satisfied and feeling full. It's the combination of fiber and natural fructose that gives them their super-food status. The fructose (natural sugar) is encased in fiber and carbo-hydrate so it satisfies a sweet tooth, but releases into your system slowly. In addition to being rich in the mineral potassium, which makes them good for hypertension, they are also richer in other min-erals than any soft fruit except strawberries. (They have twice as much vitamin C as apples.) Under-ripe or green bananas are astrin-gent and difficult to digest but can be used to relieve diarrhea and colitis. Eaten ripe—when the brown speckles begin to appear—they are sweeter, more easily digested, anti-ulcerous, and soothing to the mucus lining of the stomach.

Placing them in a closed brown paper bag will speed the ripening process.

Very Berry Pudding

The bananas lend a rich creaminess to this puréed berry treat.

Bananas, ripe with brown speckles
Berries, fresh or frozen

In a food processor or blender, purée the bananas and berries together. Continue to add fruit until you reach a consistency you like. For a deeper color and more berry flavor, just add more berries. If using frozen berries, you do not need to refrigerate before serv-ing. Otherwise, refrigerate for at least 1 hour. This looks great in a clear glass dish. Try it with a single type of berry, such as strawberry or blueberry, to create several different color puddings and layer in a parfait glass (individual or larger) for a beautiful dessert, snack, or mid-afternoon meal.

Yummy Yam Pudding

Serves 6

Served in orange shells, this delicious, vitamin-packed treat will delight your kids or your most elegant dinner guests.

3 large yams, baked and peeled
3 large oranges, juiced (save the orange shells)
1 ripe banana
2 ounces silken tofu
2 teaspoons pure maple syrup
3/4 teaspoon cinnamon
1/8 teaspoon nutmeg
1/8 teaspoon pure vanilla extract
Fresh mint sprigs, for garnish

In a blender or food processor, purée all the ingredients with enough juice to whip into a creamy, light consistency. Spoon mixture back into the orange shells. Sprinkle with cinnamon and garnish with mint. Serve warm or cold.

Blueberry Apple Banana Bread

If you like banana bread, try this wonderful variation. Biting into a blueberry is like finding buried treasure. As always, this banana bread is a great thing to make when you've got overripe bananas on your hands.

4 cups oat flour (grind oatmeal into flour in a blender or food processor
3 ripe bananas, mashed
1 cup apple juice
1 cup frozen blueberries
2 1/2 teaspoons baking powder
1 teaspoon pure vanilla extract
1/2 teaspoon cinnamon
1/4 teaspoon allspice

Preheat oven to 300°F.

In a blender or food processor, blend the bananas, apple juice, and vanilla until smooth.

In a large bowl, combine the flour, baking powder, cinnamon, and allspice. Add to the banana mixture in 2 batches, blending each time.

Return batter back in the bowl and stir in the frozen blueberries (if they thaw, the juice will run). Pour into a nonstick loaf pan that's been lightly sprayed with a nonstick spray. Sprinkle with a few rolled oats on top. Bake 50 to 60 minutes or until a knife comes out clean. Let cool before slicing and serving.

Blueberry Bonanza Smoothie

Serves 1 to 2

The color alone makes this one a hit with kids. Loaded with the antioxidant properties of blueberries and with a splash of protein from soy, this nutritious "shake" makes a great snack you can give to your kids with no guilt.

1 cup freshly squeezed organic apple or orange juice
1/2 cup fresh or organic blueberries, strawberries, or raspberries
1 tablespoon soy powder
2 to 3 ice cubes

In a blender or food processor, blend all the ingredients until creamy smooth.

• **F Y I**

Blueberries

Blueberries are one of the foods highest in antioxidants, according to researchers at Tufts University. Just 1/2 cup a day retards aging and can even reverse failing memory. I keep several packages of frozen organic blueberries on hand in my freezer so I don't run out.

Purple Grape Julius

Serves 2 to 3

Another colorful and frothy juice treat kids just love.

1 cup freshly squeezed purple grape juice
1 cup freshly squeezed orange juice
$1/2$ cup frozen red or purple seedless grapes
1 tablespoon soy powder
2 to 3 ice cubes

In a blender or food processor, combine all the ingredients and blend until creamy smooth.

• **F Y I**

Grapes

Red grapes and red grape juice have moderate antioxidant power but purple grape juice tops other juices in antioxidant activity, having 4 times more than orange or tomato.

Creamy Cashew & Apple Cinnamon Smoothie

Serves 2 to 3

$1^{1}/2$ cups apple juice
$1/2$ cup soy milk
2 ounces silken tofu
$1/4$ cup raw cashews
2 ice cubes
Cinnamon to taste

In a blender or food processor, combine all the ingredients and blend until smooth.

• F Y I
Soy Milk

Milk from the soybean is similar to cow's milk but without the choles-terol or dairy allergens. It has the same amount of protein but only 1/3 the fat, fewer calories, no cholesterol, many essential B vitamins, and 15 times as much iron. It comes in plain, vanilla, and chocolate in all natural food stores and most supermarkets. It can be used in any dish calling for cow's milk: breakfast cereal, smoothies, casseroles, soups, pudding, quick breads, pancakes, or by the glassful as a beverage. Look for organic soy milk or you can make it yourself with a soy milk machine, which is a wise investment if you consume lots of soy milk. It takes only minutes, you can use organic soybeans, and it costs less than 25 cents a quart to make. I make 1 to 2 quarts each week and add pure vanilla extract when I want vanilla flavor.

FROZEN TREATS

You can freeze many different fruits to nibble on whenever you want. Some fruits that freeze particularly well are grapes, raisins, bananas, blueberries, and medjool dates. Everyone loves these simple frozen treats.

Popsicles–a–Plenty

These popsicles are a fun variation on the simple frozen fruit treat. With no added sugar or any colorings, these natural and refreshing fruit ices are a great snack on a hot day. They'll last a month in the freezer, but I guarantee you won't have them around that long.

Popsicle molds
Fresh juice of your choice
Purified water

Fill each popsicle mold with a combination of 1/2 fruit juice and 1/2 water. Fresh juice is always the best, but any natural juice will do. Freeze and enjoy.

VARIATIONS: Try adding fresh fruit, such as berries, diced pineapple, or peaches, to the juice in the popsicle mold, and for another special treat, pour your favorite fruit smoothie into the popsicle mold and freeze.

Lemon–Coconut Sherbet

Serves 4 to 6

Your kids will think they're eating ice cream.

1 coconut
$1/3$ cup fruit concentrate
2 teaspoons fresh lemon juice
2 teaspoons fresh lemon zest from an organic lemon
Organic vanilla soy milk

Open the coconut and strain the milk through a fine mesh strainer and remove any shell pieces or fiber. Set aside.

Remove the coconut flesh. Juice it and save the pulp.

In a bowl, combine the coconut milk, coconut juice, and pulp. Add the lemon juice and zest and enough soy milk to make 2 cups. Transfer the mixture to a shallow plastic or metal dish. Freeze until solid, about 4 hours.

Using a knife or metal spatula, break the frozen mixture into 2- to 3-inch pieces and transfer to a food processor. Purée until creamy smooth. Stop occasionally to scrape the sides. Serve immediately or store in a tightly covered plastic container in the freezer. It will keep for a month in your freezer, but I can guarantee it will be gone long before then!

Chapter 18

DESSERTS

As you begin to eat a healthier diet and cleanse and detoxify your body, you'll discover that you will lose the desire to end your meal with a heavy dessert, especially one that's laden with fat and calories. ("Stressed" is "desserts" spelled backwards.) Of course, every so often everyone craves a luscious dessert, and there are even those times when you want to eat dessert instead of a meal. Well, you're in luck! The first recipe in this chapter makes a great lunch. It's so good that it's hard to believe that it's low in fat and chock full of isoflavones (from the soy), the phytonutrient that may help prevent cancer.

So here are some suggestions for a variety of different desserts you'll enjoy sharing with your family and friends. Remember, try to keep your ingredients as pure as possible, so you obtain the maximum health benefits from every meal—even dessert. À vôtre santé.*

*French for "to your health!"

Chocolate Date Peppermint Shake/Ice Cream

Serves 2 to 3

I sometimes have this positively scrumptious healthy shake for a meal or afternoon snack.

2 cups nonfat vanilla soy beverage

2 small or 1 large ripe frozen banana

5 to 6 medjool dates, pitted and chopped

4 to 5 ice cubes

2 tablespoons cocoa powder

1/8 teaspoon peppermint extract

THE SHAKE: Place all the ingredients in a blender and blend until creamy smooth, about 60 to 90 seconds.

THE ICE CREAM: Follow the steps for the shake, then pour the shake into ice cube trays. After they're frozen, press them through a Green Power or Green Life Juicer (see Resource Directory) to creates a delicious ice cream, though the ice actually makes it more like a sorbet. For a creamier texture, omit the ice cubes and add 1 more frozen banana and 1 more date, or use a regular vanilla soy beverage instead of nonfat. After pressing the frozen ice cubes through your juicer, you'll have a delicious chocolate date ice cream. Try serving it with a pressed frozen banana. Serve in chilled bowls.

VARIATIONS: Instead of peppermint extract, substitute orange. Or try it without any extract. You can even include some fresh peppermint or spearmint herbs.

To add more nutrients (and protein) to the shake or ice cream, add 1 heaping tablespoon of Living Food (see Resource Directory) to the above recipe.

Pour lite coconut milk into ice cube trays and freeze. Press together with the Chocolate Date Ice Cream for a delicious combination.

Frozen Fruit Treats

Serves 2

Here's another simple way to get more fresh fruit into your diet. It's hard to believe that these delicious desserts are actually very good for you.

2 cups of your favorite fruit, frozen, such as blueberries, strawberries, pitted black cherries, mangos, papayas, raspberries, apricots, and bananas.

Fresh fruit juices such as apple, orange, or pineapple

Fresh mint sprigs

In a blender or food processor, blend your favorite frozen fruit until smooth, adding just enough fresh squeezed juice so it blends well.

Serve immediately in chilled bowls or freeze for one hour to increase firmness before serving. Garnish with mint sprigs.

VARIATIONS: To any of these fruit ices, when you are blending, add a couple drops of pure organic extracts: peppermint, orange, almond, vanilla, lemon, etc. to vary the flavors.

Apple Walnut Pudding

Serves 3 to 6

2 cups dried apples, soaked for 8 hours in 4 cups of purified water (save the water)

1 apple, peeled, cored, and finely chopped

1 cup raw walnuts, soaked for 8 hours in 2 cups of purified water

4 drops liquid Stevia*

1 ripe banana

Cinnamon to taste

In a food processor or blender, purée all the ingredients along with the water from the soaking apples. Chill in the refrigerator. Serve cold.

*Stevia is a natural sweetener. You can find it at your health food store. It's actually an herb that's 30 times sweeter than sugar.

Raw Sunflower Apricot Cookies

Serves 6 to 8

3 cups raw sunflower seeds, soaked in purified water for 8 hours or overnight

1 cup raisins, soaked overnight or for 8 hours

1 cup unsulphured dried apricots, chopped and soaked overnight in purified water

1/2 cup raw cashew butter

1/2 cup raw almond butter

1 tablespoon pure vanilla extract

1 teaspoon almond extract

1/2 teaspoon cinnamon

1/8 teaspoon pure organic orange extract

After soaking the apricots, sunflower seeds, and raisins, drain and spread them out on two clean, dry dish towels to remove extra moisture.

In a food processor, blend all the ingredients into a nutty consistency. Transfer to a large bowl. Make equal size small balls, 1- to 11/2-inches in diameter. Press out to a 1/4-inch thickness. Cover and refrigerate for 1 to 2 hours before serving. If you have access to a low temperature dehydrator, try making them in there. They come out a little crispy but they still retain all the live enzymes and vital nutrients.

Dried Plum & Chocolate Whip

Serves 2 to 3

Dried plum is a fancy way of saying prune, but don't let that word cause you to turn the page too quickly. You will love this light, melt in your mouth dessert.

12/3 cups pitted stewed prunes

2 ounces silken tofu

2 tablespoons cocoa powder

2 tablespoons pure maple syrup

Pour boiling water over prunes, cover, and let stand for 2 hours. Save the stewing liquid. Or you can buy stewed prunes, without preservatives, in a can. In a blender or food processor, purée all the ingredients together using just enough of the cooking liquid to create a creamy, smooth consistency. Chill and serve.

VARIATIONS: Instead of the cocoa powder, substitute carob powder and try adding 1/8 teaspoon peppermint extract or orange extract.

• F Y I

Prunes

Because they are a powerhouse of both insoluble and soluble fiber, prunes, which are really dried plums, are an excellent laxative and also help to lower cholesterol. They provide a healthy dose of magnesium, calcium, potassium, beta carotene, and iron, too. Prune juice is also an effective laxative. Studies reveal that 1/2 cup of prune juice or 3 prunes a day is all it takes to establish regularity. Make sure the prunes are free of preservatives. Besides being stewed, prunes can be chopped and added to cereal or to salads as well as to grain dishes. In fact, chopped prunes can be substituted for raisins in almost any recipe. Finally, if you purée the stewed prunes in their stewing liquid, you can use this purée in recipes for baked goods in place of eggs and most of the oil. It helps bind the ingredients together and keep it moist.

Cinnamon Vanilla Poached Pears

Serves 4 to 8

This elegant dessert wins rave reviews at dinner parties or family gatherings. It's so easy and healthfully delicious—a winning combination.

4 Anjou or Bosc pears, peeled, cored, and cut in half

1 cup apple juice

1/2 cup purified water

1 (3-inch) piece vanilla bean, cut in half lengthwise

1 (1- to 2-inch) piece cinnamon stick

1 tablespoon pure maple syrup

Mint sprig

In a large skillet, combine the water and apple juice, maple syrup, and cinnamon stick. With a knife, scrape the seeds from the vanilla bean into the water. Add the bean pods, too. (Save the rest of the bean.) Over medium heat, bring the liquid to a simmer for about 3 minutes, so the vanilla flavor permeates the liquid. Add the halves to the liquid, core side up. Spoon some of the poaching liquid into the core cavity. Cover, and continue to simmer gently until the pears are tender, about 8 to 10 minutes. Cool in the liquid, then chill the pears in the refrigerator. To serve, place 1 or 2 pear halves in a bowl and top with some poaching liquid and a sprig of fresh mint.

• F Y I

Pears

There are over 3,000 varieties of pears, but only a handful are commercially popular. Perhaps the oldest cultivated fruit in the world, pears aid digestion, are an excellent source of fiber, and provide vitamin C and iron. Bartletts are juicy, tasty, and yellow in color; Comice are red-blushed yellow and not quite as juicy; Bosc are less juicy and more chewy with a russet skin; and Anjou are yellow-green and it is the only variety that will ripen in the refrigerator. Always choose firm, well-shaped pears that are free of bruises and soft spots.

Strawberry–Mango–Banana Ice Cream

Serves 2 to 3

1 very ripe mango, diced
8 large frozen strawberries
2 large frozen bananas, cut into chunks

In a blender or food processor, blend the mango. Add the strawberries and bananas until the consistency becomes just like ice cream. Serve in chilled bowls.

• T I P

Frozen Bananas

Use ripe (very spotted) bananas. They are sweeter, easier to digest, and more flavorful. Peel and freeze whole in a zip-lock freezer bag. Press out extra air before locking shut. I keep a dozen or two on hand so they're readily available for fruit ice cream and smoothies.

Sesame Banana Orange Pudding

Serves 1

1 large ripe banana
1 large medjool date, chopped
2 tablespoons raw sesame seeds

2 drops pure organic orange extract

Dash of cinnamon

In a blender or food processor, blend the banana and date together. In a nut grinder, grind the sesame seeds to create a meal. Add the sesame seed meal and extract to the banana and blend. Serve in a small chilled bowl. Garnish with a dash of cinnamon.

VARIATIONS: You can blend a few seconds longer and add a teaspoon of pure maple syrup, if you like it sweeter.

Instead of sesame seeds, substitute 1¹/2 tablespoons raw tahini (sesame paste).

Outrageous Oatmeal Cookies

Makes 20 to 24 cookies

Since these scrumptious cookies freeze well, you might want to make extra so you have them on hand for unexpected guests or for special treats.

2 cups oat flour (this can be ground fresh in a blender)

2 cups rolled oats

1 cup apple juice

¹/2 cup raisins

¹/3 cup flax seed meal (you can grind your own
    from fresh flax seeds)

¹/3 cup chopped walnuts

2 ripe bananas

¹/3 cup applesauce

1 tablespoon frozen apple juice concentrate

¹/2 teaspoon baking soda

1 teaspoon baking powder

1 teaspoon cinnamon

¹/4 teaspoon nutmeg

Preheat oven to 375°F.

In a large bowl, combine the oat flour, rolled oats, flax seed meal, baking soda, baking powder, and spices.

In a blender or food processor, purée the bananas, juice, concentrate, and applesauce.

Add the dry mixture to the apple mixture, a little at a time, while mixing. Stir in the raisins and walnuts. Drop by spoonfuls on a nonstick baking sheet. Bake in the center of the oven for about 10 minutes. (Make sure not to overbake!)

VARIATIONS: Add unsweetened dried cherries and/or shredded coconut instead of the raisins and walnuts.

• F Y I
Oats & Oat Bran

Oats and oat bran are excellent sources of soluble fiber, which is the kind of fiber that helps lower cholesterol. Oatmeal, also called rolled oats, is available as regular (or old fashioned), which cooks in about 15 minutes, and quick cooking, which takes about 5 minutes. Instant oatmeal requires no cooking and retains the nutrients, but it's hard to find it without added sugar or salt. Steel-cut, or Scotch oats (my favorite) can take 45 minutes to an hour to cook. They have a nuttier flavor and consistency. If you've never tried them, get some soon and try my recipes for oatmeal in Chapter 9 using steel-cut oats.

Nut Date Balls
Serves 6 to 8

1/2 cup raw cashews
1/2 cup almonds
1/4 cup walnuts
1/4 cup flax seed meal
1/2 cup chopped dried unsulphured black figs
1 cup chopped dates, preferably medjool
Unsweetened shredded coconut
Raw sesame seeds

In a food processor, blender, or nut grinder, grind the nuts into a meal. Add flax seed meal. Add the chopped fruit and blend so everything is well mixed. Roll into balls about the diameter of a quarter, then roll the balls in the coconut and sesame seeds. These freeze well so consider making extra so you have them on hand. These also make great snacks.

VARIATIONS: You can also add a little raw nut or seed butter to the mixture such as almond, sunflower, pumpkin, soy, cashew, or hempini. For a real treat, add some chocolate spreads or cocoa powder (see Rejuvenative Foods in the Resource Directory).

Moist & Chewy Brownies

Serves 6 to 8

You won't miss the butter, sugar, or eggs in these moist and luscious brownies.

2 cups oat flour (this can be ground in a blender)
1/2 cup carob or cocoa powder
2/3 cup vanilla soy milk
3/4 cup applesauce
1/3 cup chopped walnuts
1/3 cup chopped pitted medjool dates
1 tablespoon arrowroot
1 teaspoon baking powder
1 teaspoon pure vanilla extract
1/8 teaspoon sea salt

Preheat oven to 375°F.

In a large bowl, combine the flour, carob or cocoa powder, walnuts, dates, baking powder, arrowroot, and salt.

In a separate bowl, combine soy milk, applesauce, and vanilla. Add to the dry ingredients and combine thoroughly.

In a nonstick 8" x 8" baking pan that's been lightly sprayed with a nonstick spray, spread the brownie mixture evenly and bake for 20 to 25 minutes.

• **F Y I**

Chocolate

Chocolate, native to tropical and Central America, was believed to be a food of the gods. In Mexico, as late as 1885 cocoa beans were used as standard currency. Once the beans are removed from the pods of the cacao tree, they are roasted, chopped up, and ground into an oily paste called chocolate mass or liquor. The liquor is suspended in the cocoa butter, which is more than 50% fatty acids. To make powder, most of the cocoa butter is pressed out of the liquor. The taste of chocolate depends upon the variety of the cacao tree, the soil it was grown in, and what it is blended with, as well as the processing. Bitter chocolate is a diuretic and an antioxidant. The darker chocolate has more antioxidants and the white has none. It may help lower blood pressure and is even considered to be an aphrodisiac. It is said to release the brain chemicals responsible for the feeling of being in love. While it may have some benefits, keep in mind that it also contains theobromine which, like caffeine, can trigger various nervous symptoms, including insomnia, hyperactivity in children, anxiety, and mood swings. On the rare occasion when I eat chocolate, I try to choose organically grown cocoa beans and dark chocolate, which has no dairy added.

Cracker Jack Popcorn

A healthful variation on an old snack favorite.

3 1/2 cups air-popped popcorn
2/3 cup raw cashew pieces or soy nuts (optional)
1/3 cup barley malt syrup
1/3 cup rice syrup
1/2 teaspoon sea salt

Preheat oven to 300°F.

In a saucepan, heat the barley malt and rice syrups and sea salt together until they're hot but not boiling.

In a large bowl, mix the popcorn and nuts, then pour the syrup mixture over them. Mix by hand, being sure to lightly oil them first (this is sticky stuff).

On a large nonstick baking sheet that's been sprayed with nonstick spray, spread out the corn mixture and bake until lightly crisp, about 5 minutes. Watch it carefully to be sure it doesn't burn.

Tapioca Pudding with Toasted Almonds
Serves 3 to 4

2 cups vanilla rice milk

1/2 cup tapioca

1/3 cup chopped almonds, toasted in a dry skillet

1/4 cup maple syrup

1/2 teaspoon pure almond extract

1/8 teaspoon sea salt

In a medium saucepan, without heat, combine the rice milk, tapioca, syrup, and salt. Stir the mixture and let it stand for 5 minutes before setting on the heat. Then, bring it to a full boil over medium heat, stirring constantly. Remove from the heat. Stir in the almond extract. Pour into 3 or 4 dessert cups. Sprinkle toasted nuts over pudding mixture. Serve warm or cold.

Frozen Coconut Berry Mint Pie
Serves 6 to 8

THE CRUST:

1 tablespoon carob or cocoa powder

1 cup walnuts

1 cup almonds

1 cup unsweetened shredded coconut

3/4 cup apple juice

1/3 cup fresh flax meal

1/4 teaspoon pure organic peppermint extract

2 tablespoons apple juice concentrate

THE FILLING:

4 cups fresh or frozen berries (blueberries, strawberries, blackberries, or raspberries)

3 ounces soft silken lite tofu

6 medjool dates, pitted and sliced

1/2 cup lite coconut milk

1 tablespoon apple juice concentrate

1/4 teaspoon pure organic peppermint extract

To make the crust, place all the ingredients in a blender or food processor and blend to combine. Transfer to a glass pie dish, and using your hands, spread evenly throughout the bottom and sides. Refrigerate.

To make the filling, place all the ingredients in a blender or food processor and purée until creamy smooth. Pour into the chilled crust and smooth it with a spatula or knife. Cover and freeze until firm, at least 2 hours.

VARIATIONS: To create a tropical pie, use a combination of fresh or frozen pineapple, mango, and papaya.

• F Y I

Berries

With an average of 50 calories per 1/2 cup, berries are a perfect weight-loss food. Whether as a fresh bowl of ripe fruit, added to smoothies, or made into fruit ices, sorbets, ice cream, or pies, it's hard to resist these colorful, delectable fruits. They're full of fiber and potassium and enough natural fructose to satisfy any sweet-craving.

Ginger Fruit Salad

Serves 3 to 4

Fresh ginger juice and lemon zest give this fruit salad a wonderful zip.

2 apples, peeled, cored, and chopped

1 orange, peeled and seeded

1 ripe banana, sliced

1 ripe pear, peeled, cored, and chopped

1 cup strawberries or other berry in season, stemmed and chopped

1 tablespoon maple syrup

1/2 teaspoon fresh lemon zest

11/2 teaspoons fresh ginger juice

Fresh mint sprigs for garnish

In a blender or food processor, purée the orange, maple syrup, lemon zest, and ginger juice.

In a bowl, combine all the fruit, toss with the purée and chill before serving. Garnish with fresh mint sprigs.

• **F Y I**
Ginger

Rich in calcium, magnesium, phosphorus, and potassium, ginger helps prevent nausea, is good for menstrual cramps, and helps improve circulation. A favorite of gourmet chefs, this root is such a versatile food that it can be juiced, sautéed, puréed, stir-fried, and simply made into a soothing tea when a sliver is mixed with some hot water and fresh lemon. I also like to add a thin sliver of fresh ginger root to other organic teas such as peppermint, chamomile, rose hips, or green tea.

Apple Lemon Crisp
Serves 5 to 6

21/2 pounds of Granny Smith apples (about 5 to 6), peeled, cored and cut in 1/2-inch-thick slices

3/4 cup golden raisins

1/3 cup sugar-free orange marmalade

1 small organic lemon (since we're using the peel, get organic)

THE TOPPING:

1 cup rolled oats

1/3 cup maple syrup granules

1/3 cup chopped almonds

1/4 cup unbleached all-purpose flour

1/4 cup Spectrum Spread, chilled*

1 tablespoon fresh flax seeds

1 tablespoon sesame seeds

1/8 teaspoon sea salt

1/8 teaspoon cinnamon

*A butter-like spread made from cold-pressed oil, Spectrum Spread has no trans-fatty acids. You can find it in the refrigerated section of your health food store.

Preheat oven to 375°F. Use an 8-inch square baking dish and spray with nonstick cooking spray.

In a bowl, combine apple slices, raisins, and marmalade so the apples are completely coated. Take half the filling and arrange in the baking dish.

Cut the lemon in thin slices, discarding the ends and seeds. Cut slices in half and arrange over the apple filling to cover most of the apples.

In a nut grinder, grind the sesame seeds and flax seeds for 15 seconds to create a meal.

In a bowl, combine the oats, flour, maple granules, cinnamon, nuts, sesame seed and flax seed meal, and salt. First with a fork and then with your fingers, mix in the Spectrum Spread. Try to moisten all the flour and oats. Spread the topping evenly over the apple filling.

Bake for 30 minutes, or until the topping is lightly browned and firm. Let it stand for 30 minutes, and serve it warm.

VARIATIONS: Substitute chopped walnuts, cashews, or hazelnuts for the almonds, and peaches, nectarines, mangos, papayas, or blueberries for the apples.

Substitute apricot, blueberry, raspberry, peach, or strawberry sugar-free jams for the marmalade and top with fruit ice cream.

Berry–Mint Coconut Protein Delight
Serves 3 to 4

11/2 cups frozen raspberries and strawberries or other favorite fruit

4 cubes of frozen low-fat coconut milk

1/2 cup (4 ounces) soft silken lite tofu

2 tablespoons apple juice concentrate

1/8 teaspoon pure organic peppermint extract

Fresh mint sprigs

In a blender or food processor, place all the ingredients and purée until smooth. Serve in chilled bowls and garnish with a sprig of fresh mint.

VARIATIONS: Instead of peppermint, try lavender, rose, almond, vanilla, or orange extracts and garnish with edible flowers (see Mountain Valley Growers in the Resource Directory).

Tropical Sorbet
Serves 3 to 4

2 cups pineapple chunks, frozen

3 frozen strawberries

1 ripe banana

1/4 cup lite coconut milk

2 tablespoons orange juice

In a food processor or blender, purée the pineapple, banana, and strawberries while slowly adding the juice and coconut milk. Stop occasionally and scrape down the sides. Blend until smooth. Spoon into dessert cups and freeze for 1 hour before serving.

• F Y I
Coconut

Coconut helps build energy and blood, contains lauric acid (which helps with calcium absorption), and has antimicrobial properties. It also has a slightly laxative effect. Because 60% of the coconut is fat, you don't want to overdo eating this tropical nut. I always buy organic milk (usually lite) and organic nonsweetened coconut that's shredded or flaked to use in recipes or as toppings because most commercial shredded coconut may contain propylene glycol and sugar. You can shred your own in a processor or with a hand grater, using freshly shelled coconut for incomparable flavor and moist richness.

Carob Frozen Banana Sticks

Serves 4

This is one of those recipes you'll want to double or triple so they're always available for a healthy dessert or snack.

4 firm small bananas

2/3 cup raw carob powder

1/2 to 2/3 cup purified water

1/8 teaspoon pure organic peppermint extract

4 popsicle sticks

Place a stick in each peeled banana.

Warm the water to 107-108° F, no hotter, so we keep this treat vitally alive. Add the peppermint oil. Stir. Add the carob powder and mix until dissolved. Dip each banana in the carob mixture (deep enough container to cover the banana—you can spoon or brush it on the areas needing extra. Wrap each coated banana in a piece of waxed paper and freeze overnight. They'll keep for 1 to 2 months in your freezer.

• **F Y I**

Carob

Carob, also referred to as Saint John's Bread, is the leguminous pod of the locust tree and approximates the taste of chocolate. Roasted and ground carob pods yield carob powder. Sweet, light, and dry, carob is alkaline in nature. It does contain tannin (as does cocoa), which reduces the absorption of protein through the intestinal wall, so use it as a special treat rather than a daily fare. Carob is an excellent source of calcium, containing more than 3 times as much as milk, ounce for ounce. It's also rich in potassium and other nutrients. It has less fat and fewer calories than chocolate and, unlike chocolate, is naturally sweet with almost 50% sugar and is free of caffeine and oxalic acids.

Part III:

Retreats & Resources

Chapter 19

3–Day Rejuvenation Retreat

What do you have to fear? Nothing. Whom do you have to fear?
No one. Why? Because whoever has joined forces with God obtains
three great privileges: omnipotence without power, intoxication
without wine, and life without death.

—St. Francis of Assisi

There was a time when people wanting to improve their health could get away for a month to "take the waters," or "a month in the country," breathing in clean mountain air. Now we've got a couple of weeks if we're lucky, and the weekend. Period.

What You'll Need:

- comfortable clothing
- a notebook and pens
- a watch or clock
- a half gallon glass container for your water
- 3 or more votive or fragrant candles
- a dry skin brush
- a portable cassette or CD player with classical or other relaxing music
- a small water fountain if you're doing the retreat at home (available at your local nursery or see Fountainside in the Resouce Directory) or nature tapes with the sound of running water

- one or two uplifting and inspiring books (yes, you'll have some time to read—my book *Choose to Live Peacefully* is a perfect companion for this retreat)

Recommended Supplements and Other Optional Products (see the Resource Directory and Chapter 20 for more information on availability and use:

- AlkaLife
- Barlean's Organic Flax Oil and Barlean's Organic Greens
- Emer'gen-C
- Bio-Strath
- Sun Chlorella tablets
- Living Food and Living Cleanse
- Kyolic
- ALL ONE
- Shiatsu-Aid Massage Board
- X-ISER—optional
- Heavenly Heat Sauna—optional
- Green Power®/Life™ Juicer—optional
- Ionizer Plus®—optional
- lots of fresh fruits and vegetables, including lemons
- ice cubes
- Most important: an open heart and a willing mind.

The way I see it, we're all suffering from too much "busyness." We barely have time to relax and cultivate relationships with our spouses, children, friends, and nature. We are under pressure to keep busy, even in our leisure hours! We want to do everything, and we want to do it all at once. We talk on the telephone while we drive, watch television while we read, conduct business while we listen to the radio. Fortunately, we *can* choose to slow it down, and that's exactly what we're going to do in this 3-day retreat. Step out of the rush of life and create an environment of peaceful calmness and relaxation. The following is the basic outline of my De-Stress: Living with Calmness Retreat. It will have you looking and feeling fantastic in just 3 days. I GUARANTEE IT! For the next 3 days, you will:

- Release tension from both body and mind
- Appreciate the joy of *being* and not *doing*
- Release your inherent splendor and serenity
- Experience bliss in solitude
- Get in touch with your innate Divinity and unleash your power
- Experience a greater sense of gratitude, inward stillness, well-being, joy, and gratitude
- Awaken intuition and creativity
- Be infused with renewed faith and feel a strengthened oneness with God and all life

Of all the retreats that I have created for my clients and workshops, this one is my favorite. In fact I take a de-stressing retreat 3 or 4 times a year with each change of season. It is a very relaxing retreat with lots of choices of foods and activities and lots of free time, if you want it, with plenty of time for inner reflection, meditations, and what I call "Joy Activities." This retreat can be done in almost any environment where you can be alone.

Advance Planning Tip

Avoid all caffeinated foods and beverages while on this retreat. If you are a coffee drinker, I urge you to give it up gradually, starting two or three weeks prior to the retreat. Going cold turkey puts too much stress on the system, thus defeating the purpose of the retreat.

A Few Important Guidelines:

1. Set aside three days to be completely alone, and follow the course set out here from start to finish. The fact that you've chosen this program undoubtedly means that you lead a stress-filled life with very little free time just for you ("What's that?" you ask!). But for 3 days, you'll put all that aside and be totally, blissfully alone.

You can do this retreat in your own home, rent a cabin, camp out under the stars, or check into a bed and breakfast or a hotel. The point is to create an atmosphere of genuine privacy and solitude for 3 days, no matter where you find yourself. Ship the kids off to Grandma's, hire a baby-sitter, plan it when your partner is away on a business trip, or remove yourself to a quiet environment.

Some of us may have a hard time feeling safe in solitude. For those of you who do a lot of camping, for instance, sleeping alone in a tent is a wonderful experience of solitude; for others just the thought of being alone in nature is too frightening. Choose a place that makes *you* feel safe and don't judge yourself for your choice. If at any time during the retreat you experience fear, affirm: "I am loved. Everything is working out for my highest good. Out of this experience of solitude, only good will come. I am safe, secure, and at peace with myself and my world."

If you live alone and choose to stay at home for these 3 days, you *must* turn off your phone ringer and cover up your phone answering machine. If you think you'll be tempted to check messages or talk on the telephone, box them up and put them in a closet. Also, no chores! Remember, you're on a mini-vacation and you don't do chores while you're on vacation, right? Actually, you don't want to participate in any activities that will create stress for you or interfere with living with calm and joy.

2. No alcohol, nicotine, or recreational drugs. You want your mind fresh and clear for this exploration into your inner world and newly awakened outer world. Any substance that artificially stimulates you or alters your state will cloud your experience.

3. No radio or TV (with the exception of videos, which I'll explain in a moment). What you want is to close yourself off from the world, especially from the news (stressful!), and create your own world of serenity and calmness. If you decide to use your car during the 3 days, instead of turning on the radio, opt for a cassette or CD of calming music or motivational tapes.

4. Abstain from all animal products, including eggs, milk, butter, fish, fowl, beef, and pork. For 3 days you will be a vegetarian, actually a vegan. (Refer to Chapter 3 for a discussion of nutrition.) Throughout each day, you are free to eat as many fresh fruits and vegetables as you want. Fifty percent of the foods you will eat for this retreat will be raw to help lessen the stress on your body. This means no frozen or canned foods except for frozen fruit in smoothies. Fresh fruits and vegetables are the healthiest foods you can eat. They provide a treasure house of vitamins, minerals, antioxidants, fiber, and phytonutrients, are highest in water content, and give your digestive system a rest, which is one of the goals during this program.

When you're tempted to eat other than a vegan diet—and you probably will be—remind yourself that *you only have to eat this way for 3 days!* If you're going to stay at home, you might want to give away or securely put away any nonvegan foods you think might tempt you.

5. Stay away from coffee and other caffeinated drinks, such as tea, soda, or chocolate. Caffeine interferes with your body's natural energy level. Can you still do this 3-day retreat if you don't give up coffee? Yes, you can, but our goal is to take away those substances that cause stress to the body.

I'm willing to bet that after this program is over and you're feeling better than you've felt in years, you won't have the desire to return to your old habits of coffee and other addictive substances.

The Retreat

Please read through to the end of this chapter before starting the program. You'll want to try to assemble everything you'll need beforehand so that you won't have to rush around finding things at the last minute.

The Night Before: Get to bed as early as possible so you can get at least 8 hours of sleep. You don't want to be falling asleep during any of our first day breathing or relaxation exercises.

Day 1

Waking up & getting started: This first morning you'll wake up without an alarm, when your body wants you to get up. If you want to sleep in until 8 or 9 o'clock, do it.

1. Fresh air stretch & breathing. As soon as you're ready to get out of bed, go directly to the nearest window and open it. For 2 minutes do some deep breathing and easy, standing stretches. For example, stretch your arms over your head and gently bend to each side. With arms stretched out to your side and knees slightly bent, twist from your waist side to side. Then with your hands placed together in prayer position under your chin, say your…

Morning affirmation: "Good morning, Lord (if Lord doesn't feel comfortable to you, substitute with whatever does: Higher Self, Spirit, Angels, Soul, Light, etc.). I turn within and feel my deep reservoir of calmness. Today I refuse to get caught up in the frenzy of life. My life is filled with peace and I carry this peace with me wherever I go. I choose to be relaxed and experience the joy and wonder of all God's (or "Your") blessing in my life."

2. Internal water bath. After fresh air stretching, drink 2 glasses of warm water (purified) to which you've added the fresh juice of one quarter lemon and 2 drops in each glass of AlkaLife. This is an excellent internal bath and flush for your entire digestive system. Even if you're not thirsty, *please* drink this water. Throughout this retreat we're going to get you into the habit of drinking more water. (Refer to Chapter 1 for a discussion of the critical importance of proper hydration to health.)

Next, fill your half gallon glass container with pure water and 8 drops of AlkaLife. You'll drink this entire amount throughout the day (making a total of 10 drops of AlkaLife). For those of you not used to drinking water, this may be the most difficult part of the retreat. Into your half gallon container, put 6 to 8 thin slices of lemon, orange, or cucumber. This makes drinking so much water more palatable. The 2 glasses you drink upon awakening are *in addition to* the half gallon you *must* consume before the day is up. In all, you'll be drinking approximately 80 ounces of water each day. While you might resist this much water the first day, you'll thank me on the third day when you experience the noticeable radiance and smoothness in your skin.

Take your water with you everywhere. Pour from the half gallon container into a large water bottle and carry it with you if you leave. By the end of the day, before you go to sleep at night, you need to have finished the water in the half gallon container.

3. Bathe. Next, do your normal bathroom routine, use the dry skin brush as described on page 193, then shower or bathe. If you ordinarily don't shower until after your workout, wait until after your workout to do your dry skin brush. At the end of the bath or shower (and every bath and shower on this retreat), but while you're still in the shower, take 2 ice cubes and for 2 minutes rub them all over your face (including your eyelids) and neck. This helps close your pores and brings a healthy, youthful glow to your skin. (Two minutes is a long time. Set your clock where you can see it and time yourself.)

4. Dressing for the day. Put on some comfortable clothes (you will wear these each time you sit to meditate or do breathing exercises). I suggest a cotton T-shirt and sweat pants.

5. Breakfast. Breakfast literally means breaking a fast. Remember, we're having mainly fresh fruits and vegetables (with a few exceptions) for 3 days. For breakfast, you have your choice of any fresh fruit in season, but limit yourself to no more than 4 kinds. It's also best not to have a heavy meal just prior to doing breathing exercises and meditation, which we'll do shortly, so a fruit breakfast is perfect. One of my favorites is Fruit Delight: one ruby red grapefruit, one navel orange, one kiwi, three or more strawberries, and some ground almonds. (Don't buy ground almonds; they spoil easily. Just grind some up in a coffee or nut grinder when you need them.) Peel the fruit and slice it so you have 4 different slice sizes of different fruit in different colors. Arrange the fruit on a plate, taking care to make it beautiful to look at, and sprinkle with the ground almonds (1 to 2 ounces). After all, half the fun of eating is in the presentation, which also encourages you to eat more slowly and to savor each bite. And don't forget, no rushing, don't eat while standing up, and take as long as you'd like. (For other fruit breakfast ideas, see the recipes in Chapter 9.)

If you'd like a hot cup of tea, go ahead, just make sure it has no caffeine. Supplement with Barlean's Organic Greens powder, Kyolic, Emer'gen-C, Bio-Strath, and Sun Chlorella. These are all antioxidants, which help the body combat stress and boost the immune system.

I always like to get out my best china, crystal, and silverware to use during my at-home retreats. I also encourage you to have fresh flowers on the table when you eat. Remember, for these 3 days, we're going to surround ourselves with beauty. Of course, if you're out in the wilderness you may want to leave the Limoges at home, but even if you're camping, arrange your things so they are attractive and comfortable.

6. Morning breathing & meditation exercises. From our earlier discussion, you have already designated a sacred spot in your home where you can sit to meditate and keep a home altar. If you're doing this retreat in a hotel, just create a sacred corner. If you're camping outdoors, your entire environment is your sacred space, so just choose a place where you can sit comfortably and focus. On your altar, place a small clock, fresh flowers, candles, and whatever else makes this space more inspiring to you. Either sit on the floor or in a chair, facing your altar. Make sure your spine is straight. Don't slump over or rest on the back of the chair. Light some candles, if you'd like.

Let's do a few introductory breathing exercises so you become familiar with proper breathing.

The 3-part breath. One of the simpler ones, and the first one we'll do, is the 3-part breath. This is a complete breath—inhalation, pause, exhalation—that is performed with awareness. Each part is executed to the count of 4 to 6 seconds initially—if you have been a habitual thoracic (shallow) breather— gradually extending the count to 8 or even 10 as you become more proficient.

Begin inhaling through your nose, deep in your abdomen as you begin to count. Gradually feel the air expand up into your chest, and move all the way up to your collarbone. Now hold for a count of 6 to 10. When you begin to exhale, reverse the order, focusing on each stage as you deflate your lungs. Continue this breathing exercise for 5 minutes.

Alternate-nostril breathing. In this exercise, you inhale through one nostril, retain the breath, then exhale from the other nostril. Healthy people actually do breathe more through one nostril than the other, alternating every couple of hours. This focused alternate-nostril breathing helps balance the use of both hemispheres of the brain and increases concentration. Here is a description of one round:

- Exhale completely, breathe in through the left nostril, holding the right closed with your right thumb.
- Hold the breath, closing both nostrils.
- Breathe out through the right nostril, keeping the left closed with your ring finger.
- Breathe in through the right nostril, keeping the left nostril closed.
- Hold the breath, closing both nostrils.

- Breathe out through the left nostril, keeping the right closed with your thumb.

Do this breathing exercise for another 5 minutes. When you've finished both of these, you will be feeling very relaxed and calm.

The Stillness Meditation. Although you'll do this right now sitting at your altar, this is also a great one to do out in nature. The Stillness Meditation helps to quiet restless thoughts and brings a wonderful calmness.

First, relax the body by inhaling and tensing all over—feet, legs, back, arms, neck, face—then exhaling and relaxing completely. Repeat this several times.

Now, observe the natural flow of your breath. Do not control the breath in any way. Simply follow it with your attention. Each time you inhale, think "still," each time you exhale, think "ness." Repeating "still … ness" with each complete breath helps focus the mind and prevents your attention from wandering from the present moment.

During the pauses between inhalation and exhalation, stay in the present moment, calmly observing whatever is in front of you. If thoughts of the past or future disturb you, just calmly, patiently bring your attention back to what is before you, repeating "still … ness" with your breathing. You can use this meditation whenever you want to feel this calmness, indoors or outdoors, with eyes open or closed. For now, do it for at least 15 minutes, even up to an hour, if you feel so inclined. Remember, you're not in any rush today. You don't have to be anywhere. You have all the time in the world.

When you've finished with the Stillness Meditation, take 3 long, slow, deep breaths and end with the prayer "Thank you, God." The great 13th-century mystic Meister Eckhart once said that if the only prayer you ever say is, "Thank you, God," that is enough.

7. Exercise. It's time to get moving. Physical exercise is one of the most effective means of reducing stress and tension. In fact, studies have shown that a single dose of exercise works better than tranquilizers to alleviate symptoms of anxiety and tension, without any of the undesirable side effects. Your body loves this type of activity even though your mind may sometimes resist.

I recommend that you find some place out in nature, in a beautiful environment, where you can take a walk or hike, skate or cycle. This might mean driving somewhere. That's okay. You'll still be alone and enjoying the peace of your own company. When I take this retreat I drive a few minutes from my home for a hike in the nearby mountains; it's my favorite exercise because I get a great workout and I'm outdoors in a magnificent environment.

If inclement weather prevents you from working out outdoors, and if you'd prefer to go to your gym to use a treadmill or take a yoga class, do it. Or create a way to get an aerobic workout at home or in a hotel. You'll figure something out. But please don't skip this activity. Your body needs this aerobic workout as an effective way to reduce stress.

If you do go to the gym, try, as much as is possible, to stay in your own world without talking to anyone. Save your energy. If you need to, put on some headphones, even if you're not listening to anything, just so others won't talk to you. After your workout, make sure you do some sit-ups and push-ups, and get in some stretching exercises, too. (Refer to Chapter 4 for specific exercises.)

Upon your return home, if you have a juicer, make some fresh juice (recipes in Chapter 8). The combination of orange, grapefruit, and pineapple is excellent after working out, as it helps reduce inflammation. If you don't have a juicer, either skip the juice or buy some freshly-squeezed juice.

8. Journal writing. After you've freshened up, take your notebook, sit in a comfortable place, and answer the following *Self-Discovery Questions and Action Choices*:

- What does it mean to me to be healthy: physically, emotionally, and spiritually?
- Here is a list of at least 5 things I love about myself:
- The following is a list of some things I am going to change to improve myself:
- Because I must take myself with me everywhere I go, I now choose to start loving myself unconditionally and consistently. Here's how:

9. Mid-day affirmation: Now, take a few minutes to mentally picture yourself as the exquisite person you are, emphasizing your many positive qualities. Say aloud: "I am a powerhouse of Divine energy and vitality. I choose to find myself more attractive than ever before. I am wonderful."

10. Lunch. I bet you're hungry now. Since we're focusing on fresh fruits and vegetables, create (or order if you're in a hotel) a large beautiful salad with lots of your favorite vegetables, such as dark leafy greens, spinach, tomatoes, green onions, colorful bell peppers, sprouts, carrots, avocados, celery, etc. Remember, this is the one retreat without designated recipes. I don't want you to get all stressed out about eating according to plan. I want you to be able to adopt this program whether you're at home, in a hotel, or camping in the wilderness somewhere (see the recipes in Chapters 11 and 12).

Because 50% of your diet will be raw, living foods during this retreat, a salad for lunch is easy. Sprinkle some raw sunflower or pumpkin seeds on the salad if you want. Along with the salad, you might add a sweet potato or yam, or some lightly steamed vegetables such as asparagus, broccoli, cauliflower, and carrots, or some soup. Remember to create a meal that is satisfying, delicious, and beautiful.

Take a package of Emer'gen-C (raspberry is great for this) blended with some ALL ONE, Living Food, 1 tablespoon Barlean's Flax Oil and Greens powder, Bio-Strath, and some Sun Chlorella tablets. You can use juice, water, or soy beverage, and add a frozen banana to make it more like a shake.

11. Afternoon delight. After lunch you have some free time. Pick from the list of Joy Activities (see page 442) some things to do that are not too strenuous and keep you home. Listen to music, read a book, take a bubble bath, work on a hobby, write in your gratitude journal, do some yoga, take a nap, or have a massage. At some point, however, during the afternoon, I invite you to just sit and "be" for a while. Gaze out a window if the scenery is beautiful, look at a painting (landscapes or expansive water or glistening scenes seem to work best to relax mind and body), or just close your eyes. I've been known to sit motionless for an hour or two gazing at one of my favorite paintings or photographs. When the time is up, I'm revived, revitalized, and filled with lots of creative ideas.

12. Late afternoon reflection. Walk or drive to a special place out in nature where you can sit, soak in the beauty all around you, do some deep breathing exercises, enjoy the peace of your own company, and reconnect with the Divinity within you and all around you. Every day during the retreat, you'll spend some quality time out in nature. Next to meditation, this is one of the best ways to experience deep relaxation and calmness.

Don't forget to take your water with you and some snacks such as fresh fruit, fresh juice, raw vegetables, or a few different nuts and seeds. I make my own trail mix using all raw and unsalted almonds, sunflower seeds, pumpkin seeds, pine nuts, brazil nuts, walnuts, cashews, dried cherries, dried apple pieces, and raisins. This is very filling and also high in fat, so eat it sparingly.

So, find a place within driving or walking distance where you can go for an hour or two this afternoon. Maybe the beach or a local park, maybe a flower garden or pond, stream, or lake near you or maybe your backyard garden. Make sure it's a natural environment and one in which you can be alone and undisturbed.

When we are out in nature, we are in touch with and surrounded by beauty, magnificence, and tranquility. This healing environment imbues us with the life force, unleashes our inner power, and lifts our spirit, giving us a more positive perspective on our lives and the divine nature of everything.

There are three things you'll do during your time in this natural environment.

a. Take a 15-minute nature stroll. For 15 minutes, just gently stroll, peacefully and quietly. Pay attention to everything, from what you see around you, to your feet touching the earth, to the fragrances in the air. If you can walk barefoot, all the better. See what objects seem to speak to you. Notice how you feel, what you're thinking. When you notice your mind wandering, gently bring it back to the present moment and experience your immediate environment with all of your senses.

b. Watch a bird or insect. For the next 15 minutes, pick some insect or bird to watch. Get as close to the object of your attention as you can. See through your heart instead of your eyes. What do you hear? As you're intently observing, be sure to breathe slowly and deeply. Let go of any feeling you might have of looking silly and feeling self-conscious. Be willing to connect with the insect or bird on a deep level and see what transpires. I do this often during my hikes with rabbits, birds, frogs, deer, raccoons, owls, etc. They'll cross my path and, when I'm alone and don't need to be concerned about slowing up a companion hiker, I'll stop, squat down and watch quietly, sometimes whispering to them. Sometimes they just keep walking away and other times I feel they are communicating with me. It's a wonderful experience.

c. Practice mindfulness. After watching the insect or bird, just quietly sit and do nothing. Just be. Observe whatever goes through your mind, not reacting or becoming emotionally involved with the thoughts, memories, worries, or images. Be detached as you watch the play of thoughts go by. The mind is like a freeway. Don't become involved with the traffic. Be the observer. Observe and let go.

This approach, which the Buddhists call "mindfulness," helps you gain a more calm, clear, and nonreactive state of mind. For at least 30 minutes just sit and be mindful. Feel the quiet peacefulness deep in your soul. Breathe slowly and deeply whenever you think about it. Enjoy the peace of your own company. If you are so inclined, when you're finished, take some time to write in your journal about your experiences, to pray, to express gratitude. To thank God. (Don't forget to drink your water, too!)

13. Dinner & sunset. Take time to watch the sunset tonight. If it's June, July, or August, and it won't be setting for a few hours, go enjoy a nice dinner first; if it's due to set shortly, find a place that gives you the best view and go there now. Then, when you're ready for dinner, create a delicious vegan meal for yourself, or order one at your hotel or at a restaurant.

If you go out to a restaurant, sit by yourself and enjoy the quiet solitude. Have another salad with some different vegetables in it. Along with the salad, have some steamed vegetables and a baked potato with salsa and a few avocado slices instead of butter or sour cream. Or have some brown rice or other grain to accompany your salad. Eat slowly and deliberately, savoring every bite. Take Sun Chlorella tablets and Emer'gen-C with dinner.

14. Evening comforts. Finish off the evening with something from the list of Joy Activities (page 442). Maybe you feel like seeing a funny movie (at a theatre or a video rental, it's up to you). If you do, choose a movie that either makes you laugh or touches your heart or, better yet, both. Stay away from films with violence or action adventure. Let's do whatever we can to nurture that feeling of calm we've gathered all day.

You might just prefer to go home or back to the hotel and relax, take a Jacuzzi or hot oil bath, listen to some classical music, or read a book. Use a Shiatsu-Aid Massage Board nightly.

15. Evening meditation. Sometime before you go to bed, sit at your altar again for at least 15 minutes and meditate. I'd like to help you get into the habit, if you haven't already, of meditating twice a day. *Bookending your day with quiet reflection first thing in the morning and before you go to sleep at night is one of the best things you can do to live a more peaceful, calm, joyful life.* At the end of the meditation and as you're falling asleep, affirm the following:

Evening affirmation: "The spirit of God (Love, Light, etc.) within is my source, supply, and support. I draw forth the kingdom into my consciousness and the fullness of my blessings is now being made evident in my world. I stand firm in my faith in God. Miracles are a natural part of my life. I trust and I believe."

16. Bedtime. Take a Living Cleanse tablet and get to bed by 10, at the latest, so you can get at least 8 hours of sleep. Even if you're not sleepy, get into bed and read or listen to some relaxing music or other uplifting tapes. There is nothing more restorative to your body than sleep. Take advantage of this special time to get enough sleep and wipe out some of your sleep debt.

When I do a personal retreat and I stay at home, I always put my favorite sheets on the bed. I make my bed look like those you see in the magazines where the bed looks heavenly and is beckoning you to get in and stay a while. I also put 3 drops of pure lavender oil on my pillowcase to promote relaxation, deep sleep, and sweet dreams (see aromatherapy in Chapter 7).

Day 2

1. Morning. Begin the day as you did Day 1: stretch and breathe by an open window for 2 minutes, take an internal water bath, bathe, then dress in comfortable clothes, eat some fresh fruit for breakfast, and sit at your altar to meditate. Substitute this ...

Morning affirmation: "Peacefully and calmly I relax in God's light and love. I let go any thoughts of unforgiveness towards myself and others. In everything I think, feel, say, and do, I let my calmness and kindness shine.

2. Breathing & meditation exercises. This morning's "White Light" meditation recharges your energy field and nourishes creativity and tranquility. Meditate for at least 20 minutes. If you want to go longer, that's fine.

White Light Meditation

- Sit in a straight-backed chair with spine erect and feet flat on the floor. (You can also sit cross-legged on the floor but always keep your spine straight when you meditate.) Fold your hands together in your lap, or hold them in prayer position. Eyes may be open or closed. If you'd like, light a candle or play some gentle meditative music.

- Feel yourself relaxing as you take several long, slow deep breaths. Imagine a beautiful white light completely surrounding you. This is your protection as you open sensitive energy centers. In fact, you can do this with any of your meditations.

- For about 10 minutes, as you breathe slowly and deeply, gently concentrate on a single idea, candle flame, picture, or word (such as peace, love, stillness, God, Jesus). Select something that is meaningful, uplifting, and spiritual to you. You could even focus on some peaceful music.

- If your mind wanders from your object of focus, gently bring it back to your awareness.

- After 10 minutes, separate your hands and turn them palms up in your lap. If your eyes are open, close them.

- Relax your hold on the object of concentration and shift your mind into neutral. Remain passive yet alert for 10 or more minutes (as long as you want). Gently observe and be mindful of any thoughts or images as they may float by. Just remain still and detached and be with whatever you are experiencing. When you notice your breath getting shallow, begin again to take long, slow deep breaths.

- When the time seems right for you, open your eyes, close your palms, and again imagine that you are surrounded completely by a white light. This is your continued protection as you go about your daily activities with peace and joyfulness.

At other times during the day, allow a sense of light and love to flow from within your being and fill your entire body. It's very easy to do, and it puts you into a meditative state.

Meditation is all about breaking through the everyday world of tension and thought to create inner peace, calm, insight. Find the method or methods that suit you best.

3. Morning exercise. Just like yesterday, get your body moving any way that works best for you. I encourage you, once again, to get outdoors, out in nature, to walk, hike, be by yourself without lots of outer noise and distractions. Don't forget to drink lots of water.

4. Morning juice snack. Next, get or make some fresh juice, this time apple and carrot blended with some vegetables such as celery, beets, and parsley. In this combination, add some fresh ginger and half a lemon.

If you'd prefer a blender drink, here's one I make often:

3/4 cup water

1 ripe, frozen banana

1/2 cup fresh fruit in season such as strawberries, blueberries, or peaches

1 tablespoon Barlean's Flax Oil and Barlean's Greens

1 heaping tablespoon of Living Food

In a blender or food processor, blend all the ingredients together until smooth. Sip slowly in your favorite glass or goblet.

5. Journal writing. After you've freshened up (make sure to dry skin brush before you shower or bathe and end with icing your face and neck), take your notebook, sit in a comfortable place, and answer the following:

1. In the past I have chosen to feel anxious about the following things: _____. I now choose to let this anxiety go.

(Although these are just words, you begin from here to reprogram your mind and strengthen your resolve to live more peacefully.)

2. Think of one person with whom you have been feeling anxious or stressed out. Close your eyes and see both of you sitting facing each other in a circle of white or pink light. Now lovingly share your feelings with that person and resolve any conflict. Finish with feeling the anxiety or stressful emotions release, seeing your hearts connect, and loving each other unconditionally.

3. I now know that the better I handle stress, the healthier and happier I'll be. Here are some ways I've handled stress in the past:

Here are the ways I now choose to deal with stress that support my immune system and well-being:

4. Sit with your eyes closed for the next few minutes, envisioning yourself as a peaceful, relaxed, healthy, successful, confident, and happy person. Now describe how that looked and felt.

5. On a separate sheet of paper, write down everything you want to release from your life that no longer supports this vision of yourself as you described in #4. List everything you can think of right now and keep this list with you during the rest of the retreat. You can add to it as you think of more things. You might add that you'll now release negative thoughts, thoughts of lack or low self-esteem, extra fat on your body, aches and pains that no longer support your healthy vision of yourself, etc. We will do something special with this list on Day 3.

6. Lunch. Create another masterpiece salad with different vegetables than you had yesterday. Always start with some dark leafy greens, organic if possible, and then add to that. (See Chapter 12 for dressings.) Remember to eat 50% or more of your meals raw and enjoy any fruits or vegetables in season that you love to eat.

You might like to experiment with some new vegetables, like kale or Swiss chard or parsnips. Take Barlean's Organic Greens powder, Emer'gen-C, Sun Chlorella, Bio-Strath, and Kyolic.

7. Early afternoon delight. Pick from the list of Joy Activities. Don't forget, if you feel tired, take a nap. Your body probably needs it!

8. Late afternoon reflection. With your water and snacks in tow, venture out to another uplifting environment where you're surrounded by beauty and will be left alone.

Walking meditation. Today you're going to do a *walking meditation*. In many traditional monastic environments, it is customary to intersperse periods of sitting meditation with walking meditation. Like sitting meditation, walking meditation is a simple practice effective for fostering calmness, relaxation, and awareness. It can be done almost anywhere and anytime when you're not rushed and you won't be interrupted. For now, select a place outdoors, weather permitting, where you can walk comfortably back and forth or in a large circle.

Try this with shoes on as well as barefoot. I particularly like doing this barefoot on some grass or on the sand at the beach. The point is to really feel the earth beneath your feet. You are not walking to get anyplace. The key is to be aware as you walk, to use the natural movement of walking to foster mindfulness and wakeful presence. This is different from yesterday's walk where you observed and communed with everything around you.

In today's walking meditation, begin by standing at the beginning of your path. Focus on your body, how you feel, and the sensation of your feet pressing against the earth. Your hands should rest easily, wherever they are comfortable. For a moment, before you begin to walk, close your eyes, breathe in slowly and deeply and become aware of your breath and "being" in the present moment. Then open your eyes and be aware of your surroundings and the relaxed feeling of your body. Remember to be fully mindful with an alert, relaxed attention to the present moment and the sensations throughout your body as you grace your walking path with your divine loving presence.

Begin to walk slowly. Focus on each step. Feel each step as it comes and be fully present with it. Notice every sensation of the walking process—your feet against the earth, how your arms move, each breath, where your thoughts wander. Like training a puppy, gently bring your thoughts back when they wander off from the present moment. You'll probably have to do this over and over, countless times, but that's just part of the process. Be gentle with yourself and simply acknowledge where you have wandered in your mind and come back to the present awareness as you take the next step.

Let yourself walk with ease, grace, and dignity. Feel each step mindfully as you lift your feet off the ground. Feel the sensations of your ankles, legs, hips, torso, neck, and face. Your pace can be very slow to brisk. Continue to walk for 10 to 20 minutes or longer.

I have incorporated walking meditation into my lifestyle for years. Whatever form you incorporate that feels right for you, you'll probably find, as I have, that after a few months of regular practice, the relaxation and calmness you feel during the meditation carries over into your daily activities. In other words, you extend your walking practice in an informal walk to or from your car, home, market, or wherever you walk. You will begin to find joy in the process of walking and being and, in this simple way, begin to be more truly aware and present and more connected to your body, heart, and mind as you walk through your daily life. With this new awareness, you'll come to understand that each day is a "holy" day.

When you start to live in and appreciate each moment you have on this earth, you will be amazed not only by how much more you enjoy life, but also by how much more you accomplish and contribute.

9. Dinner & sunset. Again, either before or after dinner, go embrace the sunset. Find a special place to view it. Let this beauty fill your heart, mind, and soul. Continually be grateful for the beauty all around you. *Thank God often.*

Dinner can be either back at home or out somewhere. If possible, create a picnic meal just for yourself with some of your favorite fruits and vegetables and commune with nature while you eat. I do this at least twice a month on the beach or at my favorite bench overlooking the ocean. There's no more beautiful way to eat a healthy meal than out in a magnificent natural setting.

10. Evening comforts. Make sure you surround yourself with beauty, calmness, tranquility, and relaxation. You may decide to head home or perhaps go to a movie. The other night I went to the Natural Science Museum in Los Angeles and experienced the 'Butterflies in Living Color' exhibit. I've always loved seeing butterflies as I often do when I hike. For 2 hours I walked in a garden of butterflies, watching their beauty and having several land on me. What a joyful, exhilarating adventure. I'll never forget it. During this De-Stress Retreat, I often visit the Getty Museum, which is just a few minutes from my home, and walk along among all the masterful paintings and other pieces of art and history. Sheer bliss! I prefer not to drive long distances when I'm on this retreat. Maybe another bubble bath or aromatherapy bath with candle light and music appeals to you most.

11. Evening meditation. For at least 15 minutes, do your deep breathing and meditation at your altar. Light a candle to symbolize the flame of peace and calmness in your heart overflowing and infusing every cell of your being.

12. Bedtime. Before going to bed, take another Living Cleanse tablet and then take a few minutes to breathe deeply at your altar before slipping into your inviting bed. Get to bed as early as possible because you're going to set your alarm early enough to see the sunrise. Put 3 drops of lavender oil on your pillow and as you go to sleep, repeat softly aloud and then silently one of your favorite affirmations and take it with you into your dreams.

Evening affirmation: "In the silence of my heart, I am at peace. In solitude, I feel God's love and guidance in my life. Today I seek out time to be alone, to enjoy the serenity of my own company."

Day 3

1. Morning sunrise & routine. Today you will be getting up early enough to watch the sunrise. In fact, I invite you to either walk or drive to a place where you get the best view. If you can't see the sunrise from where you are, visualize a spectacular one or look at a photo. For just this purpose, I have a 2 x 3 foot poster of a sunrise and sunset in my home. For those of you not used to getting up so early, I guarantee you that this sunrise experience will be one of the things you cherish the most from this retreat. As on days 1 and 2, begin with 2 minutes of stretching and breathing by an open window, internal water bath, get into comfortable clothes, watch the sunrise, eat fresh fruit for breakfast (plus Sun Chlorella, ALL ONE, Emer'gen-C, Kyolic, Barlean's Greens and Bio-Strath) and sit at your altar to meditate.

In front of the open window, after stretching, say the following:

Morning affirmation: "In this peaceful time of prayer and solitude, I lift my soul to the inspiration of Spirit and let divine wisdom fill my mind and heart. I let go of concerns for this day and the days ahead and simply bask in the glow of peace and calmness that comes from knowing my oneness with God (Spirit, Love, etc.). In God's sacred presence, I know that there is nothing to fear. With tenderness and love, God shows me the way around or through a challenge. Yet I know that God may show me more than one path, and I have freedom of choice. Which path I take is up to me. As I let go and let God guide me, I accept the gifts of divine love and understanding, encouragement and support."

2. Breathing & meditation exercise. Sit with your spine erect, eyes open or closed, palms facing up on your thighs. Breathe slowly and deeply for a few minutes focusing on your breath or some other object such as a picture, candle flame, or word. Then close your eyes, and place your focus on your third eye, the area in-between and slightly above your eyebrows. Your eyes are still closed with an inward gaze upward. Continue to breathe slowly and deeply. When your thoughts wander, gently bring them back to your breath and third eye.

Continue this process for at least 15 minutes. When finished, bring your attention back to the place you are sitting, open your eyes, and read softly aloud the following meditation prayer:

Peace meditation prayer. Love is here. God is here. Truth is here. Peace, the wonderful peace of God, is right here where I am. In this beautiful moment of eternity, I turn my attention within. I feel the peace of God (Spirit, Love, etc.) that is in me always; the peace that transcends all fear, all concern, all sense of anxiety; the peace that is everlasting. I am a center of perfect peace. Let there be peace on earth and let it begin with me.

Sweet Spirit, let me be an instrument of peace in my world. Open me to the realization that peace in the world begins with peaceful hearts. I open my heart, my mind, and all that I am to Your peace. In this moment, nothing can disturb the peace of my soul.

Every atom, cell, tissue, and fiber of my being is filled to overflowing with the peace of God. I allow that peace of God within me to come forth and bless my family, my loved ones, my friends, and my co-workers. I see and experience the peace of God in my neighborhood, my community, my city, my state, and my country. I use my God-given power of vision to see and to feel the peace of God flooding the hearts and souls of everyone on this planet. I take this moment, now to bring that vision closer to reality. I recommit myself to my own inner peace and to peace in the world in this moment of silence. AMEN

3. Exercise. Just as on days 1 and 2, go work out for as long as you want. (Remember to take your water!) As before, I encourage you to get out into the fresh air and nature for your workout, if at all possible.

4. Snack. Next, get some fresh juice or a blender drink. I recommend the Vitality Shake on page 210 or choose another from Chapter 8.

5. Journal writing. After freshening up (don't forget to dry skin brush before your shower or bath), take your notebook, sit in a comfortable place, and answer the following:

- In what ways can I simplify my home and/or office?
- What duties can I delegate to free up some time?
- How do I feel when my life is cluttered and complicated?
- Are there some relationships that complicate and clutter my life rather than enrich and enhance it?
- Does my self-esteem depend on what I have and how I live rather than who I am in my heart?
- My formula for life will be "high thinking and simple living." Here are some ways I'll begin to simplify my life, beginning immediately:
- What from my past do I need to release? What no longer serves my highest good? (Add these to the list you've been keeping.)
- What would my life look like if I carried no excess baggage from the past?

Take your list and add to it anything else you wish to release from your life—anything and everything that no longer serves you.

Now, find a way to let it go. A fireplace is an ideal place to do this. In workshops, I've used a big metal bowl (Burning Bowl Ceremony) in which we place everyone's lists and light a match to it. What joy and freedom we all experience seeing our negative, self-limiting beliefs and 'limiting ways of being' going up in ashes.

You can create your own sacred Burning Bowl Ceremony. The physical acts of writing down those things that no longer support you in living your highest potential harnesses a power within you to release the habit or emotional chain keeping you blocked. For example, you might add things to your list such as overeating, negative self-talk, criticizing, or procrastination. Add any and all things you'd like to see released from your life.

If it's not appropriate to burn your list now, hold on to it until you can do this. Make it a special ceremony. Come to it with an open heart and positive mind. Be grateful that you are being inwardly guided and empowered to live more gracefully and fully. Before you light the match, close your eyes, breath slowly and deeply, and surrender your list to God, Spirit, Higher Self (whatever you want to call it). Be willing to be healed.

As the list is burning, breathe deeply and feel your heart opening and all pressure and stress leaving your body. Relax and be still as long as you want.

6. Lunch. Pick from any of the vegetable recipes or create your own masterpiece at home or at a restaurant. Enjoy your lunch, savoring each bite. Make sure you're drinking water throughout the day and that you're on target for finishing the half gallon container before you go to sleep tonight. Take Barlean's Organic Greens powder, Emer'gen-C, Kyolic, Sun Chlorella, and Bio-Strath.

7. Afternoon delight. Pick from the "Joy" recommendations. If you haven't done so already, this is the day I really encourage you to pamper yourself. You deserve it! Have a massage. Try a facial with a manicure and pedicure, or schedule yourself for a half-day of pampering at a local spa. And if that's not your cup of tea, select any other activity, including napping, that feels perfect for you.

8. Dinner. Whether at home or elsewhere, make this an elegant meal just for you. Use linen, china, and have some fresh flowers at your table. If you're at home, try one of my recipes that's new to you. Eat slowly. (And remember your supplements.)

9. Evening comforts. Put on your favorite relaxing music. If you don't feel alert enough to meditate but you'd still like to do something to relax, this is the perfect time to practice a progressive relaxation. Sit with your back straight or lie down with your arms along your sides, palms up.

Progressive relaxation. Use whatever words or images reflect peace and relaxation for you. Imagine that a wave of golden relaxation is entering your toes. It's moving up into the arches, and up to your heels, and then your ankles. And this golden relaxing power is now moving up your calves and into your knees, relaxing them completely, then moving up to your thighs and into your hips, relaxing all the muscles and tendons. This relaxing power continues to move up into the base of your spine, moving slowly up your spine and into the back of your neck and shoulders, making them loose and limp. The wave of relaxation enters your upper arms and moves on into your forearms and hands, right through the ends of your fingertips. This golden relaxing wave moves around to the front into your facial muscles, relaxing your whole face. Your eyes are relaxed, your jaw is relaxed, and your mouth, throat, and tongue are relaxed. Your entire body is now relaxed and is filled with a golden relaxing light that feels warm and comfortable, all over. All tension is gone from your body and mind. Continue to keep your eyes closed and breathe slowly and deeply.

You can do this in a couple of minutes, but for now, please don't rush. Let it take at least 10 minutes to relax your entire body and then just stay that way for as long as you want. After a few days of doing this type of progressive relaxation, it will get easier and your body will respond more effortlessly.

10. Evening meditation. For at least 15 minutes, breathe deeply and meditate in your own special way. When finished, say the following affirmation prayer.

Evening affirmation & positive meditation prayer. Every day, each and every moment is a new opportunity to begin again, to celebrate the gift of life. There is no past or future. There is only now, a blessed moment filled with unlimited opportunities for good. I live every moment to the fullest by releasing memories that are no longer useful, by letting go of things that can limit me, and by opening my mind and heart to experiences that will uplift me and encourage me to stretch and grow. The past has no power to control me. With God (Spirit, Love, etc.), I can live fully and freely in each moment of my life.

Every thought of not being valuable, of being afraid, of uncertainty and doubt, is now cast out of my mind. My memory goes back to God alone, in whom I live, move, and have my being. A complete sense of happiness, peace, certainty, calmness, and love floods me with light. I have confidence in myself because I have confidence in God. I am sure of myself because I am sure of God.

The Spirit of Love within me knows the answer to any problem that confronts me. In calm confidence, in perfect trust, in abiding faith, and with complete peace and calmness, I let go of any problems and receive the answers.

The wisdom within me knows exactly what to do in every situation. Every idea necessary to successful living is brought to my attention. The doorway to ever increasing opportunities for self-expression is open before me. I am continuously meeting new and larger experiences. Every day brings some greater good. I prosper in everything I do. Now there is no deferment, no delay, no obstruction, or obstacle, nothing to impede the progress of right action, of Divine order, in every area of my life.

I identify myself with abundance. I surrender all fear and doubt. I let go of all uncertainty. I know there is no confusion, no lack of confidence. I know that what is mine will claim me, know me, rush to me. The Presence of God, of Love, is with me. The mind of God is my mind. The thoughts of God are my thoughts.

Spirit of Love within me, thank you for this precious gift of life. Today, and always, I choose to honor and serve you by loving myself and everyone else unconditionally and by acknowledging your Presence in everything I think, feel, say, and do. AMEN.

11. Bedtime. After the meditation and affirmation, if you're not ready to sleep, choose a simple, quiet activity such as having a hot cup of tea and curling up with an uplifting book. Then take a Living Cleanse tablet, put some lavender on your pillow, flowers on your bedside table, and drift off to sleep. Sweet Dreams.

Peace be with you.

In the days that follow, notice how relaxed, calm, and peaceful you feel and the radiant glow of your skin. I encourage you to nurture this calmness by making a habit of beginning all your days with some breathing, stretching, and meditation. When you feel the stress of the day's activities crowding in on your resolve to stay calm, here are a few things you can do:

1) Say the following Day 4 Re-Entry Affirmation:

I am filled with joy and a peaceful calmness as I sit in stillness and experience the quietude. God's (Love's, Spirit's, etc.) presence permeates my body and inspires my soul.

441

God, as I contemplate this world of plenty, I am filled with gratitude … with amazement … with joy. Thank you for the fresh ideas that open new avenues to your substance. Thank you for the unlimited possibilities of abundance.

With my heart and mind open to Your presence, I discover that I have everything I need to live fruitfully … to live prosperously … to live joyfully and peacefully. I am so grateful!

These three days of communion with You have renewed my awareness of Your loving presence and the true joy that comes with awareness, dear God. I now know that calmness is Your living breath within me, guiding me always. I hold this joy and calmness in my heart as I return my attention to the present and prepare to return to my normal life.

Thank you, God, for the gift of life.

2) Take one 2 minute deep-breathing break. I recommend that you get in the habit of doing this as a preventive measure, even every hour on the hour, except when sleeping. Deep breathing is one of the very best ways to quell stress and restore calmness.

3) Meditate. As you have experienced, meditation helps restore balance, nurtures your spirit, helps you keep things in perspective, and fosters feelings of peace. *Remember:* Stress is a fact of life, but you don't have to make it a *way* of life. You can choose to live with a peaceful calmness no matter what's happening in your life.

Joy Activities

- Watch the sunrise.
- Watch the sunset.
- Go horseback riding.
- Get a massage or use a Shiatsu-Aid Massage Board.
- Get a small water fountain (available at your local nursery or see Fountainside in the Resource Directory) and keep it running.
- Put a cucumber slice on each eye and rest for 15 minutes.
- See a movie that makes you laugh. (Steve Martin's movies are my favorite.)

- See a movie that inspires you.
- Take a bubble bath or aromatherapy bath.
- Read poetry.
- Memorize a favorite poem.
- Sleep in new sheets.
- Wear silk pajamas all day at home.
- Sip your favorite tea while gazing out your window or sitting in your garden.
- Eat a meal in your garden, at a local park, or in another beautiful, outdoor environment.
- Set a beautiful table with your best china, silver, linens, and flowers just for you.
- Treat yourself to a facial.
- Spend a few hours at a day spa.
- Hold a puppy or kitten.
- Go to a museum.
- Visit some antique stores.
- Browse a bookstore.
- Visit a flower garden.
- Work in your garden.
- Arrange fresh cut flowers and put them around your home.
- Hand pick some roses and place them on your bedside table.
- Take a bike ride.
- Plant a tree.
- Immerse yourself in a painting you love, in person, or an art book.
- Bake some healthy cookies or bread.
- Do something kind for someone else without their knowing.
- Spend 10 to 20 minutes 2 to 4 times a week basking in the sunshine with as much skin exposed to the morning or afternoon sun as possible.
- Watch a baby enjoy its world and celebrate just being alive. Let its loving energy infuse all your cells.

- Read an uplifting book.
- Go skating.
- Clean out a closet.
- Listen to classical music and do nothing else.
- Fill your bedroom with live, green plants to increase oxygen.
- Take a nap.
- Attend church, temple, or another spiritual home.
- Take someone you don't know well to lunch.
- Hug a friend.

Add your own Joy Activities here:

- _____
- _____
- _____
- _____
- _____
- _____
- _____
- _____
- _____
- _____
- _____
- _____
- _____
- _____
- _____

Chapter 20

7–Day Detox & Rejuvenate Retreat

Advance Planning Tip

I suggest that you avoid all caffeinated foods and beverages while on this retreat. If you are a coffee drinker, I recommend giving it up before you begin. Allow yourself at least 1 week without caffeine before starting so you don't experience withdrawal headaches during this program.

To prime your body for this retreat, start taking Living Cleanse (see Living Food in the Resource Directory) 3 days before the retreat begins. (Refer to the bottle for dosage information.)

Also, if you don't know how to meditate, please refer to my audio book, "Wired to Meditate" and practice for at least a few days before the retreat begins. Meditation is an important part of this retreat, so you want to be prepared.

What You'll Need:

- a gratitude journal
- a blender
- a half gallon glass container for your water
- a dry skin brush
- lots of fresh fruits and vegetables, including lemons, plus other favorite plant-based whole foods, such as sprouts, whole grains, legumes, beans, and a few raw nuts/seeds
- ice cubes
- Basic Sprouting Starter Kit from Handy Pantry (get this a few days before your program starts and begin sprouting so you'll have fresh sprouts available on day one.)
- one bottle of AlkaLife
- one bottle of Barlean's Organic Flax Oil and Barlean's Greens

- 30 packets of Emer'gen C (I like raspberry, Lite with MSM, and Triple Power for variety
- one bottle of Bio-Strath
- package of 300 Sun Chlorella tablets
- bottle of Living Food, Living Cleanse, and Living Enzymes
- small can of ALL ONE
- 1 bottle of Kyolic Aged Garlic Extract
- my book *Choose to Live Peacefully* (also in audio book)
- Shiatsu-Aid Massage Board

Optional But Helpful: These items are all wonderfully beneficial for my daily rejuvenation regime.

- Green Power® or Green Life™ Juicer
- 1 Fountainside Fountain
- X-ISER
- Thermotex heating pad
- BodySlant
- Heavenly Heat sauna or Finnleo Steam Bath
- Ionizer Plus®

This program is less structured than the 3-Day Retreat. You can even participate while still working part-time, although you'll see more positive results if you can take a week off, keep stress to a minimum, and have enough time to effectively participate in all the recommended activities without feeling rushed or pressured. So, if you can, take off a week from your normal daily responsibilities.

Because of the looser structure of this retreat, it can be done alone or with your family, your spouse, a friend, or a group of friends. Everyone can create their own time schedule or you can do meditations, nature walks, deep breathing, and meal times together. It's up to you, but just make sure you participate in all the activities.

Look through the guidelines for the 3-Day Rejuvenation Retreat (see page 417) and see which of those you can incorporate into this retreat.

Here's what you can expect from this program:

- Release toxins from your body and emotional toxins from your mind

- Lose from 2 to 5 pounds. This program has a way of helping melt fat away according to your needs.
- Supercharge your metabolism, energy, and strength
- Rev up your fat-burning enzymes and burn more calories
- Improve complexion and skin tone all over your body
- Look and feel years younger
- Nourish your body, mind, and spirit
- Release negative food habits
- Ignite your self-esteem
- Gain freedom, control of your life, and empowerment
- Reconnect with your inner peace and Higher Self

Like the 3-Day Retreat, I have a feeling that you'll really enjoy this one also. It's really not difficult if you create an environment and a schedule that supports this program. It takes discipline, but I promise you that if you stick with it for the entire week, you'll feel better than you have in years and will probably want to integrate these health- and life-enriching activities into your life on a regular basis.

The Retreat

Please read through the chapter before starting the program. Try to assemble everything you'll need beforehand rather than waiting until the last minute. Get rid of all junk food or any unhealthy food (including animal products) you think might tempt you during the retreat. 'Out of sight, out of mind' makes staying disciplined easier.

For simplicity, I will recommend the daily activities and reference the page number in the book where they're described so you can read more about the benefits. Fit these in your schedule in a way that works best for you. Unlike the 3-Day Retreat, *you* will orchestrate your day.

Each Day Engage in the Following:

1. Dry skin brush—Before you shower or bathe, use the dry skin brush all over your body, except your face. If you have a sauna, make sure to use it daily during the retreat, and dry skin brush and rinse off before taking a sauna (see page 192).

2. Water (Hydro) therapy—First thing in the morning fill up a half gallon glass container with purified water to which you've added 10 drops of AlkaLife. Have a large glass or two, first thing in the morning and then spread out the rest throughout the day. If you leave the house, always take water with you and pour from this container into a smaller bottle to carry with you. Have most of it consumed before bedtime, or else you'll be up visiting the bathroom a few times during the night. Also, if weight loss is your goal, drink a large glass of water on an empty stomach about 15 minutes before each meal. Also, get in the habit of drinking the water between meals instead of with meals so you don't dilute the digestive enzymes that are released in the saliva from chewing.

By starting with a half gallon (64-ounce) container, you get to see how much you are drinking and make sure you consume at least the 64 ounces. It's ideal to drink one half your body weight in ounces (if you weigh 140 pounds, drink 70 ounces of water) and up the amount if you are very physically active or take a sauna that day. I usually drink at least 80 ounces daily. To make the water more palatable, you can add a few drops of lemon juice or a few thin slices of cucumber, lemon, orange, grapefruit, or strawberries.

Besides drinking lots of water, make a ritual out of taking aromatherapy or other therapy baths or relaxing and invigorating showers. As you bathe or shower, think about all those things for which you are grateful and also imagine that the water is taking away all physical, mental, and emotional toxins down the drain.

End with the water as cool as you can take it, unless it's in the evening and it's close to bedtime. The increase in body temperature will help you sleep better.

And, finally, whether you bathe or shower, at the end, rub your face with a couple of ice cubes to close the pores, increase circulation to your face, and create a very healthy glow. During the final cool rinse, while standing with my back under the water, I'll ice my face, one cube in each hand, circulating the ice all around so an area doesn't get too cold. I recommend bringing 4 ice cubes in a bowl into the shower because they sometimes slide out of your hands, fall, and break.

3. Deep breathing & stretching—First thing in the morning, as soon as you get out of bed, go directly to the nearest window and open it. For 2 minutes do some deep breathing and easy stretching.

Stretch your arms over your head and gently bend to each side. With arms stretched out to your side and knees slightly bent, twist from your waist side to side. Then with your hands placed in prayer position under your chin, say your morning affirmation. For suggestions, refer to my book *Choose to Live Peacefully* or the one recommended in the 3-Day Rejuvenation Retreat on page 417.

Throughout the day, take at least 4 to 6 more deep breathing minibreaks where, for 2 to 5 minutes, you sit quietly and slowly and deeply inhale and exhale. You might begin with counts of 4 to 6 seconds (you don't need a clock; just count internally) for each inhalation and the same with exhalation. Make it a point to not only to lengthen your count time, perhaps up to 10 to 12 (without increasing your counting speed!), but also to take more breathing breaks throughout your day.

4. Sleep & rest—I can't emphasize enough that nothing is more restorative than a good night's sleep, night after night. Make this a top priority during the week and do whatever it takes to carve out at least 8 hours each night. If you want to sleep longer, do it. If you have a BodySlant, use it daily during the retreat for a deeper relaxation.

5. Sunshine—Each day expose as much of your body as possible to the sun, preferably early morning or late afternoon, especially during the summer months. Start with 10 minutes and add a minute or so each day until you reach the last day and then try to get 20 minutes, 10 minutes on each side and don't use a sun block. Healthy sunbathing boosts immunity, decreases cholesterol, revitalizes skin, and rejuvenates the body. If you don't have a backyard and can't find privacy for sunning, just get outdoors and take off whatever you can to expose as much of your body as possible (see page 181).

If there's no sun at all the week you're on this program, then visualize yourself sunbathing for the time recommended above.

6. Exercise—Each day during the program, you must engage in at least 1 hour of exercise. If you're a beginner and the most you've done is walking to your car or your office, start slowly and break up your activity during the day. Try walking for 15 minutes and then stretch for 15 minutes in the morning and again in the afternoon. If you're already physically active, feel free to do more than one hour of exercise. That's just the minimum. If you're house-bound, consider getting an X-ISER (see the Resource Directory). It makes working out easy and fun.

Once again, it doesn't matter when you fit it in, just find the right time for you. Remember, don't exercise within 2 to 3 hours of going to bed, unless it's yoga, because exercise revs up metabolism and will interfere with sleep. If you get sore from doing more exercise than usual, or if aches and pains develop from the detoxification process, use an infrared Thermotex heating pad. Refer to Chapter 4 for guidelines on how to exercise properly.

7. Meditate & pray—Two times during the day, for at least 20 minutes each session. The distinction I make between them is this: Prayer is talking to God (or whatever you might call your Source) and meditation is listening. Feel free to meditate longer, if time permits. This would certainly be the week to get in as much meditation as possible. Spacing these sessions out, such as morning and afternoon/evening works best. When I do this retreat, I usually meditate for 2 hours daily and then a couple times during the week, I'll extend one of my meditations up 2 to 4 hours. This can be done indoors or outdoors. Carve out the time and space where you won't be interrupted, barring an emergency. I like to meditate with the sound of flowing water, which is why I suggest getting a real fountain or tapes of running water before you begin the program. (If you have a copy of my book *Choose to Live Peacefully,* please refer to my chapters on meditation and prayer.)

8. Nature time—Spending time out in nature, whether a walk along the ocean, next to a lake, stream, or bay, in the mountains, at a local park, or even in your own garden nourishes your soul. Being out in nature increases the negative ions you breathe in, which naturally lifts your spirits and helps bring a feeling of well-being and vitality. During this retreat I like to take a long sunrise hike each morning and make it a Prayer Hike. I say and sing my affirmations, meditate, and consciously breathe deeply, appreciate all the beauty and wildlife around me, and get the early morning sun on my skin. What a glorious, positive way to start the day.

Each of the 7 days, spend at least 20 minutes out in nature, living in the present moment, tasting the magnificence, and appreciating the beauty all around you. You might want to do the Prayer Walk described in Chapter 1.

9. Gratitude journal—Each day, sometime before you go to sleep at night, write in a gratitude journal. List at least 7 things for which you are grateful. What you put your attention on expands and grows in your life. This practice of keeping a gratitude journal, as Oprah suggests, will change your life for the better.

10. Reading time—Carve out some time each day to read a book— something that is uplifting, empowering, and inspiring that motivates you to be the best you can be. One of the reasons I recommend my book *Choose to Live Peacefully* is because it has 40 chapters that are all relatively short in length and each one stands on its own so it's easy to pick up and read. It also offers a 40-day rejuvenation program for body, mind, and spirit.

11. Joy activities—Each day of the Retreat, participate in what I call a Joy Activity. On page 442, I listed several of these activities and I'm sure you have more to add. One day it might be planting some flowers in your yard, another day you might go to a movie that makes you laugh, or treat yourself to a few hours at a spa.

12. Visualization & affirmation—For at least 10 minutes each day, when your body is deeply relaxed, such as after your meditation and prayer time, practice visualizing one special, different goal. Visualize being healthy and fit, finding your ideal job, or being in a loving, supportive relationship. The idea is to create mental pictures of what your life would look like if this were your present reality. And as you visualize, feel the emotions of joy and thanksgiving you would feel if this were your current reality. In other words, **assume the feeling of the wish fulfilled**. And then recite some affirmations to support that goal. (Please refer to my book *Choose to Live Peacefully*, which includes affirmations.) If you don't have any memorized, just write them on a card to use when you finish your visualization. Say them out loud first, then whisper them, and finally say them internally for a few minutes. When finished with the visualization and affirmations, give thanks, turn it over to your Higher Power to orchestrate for you "this or something better," and then move on to your next adventure for the day.

13. Live from love—Most of us are our own worst enemy and if we're not judging or criticizing ourselves, we're doing this to others.

We hold grudges and forget to forgive others and ourselves. So, one of your goals during this 7 days is to come from love. Only loving thoughts are allowed. THINK LOVE! At that moment when you catch yourself being unloving toward yourself or others, stop immediately and choose another higher thought. You can't change what you don't recognize. Living from love in everything you think, feel, say, and do will enrich every area of your life, heal your body, and reconnect you with your Divine source.

14. Plant food diet—For 7 days, you will be eating a plant-based, whole foods diet. That means no animal products, such as dairy, eggs, meat, fish, fowl (have you ever wondered how it got that name?), and absolutely no white sugar or flour products, no soda, caffeine, candies, pastries, cakes, or other high-calorie, low-nutrient food. Most of the recipes in Part II of this book will work. Stick with ones that are easiest to prepare, and without chocolate (it has caffeine), and sweeteners. One of the goals during this retreat is to reeducate your taste buds, so you want to stay away from sweets with the exception of fresh fruits. Refer to Chapter 3 for more detail on a plant-based, whole foods diet. Here are a few guidelines:

- Make it your goal to eat 7 to 12 servings of fruits and vegetables a day (emphasize vegetables). Because everyone participating in this retreat is at a different level, I am offering 7 different levels from which to choose. If you have never done a rejuvenation/detox program before and/or if you eat the Standard American Diet (SAD) that's high in processed food, fat, and animal products, start with Level 1 and then, as your diet and lifestyle improves, move up the ladder one rung at a time. If you eat a diet rich in fruits and vegetables and include fish, eggs, and dairy, then begin with Level 2. If, on the other hand, you already eat a plant-based diet and lead a healthy lifestyle, you may want to start with Level 4. In other words, for the first retreat you want to start at a level one above how you usually eat and then move up.

Our goal is to detoxify our bodies, but if you try to advance too quickly, too many toxins may be released at once and you might not have such a good experience during the week. You might experience headaches, muscle ache, fatigue, or irritability. So start slowly and move up through the levels at your own pace.

- Graze. As discussed in Chapter 5, the best way to eat to support your body is to avoid huge meals, not eat late at night, and instead of three large daily meals, have smaller meals more often. Have a smaller-than-normal breakfast, lunch, and dinner (as early in the evening as possible during this retreat), plus two snacks at mid-morning and midafternoon. If you are truly hungry in the evening, then a light snack such as a piece of fresh fruit is okay. You don't want to do anything to interfere with getting a good night's sleep. Remember to eat slowly, chew your food thoroughly, set a lovely table, and sit down to eat, don't discuss problems, and keep your thoughts loving and positive.

With all of the levels, include the following supplements or foods:

- Sprouts: include fresh sprouts in at least one of your meals, such as in a salad or as a snack.

- AlkaLife: 10 drops in your half gallon of water.

- Barlean's Organic Flax Oil and Greens: 1 tablespoon daily added to your smoothie, dressing, juice, or other food.

- Sun Chlorella: take tablets on an empty stomach. If you're new to eating and living healthfully, start with 5 tablets on the first day and add 1 extra tablet per day, ending with 10 on days six and seven. For everyone else, take between 10 and 30 tablets daily, starting low and building up, as desired.

- Emer'gen-C: take 3 packets daily in water or juice spread out during the day.

- ALL ONE: 1 tablespoon daily in juice or smoothie.

- Living Food: 1 tablespoon daily in juice, smoothie, or other beverage. Living Cleanse: refer to the directions on the bottle for the amount you should take in the evening with your last glass of water. Start taking this three days before the retreat begins. Finally, take Living Enzymes with your meals.

- Kyolic: refer to the directions on the bottle.

- Vitality Shake: See recipe on page 210. The Vitality Shake already includes Living Food, Flax Oil, ALL ONE, and 2 servings of fruit. By adding some Barlean's Organic Greens powder, you'll be getting half of your supplements for the day.

- If weight loss is a goal, make the Weight Loss Express juice (see page 200) for your midmorning *or* midafternoon snack. Be creative with the combinations.

- If you need an extra Detox Boost, make a fresh juice daily with carrot, celery, beet, and parsley. If it is too potent for you, dilute it with some apple juice. You may also want to vary it by adding some ginger, lemon, or garlic. Remember, always drink your juices slowly and, unless you're using the Green Power or Green Life juicers, drink them immediately upon juicing.

- I recommend getting some cultured vegetables by Rejuvenative Foods. These are delicious, raw veggie combinations that help promote a healthy digestive tract, which is essential for radiant health and vitality.

Retreat Levels

Level 1

Choose from a variety of plant-based whole foods only and make sure that 50% of your daily diet is raw.

Level 2

Choose from a variety of plant-based whole foods only, make sure that 50% of your daily diet is raw, and pick one or two days during the week to eat only raw foods until the dinner meal, which will be at least 50% raw.

Level 3

Choose from a variety of plant-based whole foods only and eat only raw food from morning to dinner. Make sure that 50% of your dinner meal is raw food.

Level 4

Choose from a variety of plant-based whole foods only, eat all raw food from morning to dinner, make sure that 50% of your dinner meal is raw food, and pick two days during the week when you only eat raw food even through the dinner meal for two 36-hour periods on only raw food.

Living Food Retreats
Level 5

Choose from a variety of plant-based whole foods only and eat them only raw for the entire week. That means no cooked food at all! Remember, you can have lots of fresh fruits and vegetables, beautiful salads, a few seeds and nuts (limit to one ounce daily if weight loss is a goal), fresh sprouts that you've grown, including sprouted legumes, seeds and nuts, fresh juices, smoothies, etc. Be creative. Enjoy the process. Know that your body is thriving and delighting in your special attention and loving care.

Level 6

Choose from a variety of plant-based whole foods, eat them only raw for the entire week, and take one or two days during the week, such as Monday and Thursday, to consume only fresh juices and smoothies during the day, and go back to all raw foods at dinner.

Level 7

Choose from a variety of plant-based whole foods only, eat them all raw for the entire week, take one or two days to consume only fresh juices and smoothies through dinner (36-hour period) and add three additional "Super Detox & Rejuvenate" days of fresh fruit and romaine lettuce only at the beginning of the program, making it a 10-Day Retreat.

I usually do this retreat at least a couple of times a year. Start Friday morning as Day 1 and consume nothing but watermelon all day and night. Eat as much as you want. Watermelon is a cooling food and will help cleanse the liver and kidneys. On Day 2, eat only cantaloupe throughout the day and night. Cantaloupe is a warming and laxative food. Then on Day 3, nothing but papaya, which will cleanse and strengthen the entire digestive system, including the intestines. If watermelon and/or cantaloupe is not in season or not to your liking, substitute others melons. If you don't like papaya, substitute mangos or pears or a combination of apples and blueberries (or other berries in season), again, eating as much as you feel like without stuffing yourself. Place fruit on a bed of romaine lettuce and sprinkle with a little cinnamon.

These three days will deeply detoxify and rejuvenative your entire body, give your digestive system a much-needed rest, increase your energy, decrease fat and toxic build-up, break unhealthy food habits, increase your life force (chi), and deepen your meditations. This is clearly not a program you'll continue indefinitely even though you'll be feeling so good that you might want to go longer. Instead, starting with Day 4, continue on with Level 7.

(It's always prudent to check with your doctor or health practitioner before beginning a detox program. If you are diabetic, avoid the three days on just fruit.)

During these three fresh fruit only days, you don't need to take any supplements. Resume supplements on Day 4. I'm often asked if you can add these three days to the beginning of the other levels. Yes, but only with Levels 3 or higher.

Make sure to gently and lovingly ease back into your normal routine. Make sure to continue eating lots of fresh fruits and vegetables, the healthiest foods you can eat. Hopefully, you'll take many of these health- and life-enriching activities and habits with you so that your health and vitality will continue to grow in a upward direction.

Most importantly, approach the 7- and 10-Day Retreats with enthusiasm, joy, and reverence knowing that you are a miracle, that life is meant to be a celebration, and that you have the power and ability to be the best you can be: physically, mentally, emotionally, and spiritually. "If it's to be, it's up to me," is a great affirmation. Success is within your reach. Choose to take the path that leads to greatness that is you, as Robert Frost recommends in one of my favorite passages from *The Road Not Taken:*

I shall be telling this with a sigh
Somewhere ages and ages hence;
Two roads diverged in a wood, and I—
I took the one less traveled by,
And that has made all the difference.

I salute your great adventure!

Resource Directory

AERON LIFE CYCLES CLINICAL LABORATORY
(800) 631-7900, www.aeron.com
John M. Kells, co-author of the outstanding book *The HRT Solution*, is co-founder and CEO of Aeron Life Cycles Clinical Laboratories which is one of the world's most specialized hormone testing laboratories. I've been using Aeron's services for years to keep my hormones in balance.

ALKALIFE® & THERMOTEX
(888) 261-0870, www.alkalife.com
To help carry acidic wastes out of the body and relieve the cause of pain without side effects AlkaLife and Thermotex are the best solution.

ALL ONE Nutritech,
(800) 235-5727, www.all-one.com
This is a pure, high potency multiple vitamin and mineral powder that contains more than 50 important nutrients in well-balanced proportions.

AMERICAN VEGAN SOCIETY
(856) 694-2887, www.americanvegan.org
The American Vegan Society is a nonprofit, educational member-supported organization that explores compassionate living concepts. Membership includes a quarterly periodical with terrific vegan recipes, fascinating interviews, and valuable information to help you live a healthier lifestyle.

BARLEAN'S ORGANIC FLAX OIL & BARLEAN'S ORGANIC GREENS
(800) 445-3529, www.barleans.com
Barlean's Flax Oil is a superior quality and delicious tasting flax oil. The president of the company, Bruce Barlean, and his dedicated team of employees all have a commitment to excellence in producing only the best oils possible and a superlative green food powder.

BIO-STRATH
(800) 439-2324, www.bio-strath.ch
Bio-Strath is an all-natural herbal yeast product that provides a well-balanced, nutrient-rich whole food tonic that both supports and maintains balance of our body systems.

BODYSLANT, AIR-Age in Reverse
(888) AGE EASY (243-3279)
The BodySlant is a superb slant board that also functions as a bed and ottoman. I've been using one for over 30 years.

EMER'GEN-C, Alacer Corporation
www.alacercorp.com
This is a tangy non-acidic, effervescent Vitamin C drink mix that I've been

taking for more than 20 years. While it comes in many flavors, my favorites are Raspberry, Triple Power and Lite with MSM.

FINNLEO SAUNA & STEAM
(800) 346-6536, www.finnleo.com
It is the Finnleo quality and commitment to excellence that creates the perfect atmosphere to maximize the timeless therapeutic and cosmetic benefits of steam and sauna.

FOUNTAINSIDE, Bonsai World
(888) 296-8792, www.fountainside.com
This company makes the most beautiful fountains I've ever seen in a variety of sizes, designs, and prices. Each fountain is an original work of art, handcrafted from natural rocks and beautiful quartz.

GOLD MINE NATURAL FOOD COMPANY
(800) 475-3663 www.goldminenaturalfood.com
A great source for quality organic, plant-based and hard-to-find foods, including Celtic Sea Salt.

GOLDEN RATIO
(800) 345-1129, www.GoldenRatio.com
Golden Ratio has built custom massage tables for 20 years. High quality, beauty, innovation, ergonomic design, and superb customer service have earned them a worldwide reputation for excellence.

GREEN POWER® & GREEN LIFE™ JUICER/MACHINE,
Tribest Corporation, for orders, call the Whole Person Health Services: (800) 245-4691
The award-winning Green Life juicer is the one I use and recommend for anyone interested in being radiantly healthy and restoring youthful vitality. It is easy to use, assemble, disassemble, clean, and carry (it has a convenient carrying handle).

HANDY PANTRY
(800) 735-0630, www.handypantry.com
Sprouts are one of the most rejuvenating and detoxifying foods you can eat and are complete whole living foods. To get started, their "Basic Sprouting Starter Kit" is perfect.

HEAVENLY HEAT SAUNAS
(800) MY SAUNA (697-2862)
Heavenly Heat saunas are superlative portable saunas built without adhesives or synthetic materials. This sauna incorporates a flow-through air ventilation system that includes an activated carbon filter at the exit vent along with a combination of traditional and infrared heat.

IONIZER PLUS®, High Tech Health, Inc.
(800) 794-5355
This is the most advanced water ionizer and purifier on the market. It installs in minutes and it's the only one I highly recommend for anyone wanting radiant health and vitality.

KYOLIC, Wakunaga of America
(800) 421-2998, www.kyolic.com
Kyolic Aged Garlic is a remarkable nutritional supplement that I've taken for more than 30 years. It offers all the healing and salutary benefits of garlic without affecting your breath.

LIFE-FLO HEALTH CARE PRODUCTS
(888) 999-7440, www.life-flo.com
At Life-flo, they approach hormonal changes with well-researched "state-of-the-art" solutions and products that are natural, organic and ecologically sound.

LIVING FOOD, SineQuaNon
(800) 310-0729, www.sinequanon4life.com
To receive a sample of Living Food, or their other excellent products, such as Living Cleanse & Living Enzymes, or to order directly and receive *free* recipes, call the number above.

MOUNTAIN VALLEY GROWERS
(559) 338-2775, www.mountainvalleygrowers.com
Many of the recipes in this book call for fresh herbs. I get mine delivered to my door from this wonderful company, the nation's largest certified organic grower of herbs and perennials.

NATIONAL HEALTH ASSOCIATION, formally referred to as the American Natural Hygiene Society, (813) 855-6607, www.anhs.org
This health-promoting organization publishes the award-winning *Health Science* magazine. Members also receive discounts on health books, videos, cassette programs, seminars, lectures, and more.

PEACE PILGRIM, Friends of Peace Pilgrim
7350 Dorado Canyon Road, Somerset, CA 95684, www.peacepilgrim.com
To receive a free, 32-page booklet, *Steps Toward Inner Peace*; a free 216-page book titled *Peace Pilgrim*; a marvelous free video documentary titled "The Spirit of Peace;" or an inspiring newsletter, write to the above address.

PHYSICIANS COMMITTEE FOR RESPONSIBLE MEDICINE,
5100 Wisconsin Avenue, NW, Suite 404
Washington, DC , (202) 686-2210, www.pcrm.org
Become a member of PCRM and keep up with nutritional developments through their twenty-four-page quarterly magazine, *Good Medicine*.

REJUVENATIVE FOODS, (831) 462-6715
www.rejuvenative.com
This company offers some of my favorite "living" foods, including organic raw nut and seed butters, such as Tahini, Almond, Sunflower, Cashew, as well as Cultured Vegetables.

SELF-REALIZATION FELLOWSHIP, 3880 San Rafael Avenue
Los Angeles, CA 90065 (323) 225-2471
Write for information on Paramahansa Yogananda, his books, meditation, home study lessons, the locations of the Self-Realization Fellowship Centers, or a catalog of their books, tapes, quarterly magazine, and other products. I

use and recommend their award-winning week-at-a-glance calendar to use for your Gratitude Journal.

SHIATSU-AID MASSAGE BOARD
(888) 556-2117 or (253) 572-6143, www.takahashi-shiatsu.com

This is a remarkable, effective acupressure massage aid to ease or relieve aches and pains caused by the tension and stress of everyday invented by Professor George Takahashi, 6th degree black belt in the Shotokan Karate style and a Shiatsu expert.

SUN CHLORELLA, Sun Chlorella USA
(800) 829-2828, ext. 55, www.sunchlorellausa.com

Chlorella is a superlative microscopic green single-celled freshwater algae that is a pure, whole food. It is nutrient rich and contains more than 20 different vitamins and minerals, all of the essential amino acids, (including DNA and RNA) fiber, and life-giving chlorophyll. It's a terrific detoxifier and rejuvenator.

THE GRAIN & SALT SOCIETY
(800) 867-7258, www.celtic-seasalt.com

The Grain & Salt Society is your one-stop shopping resource for a variety of healthy food items you'll use daily, including Celtic Sea Salt from France.

TREE OF LIFE REJUVENATION CENTER
(520) 394-2520, www.treeofliferejuvenation.com

Founded by Gabriel Cousens, M.D., the Tree of Life Rejuvenation Center offers a variety of retreats that rejuvenate and nurture body, mind, and spirit and include juice fasting, live-food cuisine, organic gardening, massage, meditation, and all aspects of holistic health.

TRUENORTH HEALTH CENTER
(707) 792-2325

Co-founded by Dr. Alan Goldhamer and Dr. Jennifer Marano, the center offers alternative approaches to the restoration and maintenance of optimum health by focusing on diet and lifestyle changes.

UNITY VILLAGE AND RETREAT CENTER
(816) 524-3550, www.unityworldhq.org

Unity Village offers wonderful retreats ranging from one day to two weeks to rejuvenate body, mind, and spirit. The *Daily Word* is published monthly by Unity School of Christianity, Unity Village, and offers a daily inspirational message and affirmation you'll think was written just for you.

VITA MIX, (800) 848-2649, www.vitamix.com
The Vita-Mix, which I've used for decades, is a remarkable blender—and so much more—and makes eating a whole food and 'living' diet easy and fun.

X-ISER™, (888) 390-0104, www.x-iser.com
For your home or office, or to take on trips, the X-iser is the perfect piece of equipment for anyone who wants to lose fat, tone up, or take your fitness level to the top.

About the Author

Susan Smith Jones is the author of 10 books, including *Choose to Live Peacefully,* more than 500 magazine articles, and appears regularly on radio and television talk shows around the country. She holds an M.S. in kinesiology and Ph.D. in Health Sciences and has been a Fitness Instructor to students, staff, and faculty at UCLA for 30 years and works with individuals and families as a personal growth and holistic lifestyle coach.

Her inspiring message and innovative techniques for achieving total health in body, mind, and spirit have won her an enthusiastic following internationally. Susan travels year-round as a health and fitness consultant and motivational speaker. She is also founder and president of Health Unlimited, a Los Angeles-based consulting firm dedicated to the advancement of peaceful, balanced living, personal empowerment, and health and fitness education.

For more information on Susan and her work or to place an order for her books or tape albums, log on to, **www.susansmithjones.com**

Interested in a **WORKSHOP, SEMINAR, LECTURE, or KEYNOTE ADDRESS** by Dr. Susan S. Jones? If so, contact the Universal Speakers Bureau, **(800) 644-4144**.

If you would like to schedule Susan to give a motivational presentation to your corporation, community, church, or school group, please call the above number.

CELEBRATE LIFE! A best-selling series of seven cassette tapes, will educate, inspire, motivate, and empower you to develop your fullest potential. For those of you who are new to Susan's work, this is a complete program providing a wealth of practical and uplifting information you can use immediately. Those who are already familiar with her work will garner tips to fine-tune and upgrade your existing wellness lifestyle so you can live more healthfully than ever before—physically, mentally, emotionally, and spiritually.

This tape series has helped thousands of people to reclaim radiant health, joy, and vitality and reconnect with their inner power. It includes 7 tapes, 14 programs, Susan's favorite affirmations, and 6 guided meditations. To order *Celebrate Life!,* send a payment of $80.00 (U.S. check or money order—includes S & H) made payable to: Health Unlimited, PO Box 49396, Los Angeles, CA 90049. Please allow 4 weeks for delivery. (Outside the U.S., please include $95.00.)

Subject Index

Abdominals, developing, 105–108
Abused children, massage for, 186
Accountability, 49
Acidic wastes, 174
  degenerative diseases and, 175
  pain and, 176–177
Acid water, 172–173
Acupressure, 187
Adrenal compromise, 8
Adrenaline, 6
  exercise and, 87
  rushes, 8
Advanced dip exercise, 113
Aerobic exercise, 108–109
  cellulite, eliminating, 140
  machines for, 130
  metabolism and, 129–130
Aerobic riders, 130
Aeron Life Cycles, 9–10, 142
  resource information, 457
Affirmations
  and exercise, 99
  for fat loss, 43–44
  goals, supporting, 44–45
  morning affirmation, 422
  Re-Entry Affirmation, 441–442
  on 7-day detox and rejuvenate retreat, 451
  subconscious mind, repro-
    gramming, 40–42
  using, 45
African Americans, lactose
  intolerance, 64
Afterburn, 95
Afternoon activities on 3-day
  rejuvenation retreat, 427–429
Aging. See also Elderly persons
  cortisol levels and, 8–9
  enzymes and, 68–69
  estrogen-dominance and, 64
  exercise and, 91–92
  garlic and, 163, 164
  process of, 174
  sleep deprivation and, 178
  strength training and, 89–90
Ahlgrimm, Marla, 71
AIDS, massage and, 186
Air pollution, 162
Alcoholic beverages, 16, 74
  cutting consumption of, 139
  sleep and, 181
  on 3-day rejuvenation retreat, 420
Alfalfa sprouts, 152–153
Aliveness Program, 126
AlkaLife, 93, 139–140, 176, 453
  for internal water bath, 422
  resource information, 457
  skin health and, 194
Alkaline water, 172–173
  importance of, 175
  water ionizers, using, 175–176

Allen, James, vii, 52
Allergies
  flax seed oil and, 160
  milk allergies, 63
  stress and, 5
ALL ONE, 167, 453
  resource information, 457
Almond milk, 62
Alpha consciousness, 41
Alpha-linolenic acid. See
  Omega-3 fatty acid
Altering state of consciousness, 46
Alternate-nostril breathing, 424–425
Alternative Medicine Review, 63
Alzheimer's disease
  garlic and, 163, 164
  vitamin C and, 165
American College of Sports
  Medicine, 17, 131
American Diabetes Association
  diet, 60, 147
American Heart Association
  on MetLife tables, 118
  recommended diet, 60
American Journal of Clinical
  Nutrition, 80
American Vegan Society, 457
Amino acids
  in ALL ONE, 167
  in chlorella, 162
  cortisol and, 7
  in Living Food, 167
  sleep and, 181
  in sprouts, 150
Amylase, 68
Anemia, iron-deficiency, 62–63
Anger, 5
Animal products, 57–62
  avoiding, 76
  biological concentration, 61
  fiber and, 137
  on 3-day rejuvenation retreat, 420–421
Annals of Epidemiology, 121
Anorexia, 119
Anti-Aging Plan (Walfor), 135
Antibiotics in foods, 162
Antioxidants
  in ALL ONE, 167
  exercise and, 92
  in fruits and vegetables, 18, 147
  in Living Food, 167
Appetite
  curbing, 31
  exercise and, 92–93
Arachidonic acid cascade, 160
Arm exercises, 112–113
Aromatherapy, 188
Arthritis, 159
Arugula, 66
As a Man Thinketh (Allen), 52
Ascorbate acid. See Vitamin C

Ascorbic acid, 166–167
Asian Americans, lactose
  intolerance, 64
Asian diet, 57–58
"As if" acting, 40
Aspartame, 83–85
Asthma
  clothing and, 22–23
  milk allergies and, 63
Atherosclerosis, 57
  LDL (low-density lipoprotein)
    and, 88
Attitude. See also Positiveness
  power of, 50–51
Attwood, Charles, 72
Autoimmune diseases, 61

Baby weights, 83
Bach, Richard, 37
Back
  exercises, 114
  flexibility and, 101
  lower back, stretching, 104–105
Bailey, Covert, 86, 122, 123, 124, 140
Bandy, William D., 103
Barbie dolls, 119
Barlean, Bruce, 457
Barlean's Organic Flax Oil, 75, 139, 161, 453
  resource information, 457
Barlean's Organic Greens, 18, 76, 206, 418, 423, 427, 432, 433, 436, 439, 446, 453
  resource information, 457
Barnard, Neal, 71
Baseball, 131
Basic crunches, 107
Basketball, 131
Bathing on 3-day rejuvenation
  retreat, 422–423
Batmanghelidj, F., 15, 17, 71
Beauty, living in, 195–196
Becoming Vegan: The Complete
  Guide to Adopting a Healthy
  Plant-Based Diet (Davis &
  Melina), 71
Bedtime on 3-day rejuvenation
  retreat, 430
Belief, subconscious mind and, 42
Benson, Herbert, 12
Bernard, Claude, 29
Beta carotene
  bone health and, 62
  in chlorella, 162
  color of fruits/vegetables and, 81
Beta consciousness, 41
Beta-sistosterin, 157
Beutler, Jade, 71
Bicycling, 130
Bioelectric impedance test, 123

Biofeedback, 40–42
Bioflavonoids, 81
  whole foods and, 138
Biological concentration, 61
Bio-Strath, 168
  resource information, 458
Biotin, 138
Bipolar disorder, 160
Bird-watching, 428–429
Birth control pills, 122
Bladder cancer, 162
Blender drinks, 432
Blood pressure, 57
  fiber and, 149
  insulin and, 78
  monitoring, 122
  sweating and, 184
  vitamin C and, 165
Blood sugar, 9
Body
  composition of, 55
  fat, determining, 122–125
  loving care of, 49
  nurturing, 28–34
  shape of, 118–125
  temperature and sleep, 180
Body Mass Index (BMI),
  118–120
BodySlant, 12–13
  resource information, 458
  for stretching, 104
*The Body's Many Cries for
  Water* (Batmanghelidj), 16
Bone health. *See also* Osteoporosis
  potassium and, 62
Brazil nuts, 19
Breakfasts, 31
  blender drinks, 432
  on 3-day rejuvenation retreat,
  423
Breaking up exercise, 131–132
Breast cancer
  deaths from, 57
  IGF-1 (insulin-like growth
  factor-1) and, 64
  lycopene and, 148
  progesterone cream and, 143
  water consumption and, 15
Breastfeeding. *See*
  Pregnancy/nursing
Breathing
  alternate-nostril breathing,
  424–425
  cellulite, eliminating, 140
  meditation and, 14
  mindfulness of, 20
  relaxation and, 12
  on 7-day detox and rejuvenate
  retreat, 448–449
  3-part breath exercise, 424
British Medical Journal Finnish
  study, 56–57
Budgeting, 20
Bulemia, 119
Burning Bowl Ceremony, 438
Bursitis, 159

Buscaglia, Leo, 1
Busyness sickness, 3–4
Butterfly-watching, 435
Butt exercises, 114–116
B vitamins
  in alfalfa sprouts, 152
  in ALL ONE, 167
  in flax seed, 155
  nonfat milk and, 63
  in nuts, 75
  in wheat sprouts, 150
  whole foods and, 137–138
Bypass surgery, 54

Caffeinated beverages, 16
  on 3-day rejuvenation retreat,
  421
Calcium
  in alfalfa sprouts, 152
  in flax seed, 155
  in nuts, 75
  osteoporosis and, 61
  sleep and, 181
  vitamin D and, 181
Calcium ascorbate, 166
Calories, 77–80
  burn chart, 100
  exercise and, 90
  jumping jacks, safe, 105
  metabolism and, 125
  muscle mass and, 128
  restrictions on, 73
Calves, stretching, 104
Campbell, Colin, 57, 58, 59, 61
Cancer. *See also* specific types
  animal protein and, 59
  carotenoids and, 149
  color of diet and, 81
  deaths from, 57
  excess protein consumption,
  61
  exercise and, 89
  fruits and vegetables and, 147
  garlic and, 163
  IGF-1 (insulin-like growth
  factor-1) and, 64
  massage and, 186
  omega-3 fatty acid and,
  158–159
  sunlight and, 181, 182
  vitamin C and, 165
  water consumption and, 15
Candida albicans, 168
Capodilupo, Lucia, 71
Carbohydrates
  categories of, 79
  cortisol and, 7
  in flax seed, 154
  refined carbohydrates, avoiding, 73
  sleep and, 181
  stress and, 19
  water retention and, 83
  weight gain and, 78
Carbon monoxide, 162
Carotene. *See also* Beta
  carotene

  in flax seed, 155
  in sprouts, 150
Carotenoids, 81
  cancer survival and, 149
Carpeting, wool, 23
Carruthers, Malcolm, 87
Cassandra's Angel (Otto), 180
Castelli, William P., 118, 121
Cayenne pepper, 141
Celebrate Life!, 45
Cells, 55
Cellulite, 140
  massage and, 186
Celtic Sea Salt, 82–83
Center for Conservative Ther-
  apy, 458
Center for Human Nutrition,
  University of Colorado, 120
Central obesity, 121
Chair lifts, 113
Chamomile oil, 188
Checking in, 19–20
Cheese, soy, 62
Chest exercises, 113
Chewing, 76
Children
  massage for, 186
  obesity in, 124–125
  plant-based diet resources, 72
  weight of, 83
China, diet in, 57–58
China Oxford Cornell Project,
  57–58
Chlorella, 161–163
Chlorella Growth Factor (CGF),
  162–163
Chlorine, 155
Chlorophyll, 145
  in alfalfa sprouts, 152
  in chlorella, 162
  in fruits and vegetables, 18
  in Living Food, 167
  in sprouts, 150
Chocolate, 19
  on 3-day rejuvenation retreat,
  421
Choice, power of, viii
Cholesterol, 57
  animal protein and, 58
  monosaturated fats, 76
  vitamin C and, 165
Choose to Live Peacefully
  (Smith), 180, 451
Chromium
  in flax seed, 155
  whole foods and, 137–138
Cinnamon, 141
Circulatory disease, 164
Cirrhosis, 57
Citrus fruits, 81
Climate and stress, 5
Clothing
  for exercise, 93
  natural clothing, 21–23
  on 3-day rejuvenation retreat,
  423
Cobalt, 155

Coffee. *See* Caffeinated beverages
Cohen, Robert, 71
Colitis, 159
Collagen, 195
Collards, 66
Colon cancer
  deaths from, 57
  estrogen production and, 156
  fruits and vegetables and, 147
  garlic and, 164
  omega-3 fatty acid and, 158
  water consumption and, 15
Colors, 20–21
  of vegetables/fruits, 81
Commitment, 48
  to exercise, 98
  to highest vision, 2
Conscious Eating (Cousens), 69, 71
Conscious mind, 36–38
Consciousness, changing, 36–38, 40–42, 46
Constipation
  flax seed and, 154–155
  water consumption and, 15
Continuous rotation crunch, 107–108
Cooper Aerobic Center, 130
Coordination, water and, 16
Copper
  in flax seed, 155
  whole foods and, 137–138
Copper ascorbate, 166
Cortisol, 6
  exercise and, 87
  food cravings and, 10–11
  sleep deprivation and, 178
  stress, role in, 7–10
  testing levels of, 10
  weight gain, 10–11
Cotton fabrics, 22
The Courage to Be Rich (Orman), 20
Cousens, Gabriel, 69, 71, 462
Cousins, Norman, 41, 169
Crack-addicted babies, massage for, 186
Creativity in exercise, 99
CRH, 6
Criticism, letting go of, 49–50
Cross-country machines, 130
Cross-country skiing, 130
Cystic fibrosis, 160

Dairy products, 62–65. *See also* Milk
  allergies to, 63
  avoiding, 76
  iron-deficiency anemia, 62–63
  pesticide residues in, 82
Dancing, 131
Davis, Brenda, 71
Day, Jackie, 190
De-cluttering your life, 24–25
Deep tissue massage, 188
Degenerative diseases, 157–158

acidic wastes and, 175
blood circulation and, 174
Dehydration, 15
  sweating and, 184
Delta consciousness, 41
Dement, William C., 178–179, 180
Dementia, 15
Deoxypyridinoline (Dpd) bond resorption tests, 9
Department of Agriculture
  Jean Mayer Human Nutrition Research Center on Aging, Tufts University, 77
  milk products, regulation of, 64
Depression
  cortisol levels and, 9
  estrogen-dominance and, 64
  exercise and, 87
  flax seed oil and, 160
  progesterone cream and, 143
  stress and, 5–6
Dermis, 192
Desire
  being what you, 36–38
  visualization of, 43
Despres, Jean Pierre, 120
Desserts, avoiding, 76
Detox Boost, 454
Detoxification, 70, 162, 169–197
  water and, 172–173
De Vries, Herbert, 14
DHEA, 6
  and cortisol, 8, 9
  testing levels of, 10
Diabetes. *See also* Insulin
  deaths from, 57
  exercise and, 91
  flax seed oil and, 159
  fruits and vegetables for, 147
  insulin process and, 78
  milk and, 63
  refined carbohydrates and, 79
Diarrhea, 70
Dieting, 54
Digestive gas, 70
Dinner on 3-day rejuvenation retreat, 429
Discipline, 47–48
Discover the Health Equation (Fuhrman), 71, 79
Diuretics, 16
Diverticulosis, 147
Dizziness, 15
DNA (deoxyribonucleic acid), 163
Dogs, exercising with, 93–94
Do No Harm (Ohno), 71
Don't Drink Your Milk (Oski), 71
Double arm crunch, 108
Dr. Atkins diet, 77
Dr. Attwood's Low Fat Prescription for Kids (Attwood), 72
Drug-addicted babies, massage for, 186
Drugs on 3-day rejuvenation retreat, 420
Dry skin brushing, 193–194

cellulite, eliminating, 140
  on 7-day detox and rejuvenate retreat, 447
Duke, James, 158
Duncan, John, 130
Dyer, Wayne, 40
Dyno-Mill process, 163

Eating. *See also* Foods; Nutrition program
  grazing, 133–135
  process of, 32–33
  sleep and, 181
  wrong reasons for, 72
Eating disorders, 118
Eating in the Light (Virtue & Perlitz), 71
Eczema, 194
Einstein, Albert, 46, 53
Elastin, 195
Elderly persons. *See also* Aging
  massage for, 190
  strength training, 89–90
Elliptical machines, 130
Emer'gen-C, 17, 18, 93, 166, 453
  resource information, 458
  for skin, 195
Emerson, Ralph Waldo, xii, 35
Emotions
  belief and, 37
  negative emotions, 39
  as stress triggers, 5
  subconscious, power in, 43–44
Emphysema
  clothing and, 22–23
  deaths from, 57
Empowerment, 1
Endocrine events, 5
Endorphins
  laughter and, 24
  menopause symptoms and, 92
Endurance exercise, 89–90, 133
Energy
  cortisol levels and, 9
  flax seed oil and, 160
  progesterone cream and, 143
  whole foods and, 137–138
Energy Metabolism Laboratory, 77
Enkephalin, 87
Environmental Protection Agency (EPA), 171
Enzyme Nutrition, The Food Enzyme Concept (Howell), 68
Enzymes
  aging and, 68–69
  in alfalfa sprouts, 152
  in fruits and vegetables, 18
  in Living Food, 167
  raw foods and, 67–68
  weight lifting and, 128–129
Epidermis, 192
Esophagus cancer
  fruits and vegetables and, 147
  garlic and, 164
Essential fatty acids (EFAs), 156–157

thyroid gland and, 141
Essential oils, 188
Estradiol, 10
Estriol, 10
Estrogen
   for beef cattle, 64
   body fat and, 122
   cortisol levels and, 9
   exercise and, 89
   fat and, 141–142
   lignans and, 156
   phytoestrogens, 62
Estrogen-dominance, 142
Estrone, 10
Eucalyptus oil, 188
Euripides, 32
Evans, William, 89
Everyday Cooking with Dr. Dean Ornish (Ornish), 71
Evian mist, 194
Excretion, 16
Exercise, 14–15. *See also* Aerobic exercise; Flexibility; Strength training
   abdominals, developing, 105–108
   arm exercises, 112–113
   back exercise, 114
   breaking up, 131–132
   butt exercises, 114–116
   cellulite, eliminating, 140
   changing workout routine, 112
   chart for, 111
   chest/shoulders, 113
   habits, changing, 46–47
   individualizing your program, 108–112
   intensity of, 96, 132–133
   leg exercises, 114–116
   metabolism and, 90, 126, 129–130
   morning workouts, 100
   motivations for, 95, 98–99
   non-aerobic exercises, 131
   set point theory and, 73
   on 7-day detox and rejuvenate retreat, 449–450
   skin health and, 194
   skin temperature and, 192
   sleep and, 179–180
   stress and, 5
   stretching, 102–105
   target heart rate, 95–98
   techniques for, 94–95
   in 3-day rejuvenation retreat, 325–326
   tips for, 93–94
   tracking daily progress, 98
   vitality and, 87–93
   water consumption and, 17
   weight loss regime and, 69
Exercise Physiology Laboratory, University of Southern California, 14
Experiences, 41–42
Eye conditions
   carotenoids and, 149

flax seed oil and, 160

Fabrics, natural, 21–23
Fad diets, 77–78
Faith, 43
Family and stress, 5
Far-infrared (FIR) heating pads, 176–177
Fast foods, 55–56
Fasting and Eating for Health (Fuhrman), 71
Fatigue
   dehydration and, 15
   estrogen-dominance and, 64
   exercise and, 87
   flax seed oil and, 160
Fats
   avoiding, 74
   decreasing, 73
   disease and, 59
   good fats, eating, 76, 138–139
Fear
   eating and, 72
   as stress trigger, 5
Feed Your Body Right (Smith), 56, 72–73
Feelings, power of, 38–39
Fiatarone, Maria, 89, 90
Fiber, 145
   in chlorella, 162
   dairy products and, 63
   in flax seed, 154
   foods containing, 149
   in fruits and vegetables, 148
   for health, 148–150
   high-fiber diet, 16
   in Living Food, 167
   metabolism and, 137
   in nuts, 75
   from whole foods, 150
Fibroblast cells, 195
Field, Tiffany, 187
Field/ice hockey, 131
Fight Fat After Forty (Peeke), 10, 71
Fight or flight response
   flax seed oil and, 160
   sleep deprivation and, 178
Finances, 20
Finger printing, 192–193
Finnish study *(British Medical Journal)*, 56–57
Finnleo Sauna & Steam, 185
   resource information, 459
Fish oils, 158
Fit from Within (Moran), 71
Fitness trainers, 111
Flavonoids, 81
Flax for Life (Beutler), 71
Flax seed, 153–157
   Barlean's Organic Flax Oil, 75, 139, 161
   grinding, 161
   in Living Food, 167
   storing oil, 161
   using oil, 161
Flax Seed grinders, 139

Flexibility, 101–108
   stretching, 102–105
   yoga increasing, 101–102
Flinders University of South Australia, 164
Flowers, 24
Fluorine, 155
Folic acid
   in wheat sprouts, 150
   whole foods and, 138
Food additives, 162
Food and Drug Administration (FDA)
   aspartame, 83–84
   food additives, 162
   milk products, regulation of, 64
Food chain, eating down the, 81–82
Food Enzymes: The Missing Link to Radiant Health (Santillo), 69
Food Guide Pyramid, 80
The Food Revolution (Robbins), 71
Foods. *See also* Eating; Nutrition program; Plant-based diet; Raw foods; Whole foods
   aspartame in, 84
   cravings, cortisol and, 10–11
   seasoning foods, 141
   whole foods, choosing, 32
Foods That Fight Pain (Barnard), 71
Football, 131
Foot/hand reflexology, 187
Forgiveness, practicing, 39
Forti-Flax meal, 139
Fountains, 23
Fountainside, 458
Framingham Heart Study, 118
Francis of Assisi, Saint, 417
Franklin, Benjamin, 169
Frequent meals, 74
Frisbees, 97
Frisch, Rose E., 89
Frost, Robert, 456
Frugality, 39–40
Fruits and vegetables
   adding to meals, 76
   green fruits and vegetables, 81
   weight loss tips, 75
   in nutrition program, 32
   servings of, 66–67
   stress reduction and, 18–19
   as super foods, 145–148
   weight loss tips, 74–75
Fuhrman, Joel, 71, 79, 80
Fuller, Buckminster, 28

Gamma linoleic acid (GLA), 139
Gandhi, Mahatma, 153
Garlic, 163–165
Gastritis, 159
Genetics, eating and, 72
Get the Fat Out (Moran), 71

Getty Museum, Los Angeles, 435
Ginger, 141
Glucose, 178
Glycogen, 128
Goals
   fitness goals, 98
   for stretching, 103–104
   visualization of, 42–46
God-centered, ix
Goethe, Johann Wolfgang von,
   ix
Golden Ratio massage table, 189
   resource information, 458
Goldhamer, Alan, 57, 458
Gold Mine Natural Food Com-
   pany, 459
Golf, 131
   speed golf, 97–98
Grains, refined, 79–80
The Grain & Salt Society, 462
Grant, William B., 63
Gratitude, 49
   living with, 25–26
   nutrition program and, 33
Gratitude journal, 26, 49
   on 7-day detox and rejuvenate
      retreat, 451
Graves' disease, 84
Grazing, 133–135
   on 7-day detox and rejuvenate
      retreat, 453
Green fruits and vegetables. See
   Fruits and vegetables
Green Power/Green Life
   Juicer/Machine, 459
Grief and stress, 5
Guilt and stress, 5
Gymnastics, 131

Habits, changing, 46–47
Hamstrings, stretching, 102–103,
   104
Hand-eye coordination, 16
Handy Pantry
   Basic Sprouting Starter Kit, 152
   resource information, 459
Hanley, Jesse Lynn, 71
Happiness, viii
Harvard. See also Nurses Health
      Study
   School of Public Health and
      Center for Population
      Studies, 89
   vitamin C, power of, 165–166
Hatha yoga, 101
HDL (high-density lipoprotein)
   exercise raising, 88
   insulin and, 78
Headaches
   dehydration and, 15
   paying attention to, 29
   plant-based diet, changing to,
      70
Health, 29
Heart. See also Heart disease
   bypass surgery, 54
   healthy lifestyles for, 56–57

target heart rate, 95–98
Heart disease
   color of diet and, 81
   dairy products and, 63
   exercise and, 88
   Finnish study (British Medical
      Journal), 56–57
   flavonoids and, 81
   flax seed oil and, 159
   fruits and vegetables and, 147
   garlic and, 164
   Lifestyle Heart Trial, 60
   overweight and, 120
   refined grains and, 80
   vitamin C and, 165
   Waist/Hip Ratio (WHR) and, 121
Heart monitors, 96
Heating pads, far-infrared (FIR),
   176–177
Heavenly Heat saunas, 185
   resource information, 459
Heber, David, 71, 81
Heel raises, 114
Helping others, 50
Hepatitis, 159
Herbicides, 81–82
Hesperidin, 81
Hexene, 188
High-intensity exercise, 132–133
Hiking, 130
Hill, James O., 120
Hip-flexor muscles, 101
Hippocrates, vi, 29, 145
Hispanic Americans, lactose
   intolerance, 64
Homocysteine, 164
Honesty, living with, 25
Honoring yourself, 196–197
Hormone creams, 10
Hormone replacement therapy
   (HRT), 122
Hormones
   balancing, 141–142
   exercise and, 87
   as food additives, 162
   stress and, 5, 6
   testing, 9–10
Horseback riding, 131
Hot flashes, 92
Howell, Edward, 68–69
How to Get Kids to Eat Great and
      Love It! (Wood), 72
The HRT Solution (Kells &
      Ahlgrimm), 5, 71
Hu, Frank B., 91
Hull, Janet Starr, 84–85
Humor, 23–24
Hunger, feeling, 31
Hurry sickness, 3–4
Hypersensitivity diseases, 61
Hypnosis, 40–42
Hypothalamus, 6

Ice packs, 176
Ice skating, 131
Identification when exercising, 93

IGF-1 (insulin-like growth
      factor-1), 64
Ileitis, 159
Immune system
   Bio-Strath for, 168
   cortisol and, 7
   dairy products and, 63
   environmental toxins and, 162
   exercise and, 92
   garlic and, 163, 164
   psychoneuroimmunology
      (PNI), 170
   saunas and, 184
Industrial meals/chemicals,
   81–82
Infant weights, 83
Infection, vitamin C and, 165
Inflammatory conditions, 159
Injury and stress, 5
Inner power, generating, 39–40
Insect-watching, 428–429
Insoluble fiber, 149
Insomnia, 179
Inspiration, 1
Insulin
   fiber and, 148
   process of, 78
   sugar and, 73
Insulin resistance, 78–79
   dieting and, 135
Integrity, living with, 25
Intensity of exercise, 132–133
Internal water bath, 422
Intestinal cancer, 164
Intuition, nurturing, 25
Iodine
   in chlorella, 162
   in flax seed, 155
The Ion Effect (Soyka), 21–22
Ionizer Plus, 175
   resource information, 459
Ions, 21–22
Iron
   in alfalfa sprouts, 152
   in chlorella, 162
   in flax seed, 155
   sleep and, 181
   whole foods and, 137–138
Iron-deficiency anemia, 62–63
Irritability, 64

JAMA (Journal of the American
      Medical Association)
   diabetes-exercise connection,
      91
   on exercise, 91, 99
   Nurses Health Study, 88
James, William, 37
Jean Mayer Human Nutrition
      Research Center on Aging,
      Tufts University, 77
Jogging, 97, 130
John, Esther, 182
Joint health, 166–167
Jonathan Livingston Seagull
   (Bach), 37
Jones, Susan Smith, 72

Journal of the American College of Nutrition, 138
Journal of the American Heart Association, 148–149
Journals
  gratitude journal, 26, 49, 451
  on 3-day rejuvenation retreat, 426, 438–439
  on 7-day detox and rejuvenate retreat, 451
Joy activities, 442–444, 451
Judgments, letting go of, 49–50
Juice Fasting & Detoxification (Meyerowitz), 71
Juliano, 71
Jumping jacks, safe, 105
Jumping rope, 130
Junshi, Chen, 57
Junyao, Li, 57

Kale, 66
Kayaking, 97
Keller, Helen, viii
Kells, John M., 5, 7, 71, 457
Kidneys
  excess protein consumption, 61
  water consumption and, 15–16, 139–140
Kime, Zane, 143
Kindness, acting with, 26–27
Kiyasaki, Robert T., 20
Klaper, Michael, 72
Knee lift reverse crunch, 106–107
Kneeling leg curls, 114
Krueger, Albert Paul, 21–22
Kyolic Aged Garlic Extract, 163, 164–165, 453
  resource information, 460
Kyphosis, 101

LA. *See* Omega-6 fatty acid
Lamb, Lawrence, 87
Lancet, 81
Landscape pictures, 13
Langer, Stephen, 11, 18, 19
Langre, Jacques de, 71
Laughter, 23–24
Lavender oil, 180, 188
Laxatives, 154–155
LDL (low-density lipoprotein), 88
Lead in water, 162
Leafy greens, 66
Lee, John R., 64, 71, 142
Leg exercises, 114–116
Legumes, 75
Lemon oil, 188
Libido
  cortisol levels and, 9
  estrogen-dominance and, 64
  exercise and, 92
Life-Flo, 10
Lifestyle exercisers, 99
Lifestyle Heart Trial, 60
Lifestyles
  diabetes and, 91
  heart-healthy lifestyles, 56–57

Lignins/lignans, 154, 155–156
Linoleic acid. *See* Omega-6 fatty acid
Linseed. *See* Flax seed
Lipase, 68
Lipid Research Center, Laval University, 120
Lit from Within: Tending Your Soul for Lifelong Beauty (Moran), 32
Liver. *See also* Detoxification
  toxic overload, 162
  water consumption and, 139–140
Living Cleanse, 167
Living Enzymes, 69, 167
Living Food, 19, 167, 453
  resource information, 460
LNA. *See* Omega-3 fatty acid
Loneliness, 40
Longfellow, Henry Wadsworth, 11
Love
  acting with, 26–27
  living with, 50
  for yourself, 196–197
Love and Survival: The Scientific Basis for the Healing Power of Intimacy (Ornish), 143
Love Yourself Thin (Moran), 71
Lower back, stretching, 104–105
Lunch on 3-day rejuvenation retreat, 427
Lung cancer
  deaths from, 57
  fruits and vegetables and, 147
Lupus, 159
Luxuries, indulging in, 39–340
Lycopene, 148
Lymph massage, 188
Lysine, 162

Maas, James B., 180
Machines, exercising, 130
Magnesium
  in alfalfa sprouts, 152
  bone health and, 62
  in flax seed, 155
  in nuts, 75
  sleep and, 181
Manganese
  in flax seed, 155
  whole foods and, 138
Manganese ascorbate, 166
Manifest Your Destiny (Dyer), 40
Marano, Jennifer, 458
Markowitz, Elysa, 71
Massage, 20, 185–191
  cellulite, eliminating, 140
  tips for enjoying, 189–191
  variations of, 187–188
Massage tables, 189
Maximum Life Span (Walfor), 135
Mayo Proceedings, 26
Mealtime suggestions, 76
Meditation, 2, 13–14
  honoring yourself, 197

reverence, living with, 27
  on 7-day detox and rejuvenate retreat, 450
  skin health and, 195
  Stillness Meditation, 425
  subconscious mind, reprogramming, 40–42
  walking meditation, 434–435
  White Light Meditation, 431–432
Melatonin, 180
Melina, Vesanto, 71
Memory
  Bio-Strath for, 168
  garlic and, 163, 164
  water consumption and, 16
Meningitis, 159
Menopause
  beef, estrogen in, 64
  estrogen-dominance and, 142
  exercise and, 89, 92
  hot flashes, 92
  phytoestrogens and, 62
Menstrual cramps, 92
Mental health. *See also* Depression
  exercise and, 87
  flax seed oil and, 160
Meprobamate, 14
Mercury concentrations, 82
Metabolism, 117–144
  aerobic exercise and, 129–130
  alcoholic beverages, cutting, 139
  exercise and, 90, 126, 129–130
  good fats, eating, 138–139
  grazing, 133–135
  increasing, 125–144
  muscle mass and, 127–129
  spirituality and, 143–144
  strength training, 140
  sunlight and, 143, 182
  undereating, 135
  water consumption, 139–140
  weight lifting stimulating, 128–129
  whole foods and, 136–138
Metabolism, 133
Metropolitan Life Insurance weight tables, 118
Meyerowitz, Steve, 71
Milieu interieur, 29
Milk
  allergies, 63
  substitutes, 62
Milk, the Deadly Poison (Cohen), 64, 71
Mind
  conscious and subconscious mind, 36–38
  programming, 35–36
Mindfulness, 19–20
  on 3-day rejuvenation retreat, 429
Mineral ascorbates, 166–167
Minerals, 145. *See also* Trace minerals

in alfalfa sprouts, 152
in ALL ONE, 167
in chlorella, 162
in flax seed, 155
in fruits and vegetables, 18
in sea salt, 83
sleep and, 181
in sprouts, 150
Mini-trampolines, 130
Miracles, ix–x
Miscarriage, 160
Mitochondrial bioenergetics, 137–138
Molybdenum
in flax seed, 155
whole foods and, 138
Molybdenum ascorbate, 166
Monosaturated fats, 76
Monsanto, 64
Mood, vitamin D and, 182
Moran, Victoria, 32, 71
Mornings
affirmations, 422
breakfast, 31
exercise workouts, 100
Motivation for exercise, 95, 98–99
Motorcycle riding, 131
Mountain biking, 130
Mountain Valley Growers, 460
Mouth cancer, 147
Mucilage in flax seed, 154
Multiple sclerosis (MS), 160
Muscle metabolism, 125–126
Muscles. See also Strength training
abdominals, developing, 105–108
increasing muscle mass, 127–129
stress and, 11
stretching, 102–105
Music, 20
exercising to, 100
Mustard, 141

Nader, Ralph, 158
Napping, 179
National Cancer Institute, 159
National Center of Health Statistics, 117
National Health Association, 460
National Highway Traffic Safety Administration, 178
National Science Foundation (NSF), 34
Native Americans, lactose intolerance, 64
Natural Beauty and Health Magazine, 71
Natural clothing, 21–23
Natural Science Museum, Los Angeles, 435
Nature. See Outdoors
Nelson, Miriam E., 91
Nephritis, 159
Neutral water, 173
New, Susan A., 62

New England Journal of Medicine, 90
overweight and heart disease connection, 120
The New Whole Foods Encyclopedia (Wood), 71
Nickel, 155
Non-aerobic exercises, 131
Norepinephrine, 87
Norris Comprehensive Cancer Center, University of Southern California, 89
Northern California Cancer Center, 182
Northrup, Christiane, 5, 117
Nowakowski, John, 71
Nurses Health Study, 88
Body Mass Index (BMI) and, 120
diabetes-exercise connection, 91
Nursing. See Pregnancy/nursing
NutraSweet, 83–85
Nutrient density, 65–66
comparisons of foods, 146
in refined sweets, 79
Nutrition program. See also Eating
positive thoughts and, 34–35
preparation for, 30
skin health and, 194
stress and, 5
tips for, 30–34
Nuts, oils and seeds
enzymes from, 68
limiting, 75

Oat milk, 62
Obesity
central obesity, 121
in childhood, 124–125
deaths from, 57
definition of, 122
diabetes and, 91
excess protein consumption, 61
exercise and, 89
insulin resistance and, 78–79
muscle metabolism, 125–126
Ohio State University, 164
Ohno, Yoshitaka, 71
Oils. See Nuts, oils and seeds
Olive oils, 75
Omega-3 fatty acid, 139
benefits of, 158–160
deficiencies in modern diet, 157–160
in flax seed, 153–154
Omega-6 fatty acid, 139, 156–157
deficiencies in modern diet, 157–160
in flax seed, 154
The Omega-3 Phenomenon (Rudin), 157
Open knee crunch, 108
Optimism, 26
Orman, Suze, 20
Ornish, Dean, 60, 71, 143
Oski, Frank, 71

Osteoclasts, 9
Osteoporosis
cortisol levels and, 9
excess protein consumption, 61
exercise and, 88
progesterone cream and, 143
testing levels of, 10
thinness and, 120
University of Surrey study, 61–62
vitamin D and, 181
Otitis, 159
Otto, Gina, 180
Outdoors
exercising in, 97–98
scene posters, 13
on 7-day detox and rejuvenate retreat, 450
times spent, 23
Overfat, 117–118
defined, 122
Overweight, 117–118
defined, 122
Ovulation, 9
Ozone, 162

Paffenbarger, Ralph, 91–92
Pain
acidic wastes and, 176–177
massage and, 186, 190
sweating and, 184
Pancreas
enzymes and, 69
flax mucilage and, 155
in insulin process, 78
Pancreatitis, 159
Panic attacks, 9
Pantothenic acid, 138
Passionate feelings, 38
Pasta, 80
Patience, 49
Pauling, Linus, 165
Peace Pilgrim, 460
Peeke, Pamela, 10–11, 71
Peppermint oil, 188
Perimenopause, 142
Perlitz, Becky, 71
Personal Retreat Programs, xi
Perspiration, 16
Pessimism, 26
Pesticides, 81–82
in air, 162
Peto, Richard, 57
Phlebitis, 159
PH of water, 172–173
Phospholipids, 157
Phosphorus
in alfalfa sprouts, 152
in flax seed, 155
in nuts, 75
Physical Therapy, 103
Physicians Committee for Responsible Medicine, 461
Physiology of stress, 5–6
Phytoestrogens, 62
Phytonutrients, 145
in fruits and vegetables, 18, 147

in Living Food, 167
Phytoplankton, 82
Phytosterols, 157
Pillows, 180
Plant-based diet, 59–60, 65–66
  changing to, 70–73
  food chain and, 82
  heart disease and, 60
  metabolism and, 136–137
  on 7-day detox and rejuvenate
    retreat, 452–454
Plant proteins, 58–59
Plato, 25
Plié presses, 115
Pliés, 114–115
PMS (premenstrual syndrome)
  cortisol levels and, 9
  exercise and, 92
  flax seed oil and, 160
  phytoestrogens and, 62
  vitamin D and, 181
Polarity therapy, 187
Positiveness
  affirmations, phrasing, 45
  of feelings, 38–39
  nutrition program and, 34–35
  skin health and, 195
  of thoughts, 25–26
Potassium
  in alfalfa sprouts, 152
  bone health and, 62
  in flax seed, 155
  foods containing, 148
  in fruits and vegetables, 147
Potassium ascorbate, 166
Power
  of attitude, 50–51
  of emotions, 38–39
  inner power, generating, 39–40
  words, power of, 44
Power Sleep (Maas), 180
Prayer. *See* Meditation
*Pregnancy, Children, and the
  Vegan Diet* (Klaper), 72
Pregnancy/nursing
  essential oils and, 188
  miscarriage, 160
  water consumption and, 16
Preschool children, massage
  for, 186
Present tense, affirmations in,
  44–45
President's Council on Physical
  Fitness and Sports, 87
Prevention magazine, 10
Pritikin, Robert, 71
*The Pritikin Principle: The
  Calorie Density Solution*
  (Pritikin), 71
Pritikin Program, 147
ProgestaCare, 142–143
Progesterone
  cortisol levels and, 9
  creams, using, 142–143
  testing levels of, 10
Programming your mind, 35–36
Progressive relaxation, 439–440

The Promise of Sleep (Dement),
  180
Proskauer massage, 187–188
Prostaglandins, 159
Prostate cancer
  deaths from, 57
  lycopene and, 148
Prostatitis, 159
Protease, 68
Protein. *See also* Animal
    products
  in alfalfa sprouts, 152
  in chlorella, 162
  cortisol and, 7
  excess protein consumption,
    61
  in flax seed, 154
  in sprouts, 150
  stress and, 11, 18–19
Protein Power diet, 77
Protons, 21
Psychoneuroimmunology (PNI),
  170
Pure essential oils, 188
Push-aways, 113
Push-ups, 113
Pycnogenol, 81
Pythagorus, 34

Quadriceps, stretching, 104
Quercetin, 81

Race walking, 130
Racquetball, 131
Radio on 3-day rejuvenation
  retreat, 420
Raw: The UNcook Book
  (Juliano), 71
Raw foods, 67–68
  as healing, 146
  weight loss tips for, 74
Ray, Lisa, 193
Reaven, Gerald, 78–79
Recombinant bovine soma-
  totropin (rBST), 64
Rectal cancer
  garlic and, 164
  lead in water and, 162
Red leaf lettuce, 66
Re-Entry Affirmation, 441–442
Refined foods
  avoiding, 75
  grains, refined, 79–80
  set point theory and, 79
Reflective clothing for exercise,
  93
Reichian massage, 187
Rejuvenate Foods, 461
Relaxation, 12–13
  progressive relaxation,
    439–440
Relaxation response, 12
The Relaxation Response (Ben-
  son), 12
REM (rapid eye movement)
  sleep, 178
Repetition

in exercise, 98
  habits, changing, 46–47
Resource Directory, xi, 457–462
Resources for plant-based diet,
  71–72
Respiration, 16
Responsibility, 49
Retreats
  3-day rejuvenation retreat,
    417–444
  7-day detox and rejuvenate
    retreat, 445–456
Reverence, living with, 27
Reverse Aging (Whang), 177
Rewards
  for exercise, 99
  nutrition program and, 32–34
  of plant-based diet, 72
Rheumatoid arthritis, 63
Rice milk, 62
Rich Dad Poor Dad (Kiyasaki), 20
RNA (ribonucleic acid), 163
"The Road Not Taken" (Frost),
  456
Robbins, John, 71
Roberts, Susan, 77
Rock climbing, 97
Rolfing, 188
Romaine lettuce, 66
Rosemary oil, 188
Rose oil, 188
Rotation crunch, 107
Routines, establishing, 24
Rowing, 130
Rowing machines, 130
Rudin, Donald O., 157
Rush University for Health
  Aging, 165
Rutin, 81

Saccharin, 84
Saccharomyces cerevisiae, 168
Safety
  and exercise, 93
  on 3-day rejuvenation retreat,
    420
Sage oil, 188
Sailing, 97
Salads, 66, 146
Saliva hormone testing, 9
S-allyl cysteine, 165
Salt, 82–83
  in flax seed, 155
Sandalwood oil, 188
Santillo, Humbart, 69
Sapolsky, Robert, 5
Saunas, 183–185
  dry skin brushing and, 194
  for home/office use, 184–185
Schizophrenia, 160
Schweitzer, Albert, 171
Science, 135
Sea salt, 82–83
Sea Salt's Hidden Powers (Lan-
  gre), 71
Seasoning foods, 141
Seeds. *See* Nuts, oils and seeds

Selenium
  stress and, 19
  whole foods and, 138
Self-criticisms, letting go of,
  49–50
Self-mastery, 49
Self-Realization Fellowship, 461
Senses, retraining, 33–34
Sequencing food selections, 74
Serotonin, 22
The Serotonin Solution (Wurt-
  man), 19
Set point theory, 73
  refined sweets and, 79
  7-day detox and rejuvenate
    retreat, 445–456
  advance planning for, 445–447
  levels of, 454
  living foods retreat, 455–456
  7 p.m., eating after, 31
Sex appeal. *See* Libido
Sexual disorders. *See also* Libido
  flax seed oil and, 159–160
Shiatsu, 187
Shiatsu-Aid Massage Board,
  461
Shoulder exercises, 113
Side leg lifts, 115
Silicon, 155
Simplifying your life, 24–25
SineQuaNon, 167, 460
Single leg squats, 116
Skating, 131
Skiing, 131
Skin
  beautifying skin, 193–195
  conditioning of, 191–195
  flax seed oil and, 159
  functions of, 192–193
  layers of, 192
  sunlight and, 182
Skin cancer, 143
Skin fold test, 123–124
Sleep, 15, 177–181
  accidents and, 178
  bed, use of, 180
  body temperature and, 180
  delta consciousness, 41
  eating and, 181
  environment for, 180
  exercise and, 92
  on 7-day detox and rejuvenate
    retreat, 449
  skin health and, 194
  stress and, 5
  tips for improving, 179–181
Slouching, 29
Slowing down, 24–25
  eating and, 31, 75–76
  plant-based diet, changing to,
    70
Smaller meals, 73
Smith, Lendon H., 56, 72–73
Smoking, 56–57
Soccer, 131
Sodas, 74
Sodium. *See* Salt

Solidification of waste, 174
Soluble fiber, 149
Sour cream, soy, 62
Soy
  foods, 62
  milk, 62
  oils, 157
  protein, 58–59
Speed golf, 97
Sperm formation, 160
Spiegel, Karine, 178
Spinach, 66
Spirituality, 27
  exercise and, 92
  live foods and, 69
  metabolism and, 143–144
Splenitis, 159
Spock, Benjamin, 63
Spot reducing, 105
Sprouts, 66
  guide for sprouting, 151–152
  for health, 150–153
Sprout Spray, 152
Squats, 115–116
Stair climbers, 130
Standard American Diet (SAD),
  452
Starchy foods, limiting, 75
Static electricity, 22
Stationary bicycles, 130, 131
  intensity of exercise and, 132
Steam rooms, 183–185
Step classes, 130
Step/ladder climbers, 130
Sterility, 160
Steroid hormones, 6
Steve Martin: The Magic Years
  (Walker), 180
Stillness Meditation, 425
Stomach cancer
  fruits and vegetables and, 147
  garlic and, 164
Stool changes, 70
Strength training, 89–90
  cellulite, eliminating, 140–141
  individualizing program,
    109–113
  metabolism and, 140
  muscle mass and, 128
  osteoporosis and, 89
Stress, 3–4
  cortisol, role of, 7–10
  exercise and, 87–88
  flax seed oil and, 160
  physiology of, 5–6
  tips for reducing, 12–27
Stretching, 102–105
  on 7-day detox and rejuvenate
    retreat, 448–449
  on 3-day rejuvenation retreat,
    421–422
Strokes, 57
  fruits and vegetables and, 147
Strong Women Stay Young
  (Nelson), 91
Subconscious mind, 36–38
  emotions and, 43–44

reprogramming, 40–42
Subcutaneous fat, 192
Sugar
  absorption of, 79
  avoiding, 73
  blood sugar, 9
Sulfur, 155
Sun Chorella, 163, 453, 461
Sunlight, 143
  health and, 181–182
  on 7-day detox and rejuvenate
    retreat, 449
  skin health and, 193
Sunlight (Kime), 143
Sunrise experience, 436
Sunscreens, 182
Surgery and stress, 5
Sweating, 183–185
Swedish massage, 187
*Sweet Poison: How the World's
  Most Popular Artificial
  Sweetener Is Killing Us - My
  Story* (Hull), 84–85
Swimming, 130–131
Swiss chart, 66
Sylvia Skin Care Salon, 193
*Syndrome X: Overcoming the
  Silent Killer that Can Give
  You a Heart Attack* (Reaven),
  78
Synthetic fabrics, 21–23

Tae-Bo, 130
Takahashi, George, 461
Target heart rate, 95–98
Television on 3-day rejuvenation
  retreat, 420
Tendonitis, 159
Tennis, 97, 131
Testosterone, 10
Theresa, Mother, 26–27
Thermodynamics, law of, 78
Thermotex company, 177
Theta consciousness, 41
Thighs, stretching for, 104
Thinness, excessive, 120
Thin Through the Power of Spirit
  (Capodilupo), 71
Thoreau, Henry David, viii, xii, 28
Thoughts, positive, 25–26
  3-day rejuvenation retreat,
    417–444
  advance planning for, 419
  Day 1 of, 421–430
  Day 2 of, 430–436
  Day 3 of, 436–442
  guidelines for, 419–421
  Re-Entry Affirmation, 441–442
  White Light Meditation,
    431–432
  3-part breath exercise, 424
Throat cancer, 147
Thyroid gland, 141
  sunlight and, 182
Thyroid hormone, 142
Thyrotropin, 178
Thys-Jacobs, Susan, 182

Tired of Being Tired (Hanley), 71
Tonsillitis, 159
Touch Research Institute (TRI), 186–187
Toxicity
  chemicals, 81–82
  in water, 137, 162
  weight problems and, 137
Toxic overload, 162
  symptoms of, 171
Trace minerals
  in ALL ONE, 167
  in flax seed, 155
  whole foods and, 137–138
Trager massage, 187
Trampolines, mini, 130
Trans-fats, 157
Trauma and stress, 5
Treadmills, 130
Tree of Life Rejuvenation Center, 69
  resource information, 462
Triglycerides
  exercise and, 88
  insulin and, 78
Trihalomethanes, 162
Triple Power, 166–167
Trust, 49
Tryptophan, 181
Tufts University
  Jean Mayer Human Nutrition Research Center on Aging, 77
  strength training studies, 90
Turner, Tina, 31
Turn Off the Fat Genes (Barnard), 71
Twain, Mark, 43
Type 2 diabetes, 91

The Ultimate Fit or Fat (Bailey), 122, 140
Undereating, 135
Underwater weighing, 123–124
Unity Village and Retreat Center, 462
University of California, San Francisco, 60
University of Chicago sleep study, 178
University of Miami's School of Medicine, 186–187
University of Oregon, Dept. of Community Health, 138
University of Pennsylvania studies, 150
University of Southern California Exercise Physiology Laboratory, 14
  Norris Comprehensive Cancer Center, 89
University of Surrey osteoporosis study, 61–62
University of Texas Southwestern Medical Center, 147
University of Wisconsin, Madison, 24

Urinary tract cancer, 15
Urine, 74
Urine deoxypyridinoline (Dpd) bond resorption tests, 9
U.S. Centers for Disease Control and Prevention, 131
UVB rays, 182

Van Praagh, James, 28
Vedic medicine, 153
Vegetables. *See* Fruits and vegetables
Vegetable Soup/The Fruit Bowl (Warren & Jones), 72
Vegetarian Magic (Nowakowski), 71
Virtue, Doreen, 71
Visualization, 2
  of fitness goals, 98
  of goals, 42–46
  on 7-day detox and rejuvenate retreat, 451
  subconscious mind, reprogramming, 40–42
Vitality, Bio-Strath for, 168
Vitality Shake, 453
Vitamin A
  in alfalfa sprouts, 152
  in fruits and vegetables, 18
  in wheat sprouts, 150
Vitamin C, 18
  in alfalfa sprouts, 152
  bone health and, 62
  eye diseases and, 149
  in flax seed, 155
  mineral ascorbates, 166–167
  power of, 165–167
  skin health and, 195
  in wheat sprouts, 150
  whole foods and, 138
Vitamin D
  in alfalfa sprouts, 152
  skin health and, 193
  sunlight and, 181–182
Vitamin E
  in alfalfa sprouts, 152
  in flax seed, 155
  in nuts, 75
  refined foods and, 79, 80
  in wheat sprouts, 150
  whole foods and, 138
Vitamins, 145
  in ALL ONE, 167
  in chlorella, 162
  in flax seed, 155
Vita Mix, 462
Volleyball, 97
Volunteering, 50

Waist/Hip Ratio (WHR), 120–121
Walfor, Roy L., 135
Walker, Morris, 180
Walking, 130
Walking meditation, 434–435
Warming up for exercise, 94
Warming Up to Living Foods (Markowitz), 71

Warren, Dianne, 72
Waste products, 174
Water. *See also* Alkaline water
  appetite, curbing, 31
  detoxification and, 172–173
  exercise and, 93, 94
  flavorings for, 17
  internal water bath, 422
  metabolism and, 139–140
  saunas and, 184
  on 7-day detox and rejuvenate retreat, 448
  skin health and, 194–195
  stress reduction and, 15–17
  toxicity and, 137, 162
  weight loss and, 73–74
Water aerobics, 130, 131
Water retention
  estrogen-dominance and, 64
  flax seed oil and, 160
  plant-based diet, changing to, 70
  weight gain and, 83
Water skiing, 131
Web site for relaxation tape resources, 12
Weight control
  creativity and, 99
  exercise and, 90
  significant improvements and, 117–118
  tips for, 73–76
Weight gain
  big meals and, 83
  cortisol and, 10–11
  dehydration and, 15
  estrogen-dominance and, 64
  set point theory, 73
Weight lifting. *See* Strength training
Weight Loss Express, 453–454
Weight scales, 124
Weindruch, Richard, 135
Whang, Sang, 177
What Color Is Your Diet? (Heber), 71, 81
What Your Doctor May Not Tell You About Menopause (Lee), 64, 71, 142
What Your Doctor May Not Tell You About PreMenopause (Lee & Hanley), 71, 142
Wheat sprouts, 150
White Light Meditation, 431–432
White-water rafting, 97
Whitman, Walt, vii, 97
Whole foods, 136–138
  choosing, 32
  fiber from, 150
Why Zebras Don't Get Ulcers (Sapolsky), 5
Wilkie, Diana J., 186
Willet, Walter, 80
Windsurfing, 97, 131
Wired to Meditate, 13, 45
Wood, Christine, 72

Wood, Rebecca, 71
Wooden, John, 52
Wool carpeting, 23
Words, power of, 44
Wordsworth, William, 27
Worry and stress, 5
Writing affirmations, 45
Wurtman, Judith, 19

X-ISER, 100–101, 130
resource information, 462

Yeast, Bio-Strath, 168
Yoga, 14–15, 131
cellulite, eliminating, 140
flexibility, increasing, 101–102
Yogananda, Paramahansa, 37,
461
Yogurt, soy, 62
*Your Body's Many Cries for
Water* (Batmanghelidj), 71
Your Maximum Mind (Benson),
12

Zinc
in chlorella, 162
in flax seed, 155
whole foods and, 138
Zinc ascorbate, 166
The Zone Diet, 77
Zone therapy, 187
Zooplankton, 82

Recipe Index

ALL ONE in Vitality Shake, 210
Almond milk
Creamy Cinnamon Banana
Smoothie, 214
Rose Potatoes with Emerald
Green Gravy, 389
Almonds
about, 211
Candy Balls, Healthy, 394
Cucumber-Tofu Salad with
Toasted Almonds, 266
Granola, Sensational Spicy,
226–227
in High Protein Bean-Tofu
Spread, 238
Muesli, 225–226
Nut Milk, Easy, 211
Pinwheel Citrus Delight, 224
Quinoa with Soybeans, Dried
Cherries & Toasted Almonds,
356
Rice Almondine, Coconut,
343–344
Rice Pilaf, Flavorful, 387
Stuffed Dates, 392–393
Tapioca Pudding with Toasted
Almonds, 411
Anti-Cancer V-12 drink, 208–209
Antioxidant Express, 206
Antioxidant Spinach-Sweet
Potato Salad, 269
Apple butter in Health Candy
Balls, 394
Apple juice
Fruit Power Shake, 222
Mango-Butternut Squash
Soup, 306–307
Apples
about, 202, 371
Antioxidant Express, 206
Berry Apple Sauce, 370–371
Berry-Cherry Zing, 204
Bread, Blueberry Apple
Banana, 396–397
Cabbage, Apple & Turnip Salad
with Toasted Cashews, 259
Calcium Cooler, 202
Carotene Cocktail, 202
Cashew & Apple Cinnamon
Smoothie, 398

Cranberry-Apple Cooler, 213
Crisp, Apple Lemon, 413–414
Cumin Spiced Apple-Cabbage
with Toasted Walnuts, 387
Date-Apple-Berry Butter
Spread, 235–236
Dried Plum & Apple Smoothie,
212
Easy Sleepytime Cocktail, 207
Fruit Power Shake, 222
Ginger Fruit Salad, 412–413
Granola, Sensational Spicy,
226–227
Muesli, 225–226
Muffins, Banana Applesauce,
228
Natural Beauty Cocktail, 207
Oatmeal Deluxe, 229–230
Pudding, Apple Walnut, 403
Red Cabbage with Apples &
Pistachios, 327–328
Rejuvenation Tonic, 205
salads
Cabbage, Apple & Turnip
Salad with Toasted
Cashews, 259
Ginger Fruit Salad, 412–413
smoothies
Creamy Cashew & Apple
Cinnamon Smoothie, 398
Dried Plum & Apple
Smoothie, 212
spreads
Apple Butter Spread, 235
Date-Apple-Berry Butter
Spread, 235–236
Sweet Pepper-Apple Sun
Dressing, 285
Top of the Morning juice, 201
Weight Loss Express juice,
200
Applesauce
Brownies, Moist & Chewy,
409–410
Cherry, Orange, Applesauce
Deluxe, 391–392
Muffins, Banana Applesauce,
228
Oatmeal Cookies, Outrageous,
407–408

Apricots
about, 235
Chutney, Apricot-Ginger, 250
Cookies, Sunflower Apricot,
403–404
Salad, Spinach-Apricot,
261–262
Spread, 234–235
Aragon black olives, 367
Artichokes
Dip, 239
frozen artichokes hearts, 250
Hearts of Romaine, Artichokes
& Palm Salad, 259–260
Marinara Sauce, Quick & Easy
Fat-Free Garlic Roasted, 249
Millet with Artichoke Hearts
& Vegetables, 352
Pizza, Vegetable Pita, 332
Risotto with Sun-Dried Toma-
toes & Artichoke Hearts,
Roasted Garlic, 347
Stir-Fry Hearts of Palm &
Artichoke with Shiitake
Mushrooms, 330
Arugula
about, 253
Pear & Arugula Salad with
Toasted Walnuts, 258
Sun-Dried Tomato, Hijiki &
Romaine Salad, 270–271
Asian Rice, 368–369
Asparagus
about, 312
Cream of Asparagus soup,
311–312
in 4-Bean Salad, 267
Roasted Herbed Asparagus &
Potatoes, 319–320
Autumn Puree, 384
Avocados. *See also* Guacamole
about, 245
Green Goddess Dressing, 286
Guacamole, Great, 244–245
Jicama-Leek & Pepper Salad,
271–272
Living Nori Salad, 257–258
Papaya Gazpacho, 304–305
Rainbow Stuffed Peppers,
322

salads
  Jicama-Leek & Pepper
    Salad, 271–272
  Living Nori Salad, 257–258
Salsa, Sensational, 243
Sandwich, Lettuce & Veg-
  etable, 323
Soup, Fresh Corn & Avocado,
  303–304
Spread, Soybean, 248
Vegetable Wraps with Hum-
  mus Spread, 325–326
Zesty Avocado Dressing,
  282–283

Balsamic vinegar
  Dijon Vinaigrette, 275–276
  Orange Balsamic Vinaigrette,
    276
Bamboo shoots in Soba Noodle
  Salad with Garden Vegeta-
  bles, 262–263
Banana peppers, 290
Bananas, 215
  about, 215
  Berry Salad with Fruit Sauce,
    225
  Bread, Blueberry Apple
    Banana, 396–397
  Carob Frozen Banana Sticks,
    416
  Cinnamon Banana Smoothie,
    214
  Cranberry-Apple Cooler, 213
  as diet food, 395
  freezing, 210, 406
  Fruit Dressing, Fabulous, 284
  Fruit Power Shake, 222
  Ginger Fruit Salad, 412–413
  Guilt-Free Banana Split,
    394–395
  Ice Cream, Strawberry-
    Mango-Banana, 406
  Muffins, Applesauce Banana,
    228
  Oatmeal Cookies, Outrageous,
    407–408
  Peach Smoothie, 218
  puddings
    Sesame Banana Orange
      Pudding, 406–407
    Very Berry Pudding, 395
    Yam Pudding, Yummy, 396
  smoothies
    Cinnamon Banana
      Smoothie, 214
    Strawberry-Banana
      Smoothie, 217
    Tropical Fruit Smoothie, 214
  Sorbet, Tropical, 415
  Strawberry-Banana Smoothie,
    217
  Strawberry-Mango-Banana
    Ice Cream, 406
  Tofu Pancakes with, 233
  Tropical Fruit Smoothie, 214
  Vitality Shake, 210

Barlean's Organic Flax Oil
  Creamy Cherry Smoothie, 221
  Soybean Spread, 248
  Veggie Millet Spread, 237
  Veggie Smoothie, 220
  Vitality Shake, 210
Barley, 336
  about, 346–347
  Lentil-Barley-Cashew Stew, 346
Barley malt in Nut Milk, 211
Basmati rice
  about, 387–388
  Asian Rice, 368–369
  Cardamom & Parsley Basmati
    Rice, 361
  Chickpeas, Baked Basmati
    Rice with, 348–349
  Citrus Basmati Rice Pilaf &
    Mushrooms, 365–366
  Flavorful Rice Pilaf, 386–387
Bean dips
  about, 246
  Festive Black Bean Dip,
    245–246
  Spicy & Quick Nonfat Bean
    Dip, 246
Beano, 306
Beans. See also Bean dips
  about, 246, 265, 306, 336–339
  Chili, Portabello Mushroom,
    350–351
  cooking beans, tip for, 247
  digestive gas and, 337
  4-Bean Salad, 266–267
  freezing, 355
  High Protein Bean-Tofu
    Spread, 238
  Meal-in-a-Bowl White Bean
    Soup, 305–306
  soaking beans, 265, 337
  Spicy Bean Salad, 264–265
  White Bean & Tomato Casse-
    role, 341
Beets
  Anti-Cancer V-12 drink,
    208–209
  Potatoes Rose with Emerald
    Green Gravy, 389
  Top of the Morning juice, 201
  Vitality Salad, 254–255
Belgian endive, 379
  Salsa-Hummus Salad, 257
Bell peppers. See also Roasted
    peppers
  about, 290, 322–323
  Anti-Cancer V-12 drink,
    208–209
  Antioxidant Express, 206
  Antioxidant Spinach-Sweet
    Potato Salad, 269
  Apricot-Spinach Salad,
    261–262
  Black Bean Salad, Spicy,
    264–265
  in Broiled Vegetables, 320
  Brussels Sprouts Stir-Fry, 324
  Carotene Cocktail, 202

Cauliflower, Edamame & Bell
  Peppers, Roasted, 331
Chili, Portabello Mushroom,
  350–351
corn
  Creamy Spicy Herbed
    Corn, 382
  Grain Salad with Sweet
    Corn, Chilled, 366–367
  Multicolored Corn, 386
Couscous Garden Salad,
  260–261
Cucumbers, Stuffed, 381–382
Endive, Stuffed, 378–379
Fajitas, 390–391
Grain Salad with Sweet Corn,
  Chilled, 366–367
in Grilled or Roasted Veg-
  etable Packets, 317
Hearts of Romaine, Artichokes
  & Palm Salad, 259–260
High Protein Bean-Tofu
  Spread, 238
hummus
  Black Bean Hummus, 247
  Dill Roasted Yellow Pepper
    Hummus, 247
  Vegetable Wraps with
    Hummus Spread, 325–326
Italian Raspberry Dressing,
  Fat-Free, 285
Jicama-Leek & Pepper Salad,
  271–272
Living Nori Salad, 257–258
Marinara Sauce, Quick & Easy
  Fat-Free Garlic Roasted, 249
Mexican Wild Rice with
  Olives, 358–359
Multicolored Corn, 386
Natural Beauty Cocktail, 207
Noodle Vegetable Delight,
  328–329
Pizza, Vegetable Pita, 332
Rainbow Stuffed Peppers, 322
Rice Almondine, Coconut,
  343–344
roasted peppers, 238
Roasted Yellow Pepper &
  Orange Soup, Zesty, 309
salads
  Antioxidant Spinach-Sweet
    Potato Salad, 269
  Apricot-Spinach Salad,
    261–262
  Black Bean Salad, Spicy,
    264–265
  Grain Salad with Sweet
    Corn, Chilled, 366–367
  Hearts of Romaine,
    Artichokes & Palm Salad,
    259–260
  Jicama-Leek & Pepper
    Salad, 271–272
  Roasted Vegetable Salad,
    Chilled, 326–327
  Sun-Dried Tomato, Hijiki &
    Romaine Salad, 270–271

Sweet Lentil-Parsley Salad, 339–340
Sweet & Sour Black-Eyed Pea Salad, 354
Vegetable Salad, Roasted and Chilled, 326–327
Vitality Salad, 254–255
Salsa, Sensational, 243
Sandwich, Lettuce & Vegetable, 323
Sauté, Soy Thai Vegetable, 333–334
Scrambled Tofu, 231–232
Sun-Dried Tomato, Hijiki & Romaine Salad, 270–271
Sweet Lentil-Parsley Salad, 339–340
Sweet Pepper-Apple Sun Dressing, 285
Sweet & Sour Black-Eyed Pea Salad, 354
Top of the Morning juice, 201
Vegetable Lentil-Sweet Potato Cakes, 367–368
Vegetable Salad, Roasted and Chilled, 326–327
Vegetable Wraps with Hummus Spread, 325–326
Veggie Smoothie, 220
Vitality Salad, 254–255
Yukon Gold Potato Salad, 373
Beluga lentils, 264
Berries. See also specific types
about, 225, 412
Cherry-Berry Zing, 204
Ginger Fruit Salad, 412–413
Pie, Frozen Coconut Berry Mint, 411–412
Protein Delight, Berry-Mint Coconut, 414–415
Pudding, Very Berry, 395
Salad with Fruit Sauce, Berry, 225
Summer Fruit Combo, 268
Berry-Cherry Zing, 204
The Best Apple Berry Sauce, 370–371
Bibb lettuce in Couscous Garden Salad, 260–261
Black beans
about, 355
Couscous with Black Beans & Carrots, Zesty, 345
Dip, Festive Black Bean, 245–246
freezing, 355
Hummus, Black Bean, 247
Mexican Black Beans, 355
Millet with Black Beans & Vegetables, 352
Pizza, Vegetable Pita, 332
Potato Skins with Salsa, Fancy, 380
Salad, Spicy Black Bean, 264–265
in salads, 255
Southwestern Black Bean

Patties, Spicy, 363
Stew/Soup, 310–311
Blackberries
Berry Salad with Fruit Sauce, 225
Cherry, Orange, Applesauce Deluxe, 392
Pie, Frozen Coconut Berry Mint, 412
Vitality Shake, 210
Black-eyed peas in Sweet & Sour Black-Eyed Pea Salad, 354
Black peppercorns, 296
Black sesame seeds, 294
Blood pressure, 216
Blueberries
about, 397
Apple Berry Sauce, 370–371
Berry-Cherry Zing, 204
Berry Salad with Fruit Sauce, 225
Bonanza Smoothie, Blueberry, 397
Bread, Blueberry Apple Banana, 396–397
Date-Apple-Berry Butter Spread, 236
Fruit Dressing, Fabulous, 284
Orange-Blueberry Buckwheat Pancakes, 232
Pie, Frozen Coconut Berry Mint, 412
Pinwheel Citrus Delight, 224
Pudding, Very Berry, 395
in Raw Cherry, Orange, Applesauce Deluxe, 392
Vitality Shake, 210
Bok choy in Cole Slaw, Sunny Shredded Dill & Toasted Sesame, 267–268
Bouquet garni for Vegetable Broth, 299
Breadcrumbs, 341, 342
Breads
Blueberry Apple Banana Bread, 396–397
Flatbread, Herbed Garbanzo, 296–297
Muffins, Banana Applesauce, 228
Breakfasts, 223–224. See also Cereals
Banana Applesauce Muffins, 228
Berry Salad with Fruit Sauce, 225
Orange-Blueberry Buckwheat Pancakes, 232
Pinwheel Citrus Delight, 224
Scrambled Tofu, 231–232
Tofu Pancakes, 233
Broccoflower in Cauliflower-Carrot Soup with Tarragon, 314
Broccoli
about, 321
Antioxidant Express, 206

Calcium Cooler, 202
Cole Slaw with Toasted Sesame Seeds, Broccoli, 374
Curry, Cauliflower-Broccoli, 383
in 4-Bean Salad, 267
Ginger Broccoli & Shiitake Steam-Fry, 320–321
in Grilled or Roasted Vegetable Packets, 317
Marinara Sauce, Quick & Easy Fat-Free Garlic Roasted, 249
Potassium-Powered Broth, 300
Sauté, Soy Thai Vegetable, 333–334
Soba Noodle Salad with Garden Vegetables, 262–263
Top of the Morning juice, 201
Broccoli sprouts
Anti-Cancer V-12 drink, 208–209
Antioxidant Express, 206
Broiled Vegetables, 320
Brownies, Moist & Chewy, 409–410
Brown rice
about, 344
Burgers, Grain, 349–350
Casserole, Vegetable, Rice & Lentil, 326
Coconut Rice Almondine, 343–344
cooking tips, 366
Herb Rice with Shiitake Mushrooms, Toasted, 364
Mexican Wild Rice with Olives, 358–359
red lentils and, 336
Sushi Rice Salad, 352–353
Vegetable Lentil-Sweet Potato Cakes, 367–368
Brunches. See Breakfasts
Brussels sprouts
about, 325
Chopped Brussels Sprouts Stir-Fry, 324
Buckwheat
about, 233
Orange-Blueberry Buckwheat Pancakes, 232
Bulgar in Lemon Grass Tabbouleh with Toasted Walnuts, 357–358
Burgers
Grain Burgers, 349–350
Southwestern Black Bean Patties, Spicy, 363
Vegetable Lentil-Sweet Potato Cakes, 367–368
Burritos, Nori Veggi, 318
Butter lettuce in Couscous Garden Salad, 260–261
Butternut squash
Autumn Puree, 384
Mango-Butternut Squash Soup, 306–307
Butters, fruit and nut/seed, 383

Cabbage
  Broccoli Cole Slaw with
    Toasted Sesame Seeds, 374
  Crunchy Cabbage, Apple &
    Turnip Salad with Toasted
    Cashews, 259
  Cumin Spiced Apple-Cabbage
    with Toasted Walnuts, 387
  Fennel-Dill Slaw, 379
  Potassium-Powered Broth, 300
  Red Cabbage with Apples &
    Pistachios, 327–328
  Roasted Vegetable Salad,
    Chilled, 326–327
  Shredded Rainbow Salad, 255
  Sunny Shredded Dill &
    Toasted Sesame, 267–268
  Veggie Smoothie, 220
  White Bean Soup, 305–306
Calcium Cooler, 202
Candy Balls, Healthy, 394
Cantaloupes
  about, 313
  Mixed Melon Ambrosia, 215
  Smoothie, Kiwi-Melon, 217
  Soup, Lime-Cantaloupe Soup,
    312
  Summer Fruit Combo, 268
Carbohydrates, 338
Cardamom
  about, 361
  Basmati Rice, Cardamom &
    Parsley, 361
  Energizing Tonic, 204
Carob
  about, 416
  Frozen Carob Banana Sticks,
    416
Carotene Cocktail, 202
Carrot juice
  Shiitake Mushroom Sauce, 244
  Veggie Smoothie, 220
Carrots
  about, 376
  Anti-Cancer V-12 drink,
    208–209
  Antioxidant Express, 206
  Autumn Puree, 384
  Bean-Tofu Spread, High
    Protein, 238
  Black Bean Stew/Soup,
    310–311
  Broccoli Cole Slaw with
    Toasted Sesame Seeds, 374
  Burgers, Grain, 349–350
  Carotene Cocktail, 202
  Cauliflower-Carrot Soup with
    Tarragon, 314
  Chili, Portabello Mushroom,
    350–351
  Endive, Stuffed, 378–379
  Fennel-Dill Slaw, 379
  Garbanzo, Carrot & Tomato
    Salad, 362
  Living Nori Salad, 257–258
  Marinara Sauce, Quick & Easy
    Fat-Free Garlic Roasted, 249

Millet with Garbanzo Beans &
    Vegetables, 351–352
  Miso Tofu Soup, Hot 'n Spicy,
    308
  Natural Beauty Cocktail, 207
  Noodle Vegetable Delight,
    328–329
  Pacific Rim Vegetable Stew,
    329
  Pizza, Vegetable Pita, 332
  Potassium-Powered Broth, 300
  Rainbow Stuffed Peppers, 322
  Rice Pilaf, Flavorful, 387
  salads
    Broccoli Cole Slaw with
      Toasted Sesame Seeds, 374
    Fennel-Dill Slaw, 379
    Garbanzo, Carrot & Tomato
      Salad, 362
    Living Nori Salad, 257–258
    Shredded Rainbow Salad,
      255
    Soba Noodle Salad with Gar-
      den Vegetables, 262–263
    Sunny Shredded Dill &
      Toasted Sesame Cole
      Slaw, 267–268
    Vitality Salad, 254–255
  Sandwich, Lettuce & Veg-
    etable, 323
  Sauté, Shiitake Mushrooms,
    Tofu, Carrots & Eggplant,
    334–335
  Shredded Rainbow Salad, 255
  Soba Noodle Salad with
    Garden Vegetables, 262–263
  soups
    Black Bean Stew/Soup,
      310–311
    Cauliflower-Carrot Soup
      with Tarragon, 314
    Miso Tofu Soup, Hot 'n
      Spicy, 308
    Potassium-Powered Broth,
      300
    Split Pea Soup, Curried, 313
    White Bean Soup, 305–306
  Split Pea Soup, Curried, 313
  spreads
    Bean-Tofu Spread, High
      Protein, 238
    Garbanzo, Carrot & Tomato
      Salad, 362
    Tahini-Carrot Spread,
      236–237
    Veggie Millet Spread, 237
  Sunny Shredded Dill &
    Toasted Sesame Cole Slaw,
    267–268
  Sushi Rice Salad, 352–353
  Sweet & Spicy Organic Baby
    Carrots, 375–376
  Tahini-Carrot Spread, 236–237
  Top of the Morning juice, 201
  Vegetable Broth, 298–299
  Vegetable Lentil-Sweet Potato
    Cakes, 367–368

Veggie Millet Spread, 237
  Vitality Salad, 254–255
  Weight Loss Express juice, 200
  White Bean Soup, 305–306
Cashews
  about, 211, 375
  Barley-Lentil Cashew Stew,
    346
  Bean-Tofu Spread, High
    Protein, 238
  Candy Balls, Healthy, 394
  Crunchy Cabbage, Apple &
    Turnip Salad with Toasted
    Cashews, 259
  Curry, Cauliflower-Broccoli,
    383
  Emerald Green Sauce, 241
  Nut Date Balls, 408–409
  Nut Milk, Easy, 211
  Orange Sesame-Cashew
    Dressing, 278
  Pear Cashew Cream Dressing,
    287
  Pinwheel Citrus Delight, 224
  Popcorn, Cracker Jack,
    410–411
  Quinoa with Cashews, Dried
    Cherries & Toasted
    Almonds, 356
  Raisin-Cashew Balls, 374–375
  Sensational Spicy Granola,
    226–227
  Smoothie, Creamy Cashew &
    Apple Cinnamon, 398
  Stuffed Dates, 392–393
  Tomato Couscous with
    Cashews & Raisins, 365
  Top of the Morning Quinoa
    Cereal, 230–231
Casseroles
  Vegetable, Rice & Lentil
    Casserole, 326
  White Bean & Tomato Casse-
    role, 341
Cauliflower
  about, 314–315, 331–332
  Antioxidant Express, 206
  Carrot-Cauliflower Soup with
    Tarragon, 314
  Curry, Cauliflower-Broccoli,
    383
  in Grilled or Roasted Veg-
    etable Packets, 317
  Marinara Sauce, Quick & Easy
    Fat-Free Garlic Roasted, 249
  Roasted Cauliflower,
    Edamame & Bell Peppers,
    331
  Soba Noodle Salad with
    Garden Vegetables, 262–263
Celery
  Anti-Cancer V-12 drink,
    208–209
  Bean-Tofu Spread, High
    Protein, 238
  Black Bean Stew/Soup,
    310–311

cucumbers
   Stuffed Cucumbers, 381–382
   Tofu-Cucumber Salad with
      Toasted Pecans, 265–266
Easy Sleepytime Cocktail, 207
Emerald Green Sauce, 241
Green Goddess Dressing, 286
Jicama-Leek & Pepper Salad,
   271–272
Natural Beauty Cocktail, 207
Noodle Vegetable Delight,
   328–329
Potassium-Powered Broth, 300
Rainbow Stuffed Peppers, 322
salads
   Jicama-Leek & Pepper Salad,
      271–272
   Vitality Salad, 254–255
   Yukon Gold Potato Salad, 373
soups
   Black Bean Stew/Soup,
      310–311
   Potassium-Powered Broth,
      300
   Split Pea Soup, Curried, 313
   Vegetable Broth, 298–299
   White Bean Soup, 305–306
Split Pea Soup, Curried, 313
Top of the Morning juice, 201
Vegetable Broth, 298–299
Vegetable Lentil-Sweet Potato
   Cakes, 367–368
Vitality Salad, 254–255
Weight Loss Express juice, 200
White Bean Soup, 305–306
Yukon Gold Potato Salad, 373
Cereals
   Creamy Coconut Millet Cereal,
      228–229
   Muesli, 225–226
   Oatmeal Deluxe, 229–230
   Sensational Spicy Granola,
      226–227
   storing granola, 226–227
   Top of the Morning Quinoa
      Cereal, 230–231
Chamomile tea
   about, 207
   Easy Sleepytime Cocktail, 207
Cheese. See Soy cheese
Cheesy Sesame Salt, 294
   Burgers, Grain, 349–350
Cherries
   about, 204, 269
   Berry-Cherry Zing, 204
   Candy Balls, Healthy, 394
   Fruit Power Shake, 222
   Guilt-Free Banana Split,
      394–395
   Quinoa with Soybeans, Dried
      Cherries & Toasted Almonds,
      356
   Raw Cherry, Orange, Apple-
      sauce Deluxe, 391–392
   Smoothie, Creamy Cherry, 221
   Summer Fruit Combo, 268
   Vitality Shake, 210

Chestnuts
   about, 343
   Garlicky Quinoa with Chest-
      nuts & Toasted Pine Nuts, 342
   Millet with Chestnuts and
      Vegetables, 352
Chick peas. See Garbanzo beans
Chile peppers. See also Bell
      peppers; Jalapeño peppers
   about, 243
   Fajitas, 390–391
   Papaya Gazpacho, 304–305
Chili, Portabello Mushroom,
   350–351
Chilled Roasted Vegetable Salad,
   326–327
Chinese Cabbage Cole Slaw,
   267–268
Chips
   Kale Chips, 371–372
   No Oil Chips & Salsa, 375
Chives
   Tomato Soup, Fresh, 302
   Yukon Gold Potato Salad, 373
Chocolate
   about, 410
   Date Peppermint Chocolate
      Shake/Ice Cream, 401–402
   Dried Plum & Chocolate Whip,
      404
   Nut Date Balls with, 409
   in Nut Milk, 211
   Stuffed Dates, 393
Chromium, 339
Chutney, Apricot-Ginger, 250
Cilantro
   about, 381
   Black Bean Salad, Spicy,
      264–265
   Garlicky Quinoa with Chest-
      nuts & Toasted Pine Nuts, 342
   Guacamole, Great, 244–245
   Lemon Grass Tabbouleh with
      Toasted Walnuts, Spicy,
      357–358
   Mexican Wild Rice with Olives,
      358–359
   salad dressings
      Thousand Island, Cilantro,
         278–279
      Vinaigrette, Thousand
         Island, 274–275
   Salsa, Sensational, 243
   Tomatoes & Zucchini with
      Cilantro, 380–381
   in Tomato Soup, Fresh, 302
Cinnamon, 214
   about, 214
   Pears, Cinnamon Vanilla
      Poached, 405
   Smoothie, Creamy Cashew &
      Apple Cinnamon, 398
Citrus Basmati Rice Pilaf &
   Mushrooms, 365–366
Cloves in Energizing Tonic, 204
Coconut
   about, 216, 415

Apple Berry Sauce, 371
Candy Balls, Healthy, 394
Cashew-Raisin Balls, 374–375
Cereal, Creamy Coconut Millet,
   228–229
Nut Date Balls, 408–409
Pie, Frozen Coconut Berry
   Mint, 411–412
Rice Almondine, Coconut,
   343–344
Rice Pilaf, Flavorful, 387
Sensational Spicy Granola,
   226–227
Sherbet, Lemon-Coconut, 400
Coconut milk
   Pie, Frozen Coconut Berry
      Mint, 412
   Protein Delight, Berry-Mint
      Coconut, 414–415
rice
   Cocnut Rice Almondine,
      343–344
   Flavorful Rice Pilaf, 387
   Smoothie, Mango Coconut
      Cream, 216
   Sorbet, Tropical, 415
   Soy Thai Vegetable Sauté,
      333–334
   Stew, Pacific Rim Vegetable, 329
Coconut oil
   about, 348
   Risotto with Sun-Dried Toma-
      toes & Artichoke Hearts,
      Roasted Garlic, 347
Cole slaw
   Broccoli Cole Slaw with
      Toasted Sesame Seeds, 374
   Fennel-Dill Slaw, 379
   Sunny Shredded Dill & Toasted
      Sesame Cole Slaw, 267–268
Collard greens in Shiitake Con-
   sommé, 300–301
Colorful Summer Fruit Combo,
   268
Cookies
   Brownies, Moist & Chewy,
      409–410
   Nut Date Balls, 408–409
   Oatmeal Cookies, Outrageous,
      407–408
   Sunflower Apricot Cookies,
      403–404
Corn
   about, 304
   Brussels Sprouts Stir-Fry, 324
   Casserole, Vegetable, Rice &
      Lentil, 326
   combinations with, 336
   Creamy Spicy Herbed Corn,
      382
   Grain Salad with Sweet Corn,
      Chilled, 366–367
   Millet with Garbanzo Beans &
      Vegetables, 351–352
   Multicolored Corn, 386
   Pacific Rim Vegetable Stew, 329
   Rice Pilaf, Flavorful, 387

Roast Yukon Potatoes, Corn &
Peas, 333
Salsa, Sensational, 243
Sauté, Soy Thai Vegetable,
333–334
Soup, Fresh Corn & Avocado,
303–304
Cornmeal
Southwestern Black Bean
Patties, Spicy, 363
Vegetable Lentil-Sweet Potato
Cakes, 367–368
Couscous
about, 261, 345–346
Black Beans & Carrots, Zesty
Couscous with, 345
Garden Salad, 260–261
Grain Salad with Sweet Corn,
Chilled, 367
Tomato Couscous with
Cashews & Raisins, 365
Cracker Jack Popcorn, 410–411
Cranberries
about, 213
Cranberry-Apple Cooler, 213
Cranberry-Apple Cooler, 213
Cream of Asparagus soup,
311–312
Creamy Cherry Smoothie, 221
Creamy Cinnamon Banana
smoothie, 214
Creamy Coconut Millet Cereal,
228–229
Creamy Spicy Herbed Corn, 382
Crenshaw Melon-Kiwi
Smoothie, 217
Crimson lentils, 264
Crisp, Apple Lemon, 413–414
Croutons
freezing, 292
Herbed Croutons, 291–292
Plain Croutons, 291
Crunchy Cabbage, Apple &
Turnip Salad with Toasted
Cashews, 259
Cucumbers
about, 266
Green Goddess Dressing, 286
Natural Beauty Cocktail, 207
Sandwich, Lettuce & Veg-
etable, 323
Stuffed Cucumbers, 381–382
Sun-Dried Tomato, Hijiki &
Romaine Salad, 270–271
Tofu-Cucumber Salad with
Toasted Pecans, 265–266
Veggie Smoothie, 220
Vitality Salad, 254–255
Weight Loss Express juice, 200
Cultured vegetables, 256
Cumin, 295, 377
Spiced Apple-Cabbage with
Toasted Walnuts and Cumin,
387
Curries
Cauliflower-Broccoli Curry, 383
Split Pea Soup, Curried, 313

Daikon radish
about, 268
Cole Slaw, Sunny Shredded
Dill & Toasted Sesame,
267–268
Roasted Vegetable Salad,
Chilled, 326–327
Shredded Rainbow Salad, 255
Sun-Dried Tomato, Hijiki &
Romaine Salad, 270–271
Sushi Rice Salad, 352–353
Dandelion leaves, 253
Dates
about, 393
Apple-Date-Berry Butter
Spread, 235–236
Apricot & Prune Butter
Spreads, 235
Brownies, Moist & Chewy,
409–410
Candy Balls, Healthy, 394
Cereal, Creamy Coconut
Millet, 228–229
Chocolate Date Peppermint
Shake/Ice Cream, 401–402
Granola, Sensational Spicy,
226–227
Muesli, 225–226
Nut Date Balls, 408–409
Oatmeal Deluxe, 229–230
Pie, Frozen Coconut Berry
Mint, 412
Pudding, Sesame Banana
Orange, 406–407
Raw Cherry, Orange, Apple-
sauce Deluxe, 391–392
Rice Pilaf, Flavorful, 387
Sauce, Apple Berry, 370–371
Soup, Mango-Butternut
Squash, 306–307
spreads
Apple-Date-Berry Butter
Spread, 235–236
Apricot & Prune Butter
Spreads, 235
Stuffed Dates, 392–393
Date sugar, 393
Desserts, 401. See also Cookies;
Puddings
Brownies, Moist & Chewy,
409–410
Carob Frozen Banana Sticks,
416
Chocolate Date Peppermint
Shake/Ice Cream, 401–402
Cinnamon Vanilla Poached
Pears, 405
Crisp, Apple Lemon, 413–414
Dried Plum & Chocolate Whip,
404
Fruit Treats, Frozen, 402–403
Ginger Fruit Salad, 412–413
Pie, Frozen Coconut Berry
Mint, 411–412
Popcorn, Cracker Jack,
410–411
Popsicles-a-Plenty, 399–400

Protein Delight, Berry-Mint
Coconut, 414–415
Sherbet, Lemon-Coconut, 400
Sorbet, Tropical, 415
Dill
about, 378
Fennel-Dill Slaw, 379
Honey-Mustard Dill salad
dressing, 279
Mushrooms, Roasted Garlic &
Dill Stuffed, 377
Tofu "Cream" Sauce with, 241
Dioscorides, 379
Dips. See also Bean dips
Artichoke Dip, 239
Guacamole, Great, 244–245
Hummus Delight, 246–247
Mixed Vegetables & Dip,
383–384
Onion Dip, Quick & Easy,
239–240
Salsa, Sensational, 243
DNA (deoxyribonucleic acid), 209
Dressings. See Salad dressings
Dried fruits. See also Prunes
Candy Balls, Healthy, 394
Cereal, Creamy Coconut
Millet, 228–229
Granola, Sensational Spicy,
226–227
Oatmeal Deluxe, 229–230
Dried plums. See Prunes
Dulse in Gomasio, 294

E. coli bacteria, 214
Easy Nut Milk, 211
Easy Sleepytime Cocktail, 207
Edamame, 372
eating tips, 372–373
Millet with Edamame Beans &
Vegetables, 352
Pacific Rim Vegetable Stew,
329
Roasted Cauliflower, Edamame
& Bell Peppers, 331
in salads, 255
Eggplant
in Broiled Vegetables, 320
Pizza, Vegetable Pita, 332
Shiitake Mushrooms, Tofu,
Carrots & Eggplant Sauté,
334–335
Emerald Green Sauce, 241
Rose Potatoes with, 389
Endive
Belgian Endive Hummus-
Salsa Salad, 257
Stuffed Endive, 378–379
Energizing Tonic, 204

Fabulous Fruit Dressing, 284
Fajitas, 390–391
Fennel
about, 379
Dill-Fennel Slaw, 379
Endive, Stuffed, 378–379
Festive Black Bean Dip, 245–246

Flatbread, Herbed Garbanzo, 296–297
Flax seed
 Belgian Endive Hummus-Salsa Salad, 257
 Candy Balls, Healthy, 394
 Nut Date Balls, 408–409
 Oatmeal Cookies, Outrageous, 407–408
 Sweet Pepper-Apple Sun Dressing, 285
Flowers
 in salads, 254
 Vitality Salad, 254–255
4-Bean Salad, 266–267
Free radicals, 209
Freezing
 bananas, 210, 406
 beans, 355
 black beans, 355
 croutons, 292
 granola, 226–227
 Muesli, 226
French lentils, 264
Fruit Power Shake, 222
Fruit Treats, Frozen, 402–403

Garam Masala, 295
Garbanzo beans, 336. See also Hummus
 about, 248, 297
 Basmati Rice with Chickpeas, Baked, 348–349
 Carrot, Garbanzo & Tomato Salad, 362
 4-Bean Salad, 266–267
 Herbed Garbanzo Flatbread, 296–297
 Jasmine Rice with Chickpeas, Baked, 348–349
 Millet with Garbanzo Beans & Vegetables, 351–352
 in salads, 255
Garlic
 about, 378, 829
 Hummus, Roasted Very Garlic, 247
 Marinara Sauce, Quick & Easy Fat-Free Garlic Roasted, 249
 Mushrooms, Roasted Garlic & Dill Stuffed, 377
 Pacific Rim Vegetable Stew, 329
 Pizza, Vegetable Pita, 332
 Quinoa with Chestnuts & Toasted Pine Nuts, Garlicky, 342
 Risotto with Sun-Dried Tomatoes & Artichoke Hearts, Roasted Garlic, 347
 Roasted Garlic, 288–289
 Roasted Vegetable Salad, Chilled, 326–327
 Tomato Soup, Fresh, 302
 Vegetable Broth, 298–299
Garum Organic Black Olive Paste, 367
Gazpacho, Papaya, 304–305

Ginger, 203
 about, 203, 413
 Broccoli & Shiitake Steam-Fry, 320–321
 Brussels Sprouts Stir-Fry, 324
 Chutney, Apricot-Ginger, 250
 Energizing Tonic, 204
 Fruit Salad, Ginger, 412–413
 Miso-Ginger-Tahini Sauce, 251
 Pacific Rim Vegetable Stew, 329
 Peaceful Cocktail, 208
 Pear-Ginger Vinaigrette, 282
 Watermelon-Ginger Refresher, 221
 Winter Squash-Ginger Soup, Savory, 309–310
Gomasio, 293–294
Grains
 about, 336–339, 337–338
 Burgers, Grain, 349–350
 Chilled Grain Salad with Sweet Corn, 366–367
 whole grains, about, 369
Granolas. See Cereals
Grapefruit
 about, 224
 Peaceful Cocktail, 208
 Pinwheel Citrus Delight, 224
 Strawberry Citrus Deluxe juice, 201
 Tropical Fruit Cocktail, 203
 Ume-Grapefruit Dressing, 277
Grapes
 about, 398
 Fruit Dressing, Fabulous, 284
 Purple Grape Julius, 398
Green beans
 Asian Rice, 368–369
 Casserole, Vegetable, Rice & Lentil, 326
 4-Bean Salad, 266–267
Green Goddess Dressing, 286
Green lentils, 264
Green olives, 359
Green onions
 Apricot-Spinach Salad, 261–262
 Casserole, Vegetable, Rice & Lentil, 326
 Citrus Basmati Rice Pilaf & Mushrooms, 365–366
 Cucumbers, Stuffed, 381–382
 Grain Salad with Sweet Corn, Chilled, 366–367
 Jicama-Leek & Pepper Salad, 271–272
 Living Nori Salad, 257–258
 Millet-Tofu Salad with Toasted Pecans, 344
 Millet with Garbanzo Beans & Vegetables, 351–352
 Pacific Rim Vegetable Stew, 329
 Pizza Pizzazz, 388
 Rainbow Stuffed Peppers, 322
 Rice Almondine, Coconut, 343–344
 Roast Yukon Potatoes, Corn & Peas, 333

salads
 Apricot-Spinach Salad, 261–262
 Grain Salad with Sweet Corn, Chilled, 366–367
 Jicama-Leek & Pepper Salad, 271–272
 Living Nori Salad, 257–258
 Millet-Tofu Salad with Toasted Pecans, 344
 Shredded Rainbow Salad, 255
 Soba Noodle Salad with Garden Vegetables, 262–263
 Sun-Dried Tomato, Hijiki & Romaine Salad, 270–271
 Yukon Gold Potato Salad, 373
 Shredded Rainbow Salad, 255
 Soba Noodle Salad with Garden Vegetables, 262–263
 Sun-Dried Tomato, Hijiki & Romaine Salad, 270–271
 Yukon Gold Potato Salad, 373
Green peppercorns, 296
Green Power/Green Life Juicers, 200, 222
 for ice cream, 402
Green tea, 206
Grilled Vegetable Packets, 317–318
Guacamole
 Great Guacamole, 244–245
 Pizza Pizzazz, 388
Guilt-Free Banana Split, 394–395

Habañero chiles in Papaya Gazpacho, 304–305
Hazelnuts, Dried Cherries & Toasted Almonds, Quinoa with, 356
Hearts of palm
 about, 330–331
 Hearts of Romaine, Artichokes & Palm Salad, 259–260
 Millet with Hearts of Palm and Vegetables, 352
 Stir-Fry Hearts of Palm & Artichoke with Shiitake Mushrooms, 330
Hearts of Romaine, Artichokes & Palm Salad, 259–260
Herbed Croutons, 291–292
Herbed Garbanzo Flatbread, 296–297
Herb Rice with Shiitake Mushrooms, Toasted, 364
High Protein Bean-Tofu Spread, 238
Hijiki, 271
 Sun-Dried Tomato, Hijiki & Romaine Salad, 270–271
Hippocrates, 378, 379
Honeydew melons
 Mixed Melon Ambrosia, 215
 Smoothie, Kiwi-Melon, 217
 Soup, Lime-Melon, 312
 Summer Fruit Combo, 268
Honey-Mustard Dill salad dressing, 279

Horseradish, wasabi, 258
Hummus
    Belgian endive, 379
    Salsa-Hummus Salad, 257
    Delight, 246–247
    Sandwich, Lettuce & Veg-
        etable, 323
    Vegetable Wraps with Hum-
        mus Spread, 325–326
Hungarian peppers, 290

Iceberg Lettuce & Vegetable
    Sandwich, 323
Ice creams, 222
    Chocolate Date Peppermint
        Shake/Ice Cream, 401–402
    Strawberry-Mango-Banana
        Ice Cream, 406
Indian saffron. *See* Turmeric
Insulin, 339
Italian Raspberry Dressing, Fat-
    Free, 285

Jalapeño peppers
    Corn, Creamy Spicy Herbed,
        382
    Guacamole, Great, 244–245
    Hummus, Spicy, 247
    Jicama-Leek & Pepper Salad,
        271–272
    Millet-Tofu Salad with Toasted
        Pecans, 344
    Pizza, Vegetable Pita, 332
    Roasted Yellow Pepper &
        Orange Soup, Zesty, 309
    Salsa, Sensational, 243
    Southwestern Black Bean
        Patties, Spicy, 363
Japanese horseradish, 258
Jasmine Rice with Chickpeas,
    Baked, 348–349
Jicama
    about, 272
    Brussels Sprouts Stir-Fry, 324
    Leek-Jicama & Pepper Salad,
        271–272
    Living Nori Salad, 257–258
    Rainbow Stuffed Peppers, 322
    Shredded Rainbow Salad, 255
    Vitality Salad, 254–255
Juicing, 199
    Anti-Cancer V-12 drink,
        208–209
    Antioxidant Express, 206
    Blueberry Bonanza Smoothie,
        397
    Calcium Cooler, 202
    Carotene Cocktail, 202
    Cashew & Apple Cinnamon
        Smoothie, 398
    Cranberry-Apple Cooler, 213
    Creamy Cherry Smoothie, 221
    Easy Sleepytime Cocktail, 207
    Fruit Power Shake, 222
    Kiwi-Melon Smoothie, 217
    Mango Coconut Cream
        Smoothie, 216

Mixed Melon Ambrosia, 215
Natural Beauty Cocktail, 207
nut milks
    Easy Nut Milk, 211
    Smoothie, 212
Peaceful Cocktail, 208
Peach Smoothie, 218
Purple Grape Julius, 398
Rejuvenation Tonic, 205
slushes, fresh fruit, 222
Strawberry Citrus Deluxe
    juice, 201
Top of the Morning juice, 201
Tropical Fruit Cocktail, 203
Tropical Fruit Smoothie, 214
Veggie Smoothie, 220
Very Strawberry-Banana
    Smoothie, 217
Vitality Shake, 210
washing produce for, 199–200
Watermelon-Ginger Refresher,
    221
Weight Loss Express, 200

Kale
    about, 372
    Anti-Cancer V-12 drink,
        208–209
    Calcium Cooler, 202
    Chips, Kale, 371–372
    Shiitake Consommé with
        Greens, 300–301
Ketchup, Homemade Sunny, 242
Kidney Beans & Vegetables,
    Millet with, 352
Kids' meals
    Bonanza Smoothie, Blueberry,
        397
    Bread, Blueberry Apple
        Banana, 396–397
    Candy Balls, Healthy, 394
    Creamy Cashew & Apple
        Cinnamon Smoothie, 398
    Flavorful Rice Pilaf, 386–387
    Guilt-Free Banana Split,
        394–395
    Multicolored Corn, 386
    Pizza Pizzazz, 388
    Popsicles-a-Plenty, 399–400
    Potatoes Rose with Emerald
        Green Gravy, 389
    Raw Cherry, Orange, Apple-
        sauce Deluxe, 391–392
    Salad with Twist of Lemon, 390
    Sensational Spaghetti Squash,
        389–390
    Sherbet, Lemon-Coconut, 400
    Stuffed Dates, 392–393
    Sweet Potato Home Fries, 385
Kim Chi, 256
Kiwi
    Pinwheel Citrus Delight, 224
    Smoothie, Kiwi-Melon, 217
    Tropical Fruit Cocktail, 203
Kombu
    Asian Rice, 368–369
    beans with, 337

Cardamom & Parsley Basmati
    Rice, 361
Chili, Portabello Mushroom,
    350–351
Miso Tofu Soup, Hot 'n Spicy,
    308
Sweet Lentil-Parsley Salad,
    339–340
Vegetable Broth, 298–299
White Bean Soup, 306
Kuzu in Carrot-Tahini Spread,
    236–237
Kyolic, 829

Leeks
    about, 272
    Jicama-Leek & Pepper Salad,
        271–272
    Potato Leek Soup, 307
    Vegetable Broth, 298–299
Legumes, 336–339. *See also*
    Beans; Lentils
Lemonaise Spread, 239
    Ranch Dressing, 286–287
Lemon balm tea, 208
Lemon Grass Tabbouleh with
    Toasted Walnuts, Spicy,
    357–358
Lemons
    Crisp, Apple Lemon, 413–414
    juicing lemons, 274
Lemonaise Spread, 239
    Mustard Lemon dressing, 277
    Salad with Twist of Lemon, 390
    Sherbet, Lemon-Coconut, 400
    Tahini, Lemon, 279–280
Lentils
    about, 264, 340–341
    Barley-Lentil Cashew Stew,
        346
    Casserole, Vegetable, Rice &
        Lentil, 326
    Curried Lentil Soup, 313
    Parsley Lentil Salad, 263–264
    Pizza, Vegetable Pita, 332
    Sweet Lentil-Parsley Salad,
        339–340
    Vegetable Lentil-Sweet Potato
        Cakes, 367–368
Lettuce. *See also* Romaine lettuce
    about, 323–324
    Sandwich, Lettuce & Veg-
        etable, 323
Lima beans
    about, 360
    Millet with Lima Beans &
        Vegetables, 352
    Quinoa with Lima Beans,
        Dried Cherries & Toasted
        Almonds, 356
    Sauté, 360
Lime-Cantaloupe Soup, Chilled,
    312
Living Food
    Cranberry-Apple Cooler, 213
    Creamy Cinnamon Banana
        smoothie, 214

Fruit Power Shake, 222
Rejuvenation Tonic, 205
Veggie Smoothie, 220
Vitality Shake, 210
Living Nori Salad, 257–258
Lutein, about, 209

Mangos
about, 307
in Apple Berry Sauce, 371
Coconut Cream and Mango
Smoothie, 216
Ice Cream, Strawberry-Mango-
Banana, 406
Pie, Frozen Coconut Mango,
412
Salsa, Sensational, 243
Soup, Butternut Squash-
Mango, 306–307
Strawberry-Mango-Banana Ice
Cream, 406
Tropical Fruit Smoothie, 214
Vitality Shake, 210
Manzanilla olives, 367
Maple syrup
in Nut Milk, 211
Rejuvenation Tonic, 205
Marinara sauces
Quick & Easy Fat-Free Garlic
Roasted Marinara Sauce, 249
Simple & Super Marinara
Spaghetti Squash, 316–317
Marinated Baked Tofu Slices,
353–354
Maui onions, 290
Cream of Asparagus Soup,
311–312
Curry, Cauliflower-Broccoli, 383
Endive, Stuffed, 378–379
Multicolored Corn, 386
Split Pea Soup, Curried, 313
Meal-in-a-Bowl White Bean Soup,
305–306
Medjool dates, 393
Melons. See also Cantaloupes;
Honeydew melons
about, 215, 313
Mixed Melon Ambrosia, 215
Smoothie, Kiwi-Melon, 217
Mexican Black Beans, 355
Mexican Wild Rice with Olives,
358–359
Milk. See Nut milks; Soy milk
Millet
about, 228–229, 345, 352
Burgers, Grain, 349–350
Cereal, Creamy Coconut Millet,
228–229
Garbanzo Beans & Vegetables,
Millet with, 351–352
Grain Salad with Sweet Corn,
Chilled, 367
in salads, 255
Spread, Veggie Millet, 237
Tofu-Millet Salad with Toasted
Pecans, 344
Mint

Lemon Grass Tabbouleh with
Toasted Walnuts, Spicy,
357–358
Tahini Mint Dressing, 281
Tofu "Cream" Sauce with, 241
in Tomato Soup, Fresh, 302
Mirin, 251
Miso, 220
about, 220, 308
Cucumber-Tofu Salad with
Toasted Pecans, 265–266
Emerald Green Sauce, 241
Ginger-Miso-Tahini Sauce, 251
Soup, Hot 'n Spicy Miso Tofu,
308
Spread, Veggie Millet, 237
Veggie Smoothie, 220
Walnut-Miso Dressing/Topping,
283–284
Misto/Misto-style spray bottles,
291
Mixed Melon Ambrosia, 215
Mountain Valley Growers, 255
Muesli, 225–226
freezing, 226
Parfait, 392
Muffins, Banana Applesauce, 228
Multicolored Corn, 386
Mushrooms. See also Portabello
mushrooms; Shiitake mush-
rooms
about, 244
Barley-Lentil Cashew Stew, 346
in Broiled Vegetables, 320
Citrus Basmati Rice Pilaf &
Mushrooms, 365–366
Couscous Garden Salad,
260–261
Garlic & Dill Stuffed Mush-
rooms, Roasted, 377
Marinara Sauce, Quick & Easy
Fat-Free Garlic Roasted, 249
Marinara Spaghetti Squash,
Simple & Super, 316–317
Pizza, Vegetable Pita, 332
Rice Almondine, Coconut,
343–344
Scrambled Tofu, 231–232
Soy Thai Vegetable Sauté,
333–334
Vegetable Wraps with Hummus
Spread, 325–326
Mustard
Dill Honey-Mustard salad
dressing, 279
Lemon Mustard dressing, 277
Mustard greens
about, 253
Shiitake Consommé with
Greens, 300–301

Native Forest Organic Hearts of
Palm, 331
Natural Beauty Cocktail, 207
Never-Fail Herb Vinaigrette, 275
Noodle Vegetable Delight,
328–329

Nori
Salad, Living Nori, 257–258
Sushi Rice Salad, 352–353
Veggie Burritos, 318
Northern beans. See Beans
Nut milks
Basic Nut Milk Smoothie, 212
Creamy Cherry Smoothie, 221
Easy Nut Milk, 211
Kiwi-Melon Smoothie, 217
Mango Coconut Cream
Smoothie, 216
Nut Milk, Easy, 211
Peach Smoothie, 218
Nutritional yeast. See Yeast
Nuts. See also specific types
Date Balls, Nut, 408–409
Sensational Spicy Granola,
226–227

Oat bran, about, 408
Oatmeal Deluxe, 229–230
Oats
about, 230, 408
Cashew-Raisin Balls, 374–375
Cookies, Outrageous Oatmeal,
407–408
Muesli, 225–226
Oatmeal Deluxe, 229–230
Sensational Spicy Granola,
226–227
Olive oil, 359
Olives
about, 359
buying olives, tips for, 367
Endive, Stuffed, 378–379
Grain Salad with Sweet Corn,
Chilled, 366–367
in High Protein Bean-Tofu
Spread, 238
Mexican Wild Rice with Olives,
358–359
Pizza
Pizzazz, 388
Vegetable Pita, 332
Yukon Gold Potato Salad, 373
One-Day Cleanse, 205
Onions
about, 240, 290
Anti-Cancer V-12 drink, 208–209
Barley-Lentil Cashew Stew, 346
Black Bean Stew/Soup, 310–311
Burgers, Grain, 349–350
Corn, Creamy Spicy Herbed,
382
Dip, Quick & Easy, 239–240
Fajitas, 390–391
Fennel-Dill Slaw, 379
Garlicky Quinoa with Chestnuts
& Toasted Pine Nuts, 342
Green Goddess Dressing, 286
in Grilled or Roasted Vegetable
Packets, 317
Guacamole, Great, 244–245
Hummus, Roasted Onion, 247
Italian Raspberry Dressing, Fat-
Free, 285

Lemon Grass Tabbouleh with Toasted Walnuts, Spicy, 357–358
Lima Bean Sauté, 360
Marinara Sauce, Quick & Easy Fat-Free Garlic Roasted, 249
Millet with Garbanzo Beans & Vegetables, 351–352
Noodle Vegetable Delight, 328–329
Pacific Rim Vegetable Stew, 329
Pizza, Vegetable Pita, 332
Potassium-Powered Broth, 300
Red Cabbage with Apples & Pistachios, 327–328
Roasted Onions, 289
Roasted Vegetable Salad, Chilled, 326–327
Roasted Yellow Pepper & Orange Soup, Zesty, 309
Salsa, Sensational, 243
Sandwich, Lettuce & Vegetable, 323
Scrambled Tofu, 231–232
Sweet & Sour Black-Eyed Pea Salad, 354
Tomatoes & Zucchini with Cilantro, 380–381
Vegetable Broth, 298–299
Vegetable Wraps with Hummus Spread, 325–326
Orange bell peppers. *See* Bell peppers
Orange juice
Fruit Power Shake, 222
Kiwi-Melon Smoothie, 217
Mango Coconut Cream Smoothie, 216
Orange Sesame-Cashew Dressing, 278
Purple Grape Julius, 398
Quinoa with Soybeans, Dried Cherries & Toasted Almonds, 356
Ume-Orange Dressing, 277
Oranges
Dressing, Sesame-Cashew Orange, 278
Fruit Power Shake, 222
Ginger Broccoli & Shiitake Steam-Fry, 320–321
Ginger Fruit Salad, 412–413
Granola, Sensational Spicy, 226–227
Pancakes, Orange- Blueberry Buckwheat, 232
Pinwheel Citrus Delight, 224
Pudding, Sesame Banana Orange, 406–407
Raw Cherry, Orange, Applesauce Deluxe, 391–392
Roasted Yellow Pepper & Orange Soup, Zesty, 309
Strawberry Citrus Deluxe juice, 201
Vinaigrette, Balsamic Orange, 276

yams
Dressing, 281–282
Pudding, Yummy Yam, 396
Osteoporosis, 216

Pacific Rim Vegetable Stew, 329
Palm oil, 348
Pancakes
Orange-Blueberry Buckwheat Pancakes, 232
Tofu Pancakes, 233
Papaya
Apple Berry Sauce, 371
Gazpacho, Papaya, 304–305
Pie, Frozen Coconut Papaya, 412
Smoothie, Tropical Fruit, 214
Vitality Shake, 210
Parfait, Muesli, 392
Parsley
about, 292
Anti-Cancer V-12 drink, 208–209
Burgers, Grain, 349–350
Cardamom & Parsley Basmati Rice, 361
Carotene Cocktail, 202
Cumin Spiced Apple-Cabbage with Toasted Walnuts, 387
Easy Sleepytime Cocktail, 207
Lentil Parsley Salad, 263–264
Sweet Lentil-Parsley Salad, 339–340
Tofu "Cream" Sauce with, 241
in Tomato Soup, Fresh, 302
Top of the Morning juice, 201
Veggie Millet Spread, 237
Weight Loss Express juice, 200
Parsnips
about, 256
in High Protein Bean-Tofu Spread, 238
Shredded Rainbow Salad, 255
Soup, Sweet Squash and Parsnip, 303
Vegetable Broth, 298–299
Peaceful Cocktail, 208
Peaches, 218
about, 218
Smoothie, Peach, 218
Vitality Shake, 210
Peanut butter in Soy Thai Vegetable Sauté, 333–334
Pears, 218
about, 218
Arugula & Pear Salad with Toasted Walnuts, 258
Cashew Pear Cream Dressing, 287
Cinnamon Vanilla Poached Pears, 405
ginger
Salad, Ginger Fruit, 412–413
Vinaigrette, Ginger-Pear, 282
Peaceful Cocktail, 208
salads
Arugula & Pear Salad with Toasted Walnuts, 258

Ginger Fruit Salad, 412–413
Smoothie, 218
Summer Fruit Combo, 268
Vinaigrette, Ginger-Pear, 282
Peas
Casserole, Vegetable, Rice & Lentil, 326
Millet with Garbanzo Beans & Vegetables, 351–352
Rice Pilaf, Flavorful, 387
Roast Yukon Potatoes, Corn & Peas, 333
Pecans
Cucumber-Tofu Salad with Toasted Pecans, 265–266, 266
Guilt-Free Banana Split, 394–395
Millet-Tofu Salad with Toasted Pecans, 344
Sensational Spicy Granola, 226–227
Stuffed Dates, 392–393
Top of the Morning Quinoa Cereal, 230–231
Pectin, about, 236
Peppermint, 205
about, 205
Chocolate Date Peppermint Shake/Ice Cream, 401–402
Energizing Tonic, 204
Pie, Frozen Coconut Berry Mint, 411–412
Protein Delight, Berry-Mint Coconut, 414–415
Pepper/peppercorns, 296
Pie, Frozen Coconut Berry Mint, 411–412
Pineapple
about, 203
in Apple Berry Sauce, 371
Banana Split, Guilt-Free, 394–395
Fruit Dressing, Fabulous, 284
Pie, Frozen Coconut Pineapple, 412
Rejuvenation Tonic, 205
Tropical Fruit Cocktail, 203
Tropical Fruit Smoothie, 214
Pine nuts
Cucumber-Tofu Salad with Pine Nuts, 266
Garlicky Quinoa with Chestnuts & Toasted Pine Nuts, 342
Sensational Spicy Granola, 226–227
Pinto beans. *See* Beans
Pinwheel Citrus Delight, 224
Pistachios
Bean-Tofu Spread, High Protein, 238
Red Cabbage with Apples & Pistachios, 327–328
Sensational Spicy Granola, 226–227
Top of the Morning Quinoa Cereal, 230–231

Pita pizzas
Pizza Pizzazz, 388
Vegetable Pita Pizza, 332
Pizzas
Pizzazz Pizza, 388
Vegetable Pita Pizza, 332
Pliny, 379
Plums, dried. See Prunes
Popcorn, Cracker Jack, 410–411
Popsicles-a-Plenty, 399–400
Portabello mushrooms
about, 351
Chili, 350–351
Marinara Spaghetti Squash,
Simple & Super, 316–317
Potassium-Powered Broth, 300
Potatoes
Cauliflower-Carrot Soup with
Tarragon, 314
Corn, Creamy Spicy Herbed, 382
Fancy Potato Skins with Salsa,
380
Leek Potato Soup, 307
Potassium-Powered Broth, 300
Roasted Herbed Asparagus &
Potatoes, 319–320
Roast Yukon Potatoes, Corn &
Peas, 333
Rose Potatoes with Emerald
Green Gravy, 389
Salad, Yukon Gold Potato, 373
Shiitake Mushroom Sauce, 244
soups
Cauliflower-Carrot Soup
with Tarragon, 314
Leek Potato Soup, 307
Potassium-Powered Broth,
300
White Bean Soup, 305–306
White Bean Soup, 305–306
Prunes, 213
about, 213, 404–405
Chocolate & Dried Plum Whip,
404
Muesli, 225–226
Sensational Spicy Granola,
226–227
Smoothie, Dried Plum & Apple,
212
Spread, 234–235
Puddings
Apple Walnut Pudding, 403
Sesame Banana Orange Pud-
ding, 406–407
Tapioca Pudding with Toasted
Almonds, 411
Very Berry Pudding, 395
Yam Pudding, Yummy, 396
Pumpkin seeds
Quinoa with Pumpkin Seeds,
Dried Cherries & Toasted
Almonds, 356
in salads, 255
Purple Grape Julius, 398

Quick High Protein Bean-Tofu
Spread, 238

Quinoa
about, 357
Burgers, Grain, 349–350
Garlicky Quinoa with Chestnuts
& Toasted Pine Nuts, 342
Grain Salad with Sweet Corn,
Chilled, 366–367
in salads, 255
Soybeans, Dried Cherries &
Toasted Almonds, Quinoa
with, 356
Top of the Morning Quinoa
Cereal, 230–231

Rainbow Stuffed Peppers, 322
Raisins
Candy Balls, Healthy, 394
Cashew-Raisin Balls, 374–375
Creamy Coconut Millet Cereal,
228–229
Muesli, 225–226
Oatmeal Cookies, Outrageous,
407–408
Oatmeal Deluxe, 229–230
Rice Pilaf, Flavorful, 387
Sensational Spicy Granola,
226–227
Sunflower Apricot Cookies,
403–404
Tomato Couscous with Cashews
& Raisins, 365
Ranch Dressing, 286–287
Raspberries
Apple Berry Sauce, 370–371
Berry Salad with Fruit Sauce,
225
Date-Apple-Berry Butter
Spread, 236
Pie, Frozen Coconut Berry Mint,
412
Pinwheel Citrus Delight, 224
Protein Delight, Berry-Mint
Coconut, 414–415
Vitality Shake, 210
Raspberry vinegar in Italian
Raspberry Dressing, Fat-Free,
285
Raw Organic Cultured Vegetable
Salad, 256
Reactive hypoglycemia, 339
Red bell peppers. See Bell peppers
Red Cabbage with Apples &
Pistachios, 327–328
Red lentils, brown rice and, 336
Red peppercorns, 296
Rejuvenation Tonic, 205
Rejuvenative Foods Raw Cultured
Vegetables, 256
Rice. See also Brown rice
Basmati Rice with Chickpeas,
Baked, 348–349
Jasmine Rice with Chickpeas,
Baked, 348–349
Risotto with Sun-Dried Toma-
toes & Artichoke Hearts,
Roasted Garlic, 347
Sushi Rice Salad, 352–353

Risotto with Sun-Dried Tomatoes
& Artichoke Hearts, Roasted
Garlic, 347
Roasted peppers, 290
Hummus, 247
Parsley Lentil Salad, 263–264
pizzas
Pizza Pizzazz, 388
Vegetable Pita Pizza, 332
roasting tips, 260
Roasted Vegetable Packets,
317–318
Roasted Vegetable Salad, Chilled,
326–327
Romaine lettuce
about, 253
Anti-Cancer V-12 drink, 208–209
Antioxidant Express, 206
Hearts of Romaine, Artichokes &
Palm Salad, 259–260
Natural Beauty Cocktail, 207
Roasted Vegetable Salad,
Chilled, 326–327
Sun-Dried Tomato, Hijiki &
Romaine Salad, 270–271
Veggie Smoothie, 220
Rose Potatoes with Emerald Green
Gravy, 389
Rutabagas with Stuffed Endive,
378–379
Rye flakes in Muesli, 225–226

St. John's Bread. See Carob
Salad dressings, 251, 253–254. See
also Vinaigrettes
Avocado Dressing, Zesty,
282–283
fat-free dressing suggestions, 287
Fruit Dressing, Fabulous, 284
Green Goddess Dressing, 286
Italian Raspberry Dressing, Fat-
Free, 285
Lemon Mustard dressing, 277
Orange Sesame-Cashew Dress-
ing, 278
Orange Yam Dressing, 281–282
Pear Cashew Cream Dressing,
287
Ranch Dressing, 286–287
Soy Dressing, Spicy, 283
for Sun-Dried Tomato, Hijiki &
Romaine Salad, 271
for Sushi Rice Salad, 352–353
Sweet Pepper-Apple Sun Dress-
ing, 285
tahini
Mint Dressing, Tahini, 281
Salsa Dressing, Tahini, 281
Tangerine-Ume Dressing,
276–277
Tangerine-Ume Dressing,
276–277
Salads. See also Cole slaw; Salad
dressings
about, 252–254
Antioxidant Spinach-Sweet
Potato Salad, 269

Apricot-Spinach Salad, 261–262
Belgian Endive Hummus-Salsa Salad, 257
Berry Salad with Fruit Sauce, 225
Black Bean Salad, Spicy, 264–265
Chilled Roasted Vegetable Salad, 326–327
Couscous Garden Salad, 260–261
Crunchy Cabbage, Apple & Turnip Salad with Toasted Cashews, 259
Cucumber-Tofu Salad with Toasted Pecans, 265–266
4-Bean Salad, 266–267
Garbanzo, Carrot & Tomato Salad, 362
Ginger Fruit Salad, 412–413
Grain Salad with Sweet Corn, Chilled, 366–367
Hearts of Romaine, Artichokes & Palm Salad, 259–260
Jicama-Leek & Pepper Salad, 271–272
Living Nori Salad, 257–258
Millet-Tofu Salad with Toasted Pecans, 344
Miso-Walnut Dressing/Topping, 283–284
Parsley Lentil Salad, 263–264
Pear & Arugula Salad with Toasted Walnuts, 258
protein, adding, 255
Shredded Rainbow Salad, 255
Soba Noodle Salad with Garden Vegetables, 262–263
Summer Fruit Combo, 268
Sushi Rice Salad, 352–353
Sweet Lentil-Parsley Salad, 339–340
Sweet & Sour Black-Eyed Pea Salad, 354
Tangerine-Ume Dressing, 276–277
tips for, 252–254
Twist of Lemon, Salad with, 390
Vitality Salad, 254–255
Yukon Gold Potato Salad, 373
Salsa
Belgian Endive Hummus-Salsa Salad, 257
Pizza Pizzazz, 388
Sensational Salsa, 243
No Oil Chips & Salsa, 375
Tahini Salsa Dressing, 281
Sandwich, Lettuce & Vegetable, 323
Sauces. *See also* Marinara sauces
Apple Berry Sauce, 370–371
Emerald Green Sauce, 241
Ketchup, Homemade Sunny, 242

Miso-Ginger-Tahini Sauce, 251
Shiitake Mushroom Sauce, 244
Tofu-Cilantro "Cream" Sauce, 240–241
Sauerkraut, Raw, 256
Sautés
Lima Bean Sauté, 360
Shiitake Mushrooms, Tofu, Carrots & Eggplant Sauté, 334–335
Soy Thai Vegetable Sauté, 333–334
Savoy cabbage in Sunny Shredded Dill & Toasted Sesame Cole Slaw, 267–268
Scotch oats, 408
Scrambled Tofu, 231–232
Seasonings
Cheesy Sesame Seasoning Salt, 294
Garam Masala, 295
Sea vegetables. *See also* Kombu; specific types
about, 319
hijiki, 270–271
Seitan in Fajitas, 390–391
Sensational Salsa. *See* Salsa
Sensational Spaghetti Squash, 389–390
Sensational Spicy Granola, 226–227
Sesame seeds
about, 294
Apricot-Spinach Salad, 261–262
Broccoli Cole Slaw with Toasted Sesame Seeds, 374
Candy Balls, Healthy, 394
Cucumber-Tofu Salad with Toasted Sesame Seeds, 266
Granola, Sensational Spicy, 226–227
Orange Sesame-Cashew Dressing, 278
Pudding, Sesame Banana Orange, 406–407
Rice Pilaf, Flavorful, 387
Sesame seed salt, 293–294
Cheesy Sesame Seasoning Salt, 294
Herbed Garbanzo Flatbread, 296–297
Sherbet, Lemon-Coconut, 400
Sherry in Risotto with Sun-Dried Tomatoes & Artichoke Hearts, Roasted Garlic, 347
Shiitake mushrooms
about, 301, 364–365
Chili, 351
Consommé with Greens, Shiitake, 300–301
Ginger Broccoli & Shiitake Steam-Fry, 320–321
Herb Rice with Shiitake Mushrooms, Toasted, 364
Marinara Spaghetti Squash, Simple & Super, 316–317

Sauté of Shiitake Mushrooms, Tofu, Carrots & Eggplant, 334–335
Stir-Fry Hearts of Palm & Artichoke with Shiitake Mushrooms, 330
Vegetable Broth, 298–299
Shiitake Mushroom Sauce, 244
Shoyu
croutons, misting, 291
Ginger Broccoli & Shiitake Steam-Fry, 320–321
Marinated Baked Tofu Slices, 353–354
Pacific Rim Vegetable Stew, 329
Stuffed Mushrooms, Roasted Garlic & Dill, 377
Shredded Rainbow Salad, 255
Slushes, fresh fruit, 222
Smoothies. *See* Juicing
Snap peas in Soy Thai Vegetable Sauté, 333–334
Soba noodles
Noodle Vegetable Delight, 328–329
Soba Noodle Salad with Garden Vegetables, 262–263
Sorbets, 222
Tropical Sorbet, 415
Soups. *See also* Potatoes
Asparagus, Cream of, 311–312
Black Bean Stew/Soup, 310–311
Cantaloupe-Lime Soup, chilled, 312
Cauliflower-Carrot Soup with Tarragon, 314
Corn & Avocado Soup, 303–304
Curried Split Pea Soup, 313
Gazpacho, Papaya, 304–305
Ginger-Winter Squash Soup, Savory, 309–310
Leek Potato Soup, 307
Mango-Butternut Squash Soup, 306–307
Meal-in-a-Bowl White Bean Soup, 305–306
Miso Tofu Soup, Hot 'n Spicy, 308
Papaya Gazpacho, 304–305
Potassium-Powered Broth, 300
Roasted Yellow Pepper & Orange Soup, Zesty, 309
Shiitake Consommé with Greens, 300–301
Split Pea Soup, Curried, 313
Sweet Squash and Parsnip Soup, 303
Tomato Basil Soup, Fresh, 301–302
Vegetable Broth, 298–299
Southwestern Black Bean Patties, Spicy, 363
Soybeans
about, 248–249, 336

Quinoa with Soybeans, Dried Cherries & Toasted Almonds, 356
Spread, 248
Soy cheese
Festive Black Bean Dip, 245–246
Pizza Pizzazz, 388
Soy milk
about, 300
Asian Rice, 368–369
Berry Salad with Fruit Sauce, 225
Cashew & Apple Cinnamon Smoothie, 398
Corn, Creamy Spicy Herbed, 382
Fruit Power Shake, 222
Kiwi-Melon Smoothie, 217
Mango Coconut Cream Smoothie, 216
Oatmeal Deluxe, 229–230
Peach Smoothie, 218
Rose Potatoes with Emerald Green Gravy, 389
Sherbet, Lemon-Coconut, 400
smoothies
Cashew & Apple Cinnamon Smoothie, 398
Creamy Cherry Smoothie, 221
Kiwi-Melon Smoothie, 217
Peach Smoothie, 218
Soy nut butter
Dressing, Spicy Soy, 283
Sauté, Soy Thai Vegetable, 333–334
Soy nuts, 410–411
Soy Thai Vegetable Sauté, 333–334
Soy yogurt
about, 390
Apricot-Spinach Salad, 261–262
Banana Split, Guilt-Free, 394–395
Cream of Asparagus Soup, 311–312
Dried Plum & Apple Smoothie, 212
Mango Coconut Cream Smoothie, 216
Muesli Parfait, 392
Onion Dip, Quick & Easy, 239–240
Peach Smoothie, 218
Ranch Dressing, 286–287
Salad with Twist of Lemon, 390
smoothies
Dried Plum & Apple, 212
Mango Coconut Cream, 216
Peach, 218
Strawberry-Banana, 217
Strawberry-Banana Smoothie, 217
Stuffed Mushrooms, Roasted Garlic & Dill, 377
Yukon Gold Potato Salad, 373

Spaghetti squash
Marinara Spaghetti Squash, Simple & Super, 316–317
Sensational Spaghetti Squash, 389–390
Spectrum Naturals salad dressings, 251, 287
Spectrum Spread, 413–414
Spicy & Quick Nonfat Bean Dip, 246
Spinach
about, 242, 262, 269–270
Anti-Cancer V-12 drink, 208–209
Antioxidant Spinach-Sweet Potato Salad, 269
Apricot-Spinach Salad, 261–262
Calcium Cooler, 202
Carotene Cocktail, 202
Couscous Garden Salad, 260–261
Emerald Green Sauce, 241
Pizza, Vegetable Pita, 332
Sun-Dried Tomato, Hijiki & Romaine Salad, 270–271
washing, 253
Spinach juice in Shiitake Mushroom Sauce, 244
The Splendid Grain (Wood), 338
Split Pea Soup, Curried, 313
Spreads
Apple Butter Spread, 235
Apricot Spread, 234–235
Carrot-Tahini Spread, 236–237
Date-Apple-Berry Butter Spread, 235–236
High Protein Bean-Tofu Spread, 238
Lemonaise Spread, 239
Prune Butter Spread, 234–235
Soybean Spread, 248
Veggie Millet Spread, 237
Sprouts. See also Broccoli sprouts
bean sprouts, 337
Rainbow Stuffed Peppers, 322
Sandwich, Lettuce & Vegetable, 323
sunflower sprouts in Vitality Salad, 254–255
Squash. See also Spaghetti squash
about, 310
Ginger-Winter Squash Soup, Savory, 309–310
in Grilled or Roasted Vegetable Packets, 317
in High Protein Bean-Tofu Spread, 238
Mango-Butternut Squash Soup, 306–307
Marinara Sauce, Quick & Easy Fat-Free Garlic Roasted, 249
Pacific Rim Vegetable Stew, 329
Pizza, Vegetable Pita, 332
soups
Ginger-Winter Squash Soup, Savory, 309–310

Mango-Butternut Squash Soup, 306–307
Sweet Squash & Parsnip Soup, 303
Sweet Squash & Parsnip Soup, 303
Vegetable Wraps with Hummus Spread, 325–326
Steel-cut oats, 408
Stevia, 403
Stews
Barley-Lentil Cashew Stew, 346
Black Bean Stew/Soup, 310–311
Pacific Rim Vegetable Stew, 329
Stir-fry
Chopped Brussels Sprouts Stir-Fry, 324
Hearts of Palm & Artichoke with Shiitake Mushrooms Stir-Fray, 330
Strawberries
about, 201
Apple Berry Sauce, 370–371
Banana Split, Guilt-Free, 394–395
Berry-Cherry Zing, 204
Berry Salad with Fruit Sauce, 225
Fruit Dressing, Fabulous, 284
Fruit Power Shake, 222
Ginger Fruit Salad, 412–413
Ice Cream, Strawberry-Mango-Banana, 406
Mixed Melon Ambrosia, 215
Peaceful Cocktail, 208
Pie, Frozen Coconut Berry Mint, 412
Protein Delight, Berry-Mint Coconut, 414–415
Pudding, Very Berry, 395
in Raw Cherry, Orange, Applesauce Deluxe, 392
Smoothie, Very Strawberry-Banana, 217
Sorbet, Tropical, 415
Spread, Date-Apple-Berry Butter, 236
Strawberry Citrus Deluxe juice, 201
Tropical Fruit Cocktail, 203
Vitality Shake, 210
Stuffed Endive, 378–379
Stuffed Peppers, Rainbow, 322
Summer Fruit Combo, 268
Sun-dried tomatoes
Couscous with Cashews & Raisins, 365
Pizza, Vegetable Pita, 332
Risotto with Sun-Dried Tomatoes & Artichoke Hearts, Roasted Garlic, 347
Salad, Sun-Dried Tomato, Hijiki & Romaine, 270–271
Sunflower seeds, 255
Bean-Tofu Spread, High Protein, 238
Candy Balls, Healthy, 394

Cookies, Apricot Sunflower
  Cookies, 403–404
Emerald Green Sauce, 241
Granola, Sensational Spicy,
  226–227
Herb Rice with Shiitake
  Mushrooms, Toasted, 364
Muesli, 225–226
Oatmeal Deluxe, 229–230
Quinoa with Sunflower Seeds,
  Dried Cherries & Toasted
  Almonds, 356
Salad, Apricot-Spinach,
  261–262
Sweet Pepper-Apple Sun
  Dressing, 285
Sunflower sprouts in Vitality
  Salad, 254–255
Sunny Shredded Dill & Toasted
  Sesame Cole Slaw, 267–268
Sushi Rice Salad, 352–353
Sweet Lentil-Parsley Salad,
  339–340
Sweet Pepper-Apple Sun Dress-
  ing, 285
Sweet potatoes
  about, 270
  Antioxidant Spinach-Sweet
    Potato Salad, 269
  Home Fries, 385
  Vegetable Lentil-Sweet Potato
    Cakes, 367–368
Sweet & Sour Black-Eyed Pea
  Salad, 354
Sweet Texas onions, 290
Swiss chard in Shiitake Con-
  sommé, 300–301

Tabbouleh with Toasted Walnuts,
  Spicy Lemon Grass, 357–358
Tahini
  about, 237, 280
  Artichoke Dip, 239
  Bean-Tofu Spread, High
    Protein, 238
  Carrot-Tahini Spread, 236–237
  Cashew-Raisin Balls, 374–375
  Cucumbers, Stuffed, 381–382
  Endive, Stuffed, 378–379
  Lemon Tahini, 279–280
  Mint Dressing, 281
  salad dressings
    Mint Dressing, 281
    Salsa Dressing, Tahini, 281
    Tangerine-Ume Dressing,
      276–277
  Soybean Spread, 248
  spreads
    Bean-Tofu Spread, High
      Protein, 238
    Carrot-Tahini Spread,
      236–237
    Soybean Spread, 248
  Tangerine-Ume Dressing,
    276–277
Tamari
  croutons, misting, 291

Ginger Broccoli & Shiitake
  Steam-Fry, 320–321
Miso Tofu Soup, Hot 'n Spicy,
  308
Sauté, Soy Thai Vegetable,
  333–334
Tangerines
  Strawberry Citrus Deluxe
    juice, 201
  Ume-Tangerine Dressing,
    276–277
Tapioca Pudding with Toasted
  Almonds, 411
Tarragon
  about, 315
  Cauliflower-Carrot Soup with,
    314
Teas
  Antioxidant Express, 206
  Easy Sleepytime Cocktail, 207
  ginger tea, 203
  Peaceful Cocktail, 208
Thai Vegetable Sauté, 333–334
Thyme, 299
Tofu
  about, 232
  Artichoke Dip, 239
  Black Bean Stew/Soup, 311
  Cashew & Apple Cinnamon
    Smoothie, 398
  Cauliflower-Carrot Soup with
    Tarragon, 314
  Cilantro Thousand Island, 278
  Cilantro-Tofu "Cream" Sauce,
    240–241
  Creamy Cherry Smoothie, 221
  Cucumber-Tofu Salad with
    Toasted Pecans, 265–266
  High Protein Bean-Tofu
    Spread, 238
  Lemon Mustard Dressing,
    277
  Marinara Sauce, Quick & Easy
    Fat-Free Garlic Roasted, 249
  Marinated Baked Tofu Slices,
    353–354
  Millet-Tofu Salad with Toasted
    Pecans, 344
  Miso Tofu Soup, Hot 'n Spicy,
    308
  Noodle Vegetable Delight,
    328–329
  Pancakes, 233
  Pie, Frozen Coconut Berry
    Mint, 412
  Pizza, Vegetable Pita, 332
  Protein Delight, Berry-Mint
    Coconut, 414–415
  Ranch Dressing, 286–287
  salads, 255
    Cucumber-Tofu Salad with
      Toasted Pecans, 265–266
    Millet-Tofu Salad with
      Toasted Pecans, 344
  Sauté, Soy Thai Vegetable,
    333–334
  Scrambled Tofu, 231–232

Shiitake Mushrooms, Tofu,
  Carrots & Eggplant Sauté,
  334–335
smoothies
  Creamy Cashew & Apple
    Cinnamon Smoothie, 398
  Veggie Smoothie, 220
soups
  Black Bean Stew/Soup, 311
  Cauliflower-Carrot Soup
    with Tarragon, 314
  Tomato Soup, Fresh, 302
Tomato Soup, Fresh, 302
Veggie Millet Spread, 237
Veggie Smoothie, 220
Yam Pudding, Yummy, 396
Tomatoes. *See also* Sun-dried
  tomatoes
  about, 242–243, 293
  Anti-Cancer V-12 drink,
    208–209
  Carotene Cocktail, 202
  couscous
    Cashews & Raisins and
      Tomatoes, Couscous with,
      365
    Garden Salad, Couscous,
      260–261
  Fajitas, 390–391
  Fresh Tomato Basil Soup,
    301–302
  Garbanzo, Carrot & Tomato
    Salad, 362
  Guacamole, Great, 244–245
  Lemon Grass Tabbouleh with
    Toasted Walnuts, Spicy,
    357–358
  Marinara Sauce, Quick & Easy
    Fat-Free Garlic Roasted, 249
  Mexican Wild Rice with
    Olives, 358–359
  Pacific Rim Vegetable Stew,
    329
  peeling tomatoes, 292–293, 302
  Pizza, Vegetable Pita, 332
  Potato Skins with Salsa, Fancy,
    380
  Rainbow Stuffed Peppers, 322
  Roasted Vegetable Salad,
    Chilled, 326–327
  salads
    Couscous Garden Salad,
      260–261
    Garbanzo, Carrot & Tomato
      Salad, 362
    Roasted Vegetable Salad,
      Chilled, 326–327
    Sun-Dried Tomato, Hijiki &
      Romaine Salad, 270–271
    Sweet & Sour Black-Eyed
      Pea Salad, 354
    Vitality Salad, 254–255
  Salsa, Sensational, 243
  Sandwich, Lettuce & Veg-
    etable, 323
  Sauté, Lima Bean, 360
  seeding tomatoes, 302

Soup, Fresh Tomato Basil, 301–302
Sun-Dried Tomato, Hijiki & Romaine Salad, 270–271
Sweet & Sour Black-Eyed Pea Salad, 354
Vitality Salad, 254–255
White Bean & Tomato Casserole, 341
Zucchini & Tomatoes with Cilantro, 380–381
Top of the Morning juice, 201
Top of the Morning Quinoa Cereal, 230–231
Tribest Corporation, 200
Tropical Fruit Cocktail, 203
Tropical Fruit Smoothie, 214
Turmeric
    about, 362
    in Cardamom & Parsley Basmati Rice, 361
Turnips
    about, 259
    Crunchy Cabbage, Apple & Turnip Salad with Toasted Cashews, 259
    Vegetable Broth, 298–299
Turtle beans. See Black beans

Umeboshi, Tangerine-Ume Dressing, 276–277

Vegetable Broth, 298–299
    about, 353
Vegetable entrées
    Broiled Vegetables, 320
    Brussels Sprouts Stir-Fry, 324
    Casserole, Vegetable, Rice & Lentil, 326
    Cauliflower, Edamame & Bell Peppers, Roasted, 331
    Ginger Broccoli & Shiitake Steam-Fry, 320–321
    Lettuce & Vegetable Sandwich, 323
    Marinara Spaghetti Squash, Simple & Super, 316–317
    Noodle Vegetable Delight, 328–329
    Nori Veggi Burritos, 318
    Pacific Rim Vegetable Stew, 329
    Pizza, Vegetable Pita, 332
    Rainbow Stuffed Peppers, 322
    Red Cabbage with Apples & Pistachios, 327–328
    Roasted Herbed Asparagus & Potatoes, 319–320
    Roast Yukon Potatoes, Corn & Peas, 333
    Soy Thai Vegetable Sauté, 333–334
    Vegetable Packets, Grilled or Oven-Roasted, 317–318
    Vegetable Wraps with Hummus Spread, 325–326

Vegetable Lentil-Sweet Potato Cakes, 367–368
Vegetable Packets, Grilled or Oven-Roasted, 317–318
Vegetable Wraps with Hummus Spread, 325–326
Veggie Millet Spread, 237
Veggie Smoothie, 220
Vegi Delite, 256
Very Strawberry-Banana Smoothie, 217
Vidalia onions, 290
    Multicolored Corn, 386
Vinaigrettes
    Balsamic Vinaigrette for Two, 275–276
    basic vinaigrette, 273–274
    French Vinaigrette, 274
    Never-Fail Herb Vinaigrette, 275
    Orange Balsamic Vinaigrette, 276
    Pear-Ginger Vinaigrette, 282
    Thousand Island, 274–275
Vinegars. See also Vinaigrettes
    Italian Raspberry Dressing, Fat-Free, 285
Vitality Salad, 254–255
Vitality Shake, 210

Wakame
    in Cole Slaw, Sunny Shredded Dill & Toasted Sesame, 268
    in Gomasio, 294
Walla Walla onions, 290
Walnuts
    about, 358
    Banana Split, Guilt-Free, 394–395
    Brownies, Moist & Chewy, 409–410
    Candy Balls, Healthy, 394
    Cumin Spiced Apple-Cabbage with Toasted Walnuts, 387
    Dates, Stuffed, 392–393
    Granola, Sensational Spicy, 226–227
    Lemon Grass Tabbouleh with Toasted Walnuts, Spicy, 357–358
    Miso-Walnut Dressing/Topping, 283–284
    Muesli, 225–226
    Nut Date Balls, 408–409
    Oatmeal Cookies, Outrageous, 407–408
    Pear & Arugula Salad with Toasted Walnuts, 258
    Pinwheel Citrus Delight, 224
    Pudding, Apple Walnut, 403
    Top of the Morning Quinoa Cereal, 230–231
Wasabi, 258
Washing produce, 199–200
    salad greens, 253
Water chestnuts
    Asian Rice, 368–369

Sauté, Soy Thai Vegetable, 333–334
Soba Noodle Salad with Garden Vegetables, 262–263
Watermelon
    Ginger-Watermelon Refresher, 221
    Mixed Melon Ambrosia, 215
    seeds, toasted, 221
Wax beans in 4-Bean Salad, 266–267
Weight Loss Express juice, 200
Wheat
    about, 346–347
    Granola, Sensational Spicy, 226–227
White beans
    Casserole, White Bean & Tomato, 341
    Soup, White Bean, 305–306
White flour products, 338–339
Wild rice
    about, 360
    Mexican Wild Rice with Olives, 358–359
Wood, Rebecca, 338

Yams
    Autumn Puree, 384
    Home Fries, 385
    Orange Yam Dressing, 281–282
    Pudding, Yummy Yam, 396
    Vegetable Lentil-Sweet Potato Cakes, 367–368
Yeast
    about, 294–295
    in Gomasio, 294
Yellow bell peppers. See Bell peppers
Yellow crookneck squash in Pacific Rim Vegetable Stew, 329
Yellow ginger. See Turmeric
Yogurt. See Soy yogurt
Yukon Gold potatoes. See Potatoes

Zucchini
    in Broiled Vegetables, 320
    Burgers, Grain, 349–350
    in Grilled or Roasted Vegetable Packets, 317
    Pacific Rim Vegetable Stew, 329
    pizza
        Pizza Pizzazz, 388
        Vegetable Pita Pizza, 332
    Scrambled Tofu, 231–232
    Spread, Veggie Millet, 237
    Sweet Squash and Parsnip Soup, 303
    Tomatoes & Zucchini with Cilantro, 380–381
    Vegetable Lentil-Sweet Potato Cakes, 367–368
    Vegetable Wraps with Hummus Spread, 325–326